Amnesia

Amnesia

Clinical, Psychological and Medicolegal Aspects

2nd Edition

Edited by

C. W. M. Whitty, MA, BSc, DM, FRCP
Consultant Neurologist, Radcliffe Infirmary, Oxford;
and Clinical Lecturer in Neurology, University of Oxford

AND

O. L. Zangwill, MA, FRS
Professor of Experimental Psychology, University of Cambridge;
and Psychologist to the National Hospital, Queen Square, London

BUTTERWORTHS
LONDON - BOSTON
Sydney - Wellington - Durban - Toronto

The Butterworth Group

United Kingdom London	**Butterworth & Co. (Publishers) Ltd** 88 Kingsway, WC2B 6AB
Australia Sydney	**Butterworths Pty Ltd** 586 Pacific Highway, Chatswood, NSW 2067 Also at Melbourne, Brisbane, Adelaide and Perth
South Africa Durban	**Butterworth & Co (South Africa) (Pty) Ltd** 152–154 Gale Street
New Zealand Wellington	**Butterworths of New Zealand Ltd** 26–28 Waring Taylor Street, 1
Canada Toronto	**Butterworth & Co (Canada) Ltd** 2265 Midland Avenue, Scarborough, Ontario, M1P 4S1
USA Boston	**Butterworth (Publishers) Inc** 19 Cummings Park, Woburn, Mass. 01801

First published 1966
Second edition 1977

ISBN 0 407 00056 9
© Butterworth & Co (Publishers) Ltd 1977

Library of Congress Cataloging in Publication Data

Amnesia. – 2nd ed.

1. Amnesia
I. Whitty, Charles William Michael
II. Zangwill, Oliver Louis
6.16.8′523   RC394.A5   77-30016

ISBN 0-407-00056-9

Printed by Chapel River Press, Andover, Hants.

2 15 35

Foreword to First Edition

To those who believe that brain and mind are different aspects of the same thing, it appears natural, and wholly desirable, that the neurologist and the psychologist should be interested in the same problems, and that their enquiries should be directed towards a common goal — the interpretation of psychological order and disorder in terms of cerebral organisation.

In this field of common interest, the study of amnesia has long been of outstanding importance. Here the clinician, neurologist or psychiatrist had a good start, beginning with the observations of Korsakoff and others on the memory disorder, later shown to be associated with Wernicke's encephalopathy. Clinico-pathological correlation has progressed slowly but steadily, so that lesions in certain parts of the brain are now known to correspond with fairly well-defined patterns of derangement of memory. The psychologist has more than caught up with his colleagues by entering the clinical field, and studying in detail the disorders of memory following, for example, head injury, encephalitis, temporal lobectomy and electroconvulsive therapy. The application of psychometric tests to such patients has yielded information of much value. Parallel with this, there have been major developments in the investigation of learning and memory in animals following experimental brain lesions.

The time, therefore, is opportune for a comprehensive review of the subject, and the Editors have brought together in this volume the observations and opinions of a number of contributors qualified by their experience to present different points of view.

We may have to admit, after reading this book, that the psychological analysis of remembering still lacks precision, and that we know virtually nothing of the physiological basis for memory, but we shall not only be better informed, but better able to ask ourselves the right questions.

I am sure that this book will gain the success it deserves and I hope that it will reappear in further editions, to keep pace with the advance of knowledge in its field.

C. P. SYMONDS

Contents

Contributors

J. B. Brierley, MD, FRCPath
Neuropsychiatric Research Unit, Medical Research Council.

M. M. Feldman, BA(Hons), MPhil, MRCP, MRCPsych
Consultant Psychotherapist, Bethlem Royal and Maudsley Hospitals, London; Lecturer, Institute of Psychiatry, London

T. C. N. Gibbens, MD, FRCP, FRCPsych
Professor of Forensic Psychiatry, Institute of Psychiatry, London; Honorary Consultant Psychiatrist, Bethlem Royal and Maudsley Hospitals and the London Remand Homes

J. E. Hall Williams, LLB, LLM
Reader in Criminology, University of London, Law Department, London School of Economics; Editorial Board, the *British Journal of Criminology*; Secretary General of the International Society for Criminology; Member of the Parole Board for England and Wales

Susan D. Iversen, MA, PhD
Assistant Director of Research, The Psychological Laboratory, University of Cambridge

W. A. Lishman, BSc, MD, FRCP, FRCPsych
Honorary Consultant Physician, Bethlem and Maudsley Hospitals; Reader in Neuropsychology, Institute of Psychiatry, London

M. F. Piercy, MA
Lecturer in Psychopathology, University of Cambridge; Consultant Psychologist to Maida Vale Hospital, London

R. T. C. Pratt, MA, DM, FRCP, FRCPsych
Physician in Psychological Medicine, National Hospital for
Nervous Diseases, Queen Square and Maida Vale, London

G. Stores, MA, MB, ChB, MRCP, MRCPsych
Consultant Neuropsychiatrist and Physician in Charge of EEG
Department, Park Hospital for Children, Oxford; Clinical Lecturer
in Psychiatry, University of Oxford

C. W. M. Whitty, MA, BSc, DM, FRCP
Consultant Neurologist, Radcliffe Infirmary, Oxford; Clinical
Lecturer in Neurology, University of Oxford

Moyra Williams, BLitt, DPhil(Oxon)
Consultant Psychologist, Fulbourn Hospital and United Cambridge
Hospitals

O. L. Zangwill, MA, FRS
Professor of Experimental Psychology, University of Cambridge;
Visiting Psychologist to the National Hospitals, London

Preface to Second Edition

In the decade which has followed the publication of the first edition of this book, no major advances have occurred in our understanding of amnesia. The position remains much as Sir Charles Symonds saw it in the conclusion of his Foreword to that edition. However an increased interest in the subject and additions to the literature, both in the field of experimental psychology and clinical medicine, justify the production of a second edition.

The interests and techniques of experimental psychology have been directed to an analysis of persisting states of amnesia. While no fundamental contributions to the subject have as yet emerged, a number of theoretical concepts and models of memory and *per contra* of amnesia have been generated and are beginning to have a collateral reflection in clinical studies. In addition, studies along these lines have clarified thinking and defined more accurately some of the content and contributory factors in amnesia. They accordingly find a more central place in this volume than in its predecessor.

At the psychological level the phenomenon of 'kindling', which seems to provide evidence of a persisting change in cortical function, induced at one site by transient (albeit unphysiological) cortical activity elsewhere, may have important implications for memory mechanisms. Clinically, the delineation of the syndrome of transient global amnesia has provided a model of memory loss, totally reversible but of sufficient duration and sufficiently unalloyed with those other cognitive dysfunctions which confuse the picture in classic Korsakoff states, to justify a chapter of its own. Reconsideration has also been given by several contributors to the nature of retrograde amnesia; this has involved re-appraisal of several widely held, if somewhat ill-supported, assumptions about retrograde amnesia and what it embraces.

Inevitably, there have had to be some changes in authorship as well as in emphasis. Professor Lawrence Weiskrantz, who wrote the admirable chapter on 'Experimental Studies of Amnesia' for the original edition, took the view that there has been so much new work in this general field over the past ten years that bringing his chapter up-to-date would be a major undertaking. As he points out, there have been a number of recent texts and critical reviews relevant to experimental studies of memory, particularly in relation to animal studies, and to add further to their number might seem somewhat redundant. With great regret, the Editors agreed to accept his decision.

In place of Professor Weiskrantz's chapter, Malcolm Piercy has written a new account of 'Experimental Studies of the Organic Amnesic Syndrome' which brings together much of the psychological work to which reference is made above and attempts a critical assessment of the varied, and on occasion discrepant, theoretical interpretations to which it has given rise. His chapter provides useful groundwork for those who wish to build further upon an experimental approach to disorders of learning and memory in man.

When revision of *Amnesia* was being first considered, Dr Brenda Milner informed us that pressure of other work would make it impossible for her to revise and update her chapter on 'Amnesia following Operations on the Temporal Lobes' and she herself suggested Dr Susan Iversen as an exceptionally well-qualified person to write a fresh chapter on this topic. This Dr Iversen was fortunately willing to undertake. She has retained admirably Dr Milner's emphasis upon the effects of temporal lobe surgery and indeed expanded the chapter to take account of much recent work bearing upon temporal lobe function in man. Her chapter does much to maintain a balance between the purely psychological issues discussed by Malcolm Piercy and the predominantly neurological and clinical issues which largely preoccupy the remaining contributors.

Lastly, there have been inevitable changes in the coverage of psychogenic aspects of amnesia. Professor Erwin Stengel, who wrote the original chapter on this theme, informed us some time before his death that he did not wish to revise it for this edition and recommended us to seek another author. We were fortunate to find a worthy successor in Dr R. T. C. Pratt, who has long had a special interest in the relations between organic and psychogenic factors in disorders of memory. At the same time, we considered that it would not be inappropriate from the psychodynamic standpoint to introduce the psychoanalytic approach. Dr M. M. Feldman, who undertook this assignment at very short notice, has brought out well Freud's views on memory which are for the most part widely scattered throughout the corpus of his writings and have seldom, if ever, been brought together in a systematic manner. Although

Freud is often regarded as inimical to neurological explanation in psychology, it should not be forgotten that he himself constantly expressed the belief that the entire psychoanalytical theory of neurosis would one day have to be set on its organic foundations.

Amnesia and memory continue to have their central place in the study of human behaviour. While animal work, with its larger opportunity for controlled experiment, continues to contribute to the cognate but more limited problem of learning, the wider question of memory with its voluntary recall of past (often long past) experience remains predominantly part of the study of man. This will continue to be the heart of the problem and here some small but useful pieces of the jig-saw may have been added. The work confirms and reinforces the general viewpoint of our earlier preface that an understanding of memory and its disorders must lie within the framework of neurology.

Sir Charles Symonds' Foreword is still apposite and we are grateful both for his agreement to retain it and for his continued advice. Our thanks are again due to the Editorial staff of Butterworths for advice and guidance over technical problems; and to Mrs Marion Crouch for expert secretarial assistance.

C.W.M.W.
O.L.Z.

Preface to First Edition

There have been several recent symposia on problems of memory viewed from the neurophysiological and experimental psychological standpoint, but there has been no attempt on any scale to draw together the findings of neurology, psychiatry and clinical psychology relevant to memory and its disorders. The need exists for a work covering the whole topic of amnesia in a systematic way. Amnesia is not only of interest in itself, but also a matter of highly practical concern to many physicians, psychologists and lawyers who have not infrequently to deal with the difficult diagnostic and medicolegal problems which it may pose. After consultation with several people known to have an interest in the subject, it was decided that the best form in which to try and meet this requirement was in a book with multiple authorship. In no other way, it was felt, could the many and varied ramifications of the subject be explored at an appropriate level of expert knowledge. The editors, therefore, approached a number of people in the fields of neurology, psychiatry and psychology whose work they knew to be concerned with memory and its disorders, inviting contributions within their respective areas of specialist competence. Happily, almost all were in a position to accept and the result is the present book.

Although the editors have endeavoured to keep the scientific implications of amnesia well to the fore, they cannot deny that they have sought contributions primarily from those concerned with the subject in its clinical and pathological aspects. This policy was deliberate, and was the outcome of the present lacuna envisaged in the literature on memory. It is hoped that the volume may not only provide a broadly based survey of disorders of memory, but also stimulate those whose interests lie primarily in the scientific sphere to ask fresh questions. In particular, it is believed that far greater heed should be paid to the findings of clinical enquiry in formulating general theories of memory.

xvi

No book, not even a collective one, can wholly dispense with a point of view. While no attempt has been made to constrain the contributors in any way, it must be said that a distinctive point of view quite certainly emerges. This may be broadly described as a neurological one. By this is meant that memory is viewed as a biological capacity, if one of very considerable complexity, that may be expected to find its ultimate explanation in terms of the physical structure and functions of the central nervous system. In consequence, the approach to amnesia, whether viewed from the experimental or the clinical standpoint, is largely governed by considerations of cerebral organization and its breakdown. At the same time, it should be clearly understood that this approach implies no disregard of psychological issues or lack of appreciation of those who, like Freud, have chosen to approach the problem of memory from an exclusively psychological angle: although it is worth noting that his own earlier viewpoint was a strikingly neuro-psychological one. Indeed, psychopathological issues are considered at some length by several contributors to this volume. However, it does imply a belief that progress in our understanding of memory and its disorders is most likely to come about within the broad framework of organic neurology.

Apart from our contributors who have worked so loyally within the somewhat arbitrary framework imposed upon them, our gratitude is due to many who have helped us with advice and criticism. First and foremost, we wish to thank Sir Charles Symonds, who encouraged us from the beginning to persist with the idea of this book, and who so kindly agreed to write the Foreword. Dr. Ritchie Russell's early interest and advice was also a valuable impetus. We wish also to express our thanks to the Editorial Staff of Messrs. Butterworths for their advice and forbearance in the face of difficulties inseparable from the preparation of a book of this character. Mrs. M. B. M. Litman Goodchild, Mrs. J. Brett, Miss Susan Davies and the late Mrs. E. Goscombe gave invaluable secretarial assistance.

C.W.M.W.
O.L.Z.

1 Experimental Studies of the Organic Amnesic Syndrome

M. F. Piercy

INTRODUCTION

Since the publication of the first edition of this book, there have been numerous reports of experimental studies of the organic amnesic syndrome. This work has not only resulted in the emergence of challenging new facts but has also brought into focus a number of sources of theoretical controversy. The controversies are radical and many of the facts would have been unexpected in 1966. One consequence of this state of affairs is that any attempt to synthesize and resolve outstanding issues is at present likely to be rather polemical. Despite this danger, a review of the experimental evidence can and should go somewhat beyond a bald presentation of the empirical data. An investigator's choice of experiment is commonly determined by theoretical predilection and, in this area of research, there are considerable difficulties in avoiding tacit and possibly unjustified assumptions when experimental results are examined for their theoretical implications. Although little is to be gained from theoretical nihilism, an occasional sceptical comment on current theoretical positions may help broaden the view available to the uncommitted reader and yield some impression of the variety and quality of competing explanations.

Some previous reviews concerned with organic memory defects (Weiskrantz, 1971; Warrington and Weiskrantz, 1973) have encompassed experimental studies in animals and studies of other types of memory disorder in man such as retrograde amnesia following head injury and memory disturbance specific to a particular sensory modality. This is not attempted here. Studies of this kind, especially certain animal studies, have been cited in support of particular theories of amnesia. However, in this chapter, such indirect evidence has been sacrificed in the interests of properly accommodating recent experimental studies of the organic amnesic syndrome itself and, to a lesser extent, certain associated studies of normal memory. Theories of human amnesia which are derived from animal studies but which have not been directly tested in the human are outside the compass of this chapter. Accordingly the theoretical suggestions offered by animal experimenters such as Gaffan (1972) and Nadel and O'Keefe (1974) are not discussed here.

Influence of theories of normal memory

A prominent feature of much recent work is its close association with theories of normal memory processes. This feature produces difficulties as well as obvious advantages. On the credit side, the converging of amnesic research and normal memory research gives hope both that amnesia may clarify the nature of normal memory processes and that analysis of amnesia in terms of hypotheses arising from normal memory research may more rapidly illuminate the nature of the defect. On the debit side however, the controversial character of modern theories of normal memory presents problems when concepts derived from these theories are used in attempts to explain amnesia.

One notable example of ambiguities introduced into amnesic research by modern theories of memory is the distinction usually made between short- and long-term memory. The distinction is made in order to account for certain disjunctions in normal verbal memory relating to storage capacity, speed of forgetting and the encoding of information in memory. The evidence cannot be presented here and has been reviewed elsewhere (e.g. Baddeley and Patterson, 1971). But briefly, experimental work has given rise to a fairly widely accepted notion that two distinct processes are involved in normal human memory, at least for verbal material. One process is concerned with short-term memory and operates only when no distraction occurs between the presentation of information and its subsequent retrieval. It is a store of strictly limited capacity and this is illustrated by the limitations of immediate memory for sequence: usually 7 or 8 unrelated, ungrouped items. It is also a temporary store and this is illustrated by the rapid decay of newly acquired information when rehearsal is prevented by 30 seconds of verbal distraction occurring immediately after presentation of the information. The other process is concerned with long-term memory —

e.g. for well rehearsed information – which is far more durable and has no known limit to its storage capacity. The short-term process is concerned primarily with acoustically coded information and the long-term process with semantically coded information. Thus information in the short-term store is especially susceptible to interference from acoustically similar material whereas information in the long-term store is more susceptible to interference from semantically similar material. It has also been generally assumed that information reaches the long-term store by transfer from the short-term store.

It has been suggested both by theorists concerned with normal memory (Atkinson and Shiffrin, 1968; Wickelgren, 1973) and by investigators interested in amnesia (Warrington and Weiskrantz, 1973) that organic amnesia provides particularly convincing verification of this hypothesis concerning the structure of normal memory: in amnesia, the long-term component is severely impaired but the short-term component is said to be intact. The difficulty is that the suggestions concerning differences in coding, in capacity and in rates of forgetting, as well as the suggestion that the contents of the long-term store originated in the short-term store, are all now in question. (Baddeley and Scott, 1971; Craik and Lockhart, 1972; Schulman, 1971; Shallice and Warrington, 1970). If, therefore, an appeal is made to amnesic research to confirm the original hypothesis, the position, as Marslen-Wilson (1974) has pointed out, becomes circular. The performance of amnesics on tests of 'short-term memory' cannot readily be accepted as demonstrating dissociation of short- and long-term memory in amnesia if the distinction which these tests are alleged to reveal is not adequately justified other than by amnesic performance.

A further example of the uneasy relationship between normal memory theory and research into amnesia is provided by our ignorance concerning the processes involved in normal forgetting. Some theorists have wished to explain all human forgetting as the effect of interference (Melton, 1963; Underwood, 1957). Others would postulate processes of memory-trace decay (Wickelgren, 1970), and it has also been pointed out that trace decay could entail greater sensitivity to interference effects. It is now rather generally acknowledged that amnesics are very sensitive to interference effects and it can readily be seen that there is likely to be uncertainty as to whether increased sensitivity to interference is the cause or the consequence of the amnesic defect. It must simply be accepted that unresolved issues in research into normal human memory form the unavoidable theoretical background of recent studies of amnesia and that these introduce uncertainties into present attempts to give an account of the functional basis of the organic amnesic syndrome.

The definition of organic amnesia

Although it is the purpose of this chapter to describe and, in some degree, evaluate recent empirical studies, one methodological difficulty must be mentioned. This concerns the definition of organic amnesia and the basis on which patients are selected as suitable cases of the syndrome. At least three different procedures have been adopted: (1) Patients in whom the locus of the lesion is thought to be known with some precision are studied and the disabilities observed are ascribed to loss of the functions sustained by that cerebral region (e.g. Milner, 1970); (2) Amnesia is explicitly or tacitly defined in some way and all patients whose symptoms conform to that definition are accepted for investigation, irrespective of aetiology, (e.g. Warrington and Weiskrantz, 1970; Warrington and Baddeley, 1974); (3) Amnesia is defined in some way but the only patients accepted for investigation are those whose symptoms both conform to the definition and occur in association with a particular aetiology, even though the lesion may not be precisely known in individual cases (e.g. Butters and Cermak, 1974). These practices call for consideration of at least two possible ways in which different groups of patients may vary in their memory performance. First, patients with different lesions may have different types of memory disability even though their symptoms conform to some agreed clinical or test criterion. It has indeed already been claimed that alcoholic Korsakoff patients and postencephalitic amnesic patients each have certain memory defects which are not shared by the other group (Lhermitte and Signoret, 1972). Second, different groups of patients may vary in the severity of their amnesia. No-one has ever questioned that mild forms of amnesia are often observed and such cases are not usually included in studies of the amnesic syndrome. However, given that organic amnesia is inadequately understood and that previously unsuspected facts about amnesic performance are coming to light, it is quite possible that different patients regarded as maximally amnesic differ quantitatively in their memory capacities in such a way as to give rise to disagreements as to what amnesics can and cannot do. Finally, although it is usual to exclude from consideration patients who have intellectual disabilities additional to the amnesia, it must be remembered that if amnesia, or a particular form of amnesia, is associated with a defect in the initial encoding of information in memory, then this encoding defect might be elicited by tests which are not tests of memory (e.g. Oscar-Berman, 1972; Lhermitte and Signoret, 1972). If the discovery of such associated non-mnemonic cognitive defects resulted in these patients being excluded from consideration because they were not 'pure' cases of memory defect, then the question of the nature of amnesic defects would have been prejudged by the premature definition of amnesia.

We are therefore confronted with a variety of experimental techniques utilized by investigators with different theoretical orientations and applied to groups of patients which may or may not differ in the type and extent of the amnesia. Before inspecting this evidence, it would perhaps be sensible to enumerate briefly, and perhaps rather dogmatically, the features of the organic amnesic syndrome on which, so far, there is little or no disagreement.

The area of agreement

What amnesics cannot do

Patients designated as severely amnesic are extremely inefficient at describing on request unique events in their lives which occurred more than two or three minutes ago but subsequent to the onset of the amnesic state. Similarly, the explicit verbal recall of a list of test items such as pictures or common words is grossly defective, and when the retention interval is several minutes, commonly completely absent. When conventional methods are used, these patients are incapable of learning to a conventional criterion (e.g. two successive correct repetitions) sequential verbal material which appreciably exceeds their immediate memory span. Cumulative learning to criterion of certain other not obviously verbal sequential tasks such as tactile mazes which exceed a certain length, is also impossible. Recognition of previously shown common words, nonsense shapes and faces is also grossly defective compared with normal performance. These features yield the clinical impression that amnesic patients 'forget the incidents of their daily life as fast as they occur' (Scoville and Milner, 1957).

What amnesics can do

There is also a good measure of agreement concerning some of the mnemonic abilities which remain comparatively efficient among amnesics. Indeed the most outstanding general conclusion that can be drawn from research over the last ten years is that severely amnesic patients can, in certain ways, retain far more information than was previously suspected. There is general agreement that immediate memory as tested by the digit-span test is usually unimpaired, although there is now radical disagreement as to whether 'short-term memory' is spared. As early as 1962, Milner demonstrated that a severely amnesic patient with bilateral surgical lesions of the hippocampus was capable of learning a mirror drawing task. There was clear evidence of cumulative learning both within and between three daily sessions. Performance at the beginning of each session was at the level attained at the end of the previous day's session (*see* Chapter 6). In the same patient, Corkin (1968) demonstrated learning and retention of three further motor skills, although the performance of the control subjects included in her experiment made it clear that the patient's learning was less efficient. The performance of the same patient on maze learning is described in Chapter 6 where it is made clear that capacity for cumulative learning is inversely related to the length of the maze. Starr and Phillips (1970) obtained similar maze-learning results from a patient who was severely amnesic, but otherwise undemented, six years after an episode of herpes encephalitis. Learning was slower than the normal but there was clear evidence of learning and of savings on relearning. The same patient, who could play the piano, was taught a new melody and the following day could reproduce the piece after being prompted with the first few bars.

Relatively efficient learning and retention demonstrated in amnesic patients has not been confined to the acquisition of skills involving motor performance. Warrington and Weiskrantz (1968b) demonstrated that, under certain conditions of testing, severely amnesic patients were able to retain both pictorial and verbal information. Their technique was based on Williams' (1953) methods of progressive prompting and, in one experiment, they used items from Gollin's (1960) test in which picture perception is examined by presenting fragmented versions of pictures of single objects. There were five versions of each picture, starting with the most fragmented version and ending with the complete line drawing. Studying six amnesic subjects working with ten sets of pictures, they demonstrated cumulative learning of this task between sessions on the same day and significant savings between successive days as measured by an error score. A non-specific practice effect was excluded by subsequently observing performance on a fresh set of fragmented pictures. Scores on this set were comparable with the original performance on the experimental set. Similar savings between days was observed on a test of fragmented words which were prepared by photographing words through patchwork filters of varying density (*Figure 1*).

In a further experiment, these authors were able to show that the facilitating effect of this partial cueing on amnesic memory did not depend solely on the perceptual character of the task (Weiskrantz and Warrington, 1970b). Amnesic patients could be taught to identify a short list of 5-letter words in response to the first two letters of each word. Training involved presenting graded cues of this kind, including if necessary the whole word, until each word was recognized from its first two letters alone. After a one-hour retention interval, the procedure was repeated and significant savings were observed for both amnesics and controls on the first trial of relearning compared with the first trial of original learning.

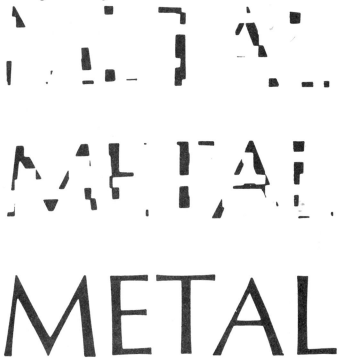

Figure 1. Example of fragmented word (Warrington and Weiskrantz, 1968b. Reproduced by permission.)

The work so far described, is unlikely to be challenged insofar as it is presented descriptively. Few would disagree that, under the conditions of these experiments, amnesic patients are able to utilize information which has been held in store over a considerable period of time. Disagreements arise only in explaining why these rather than other memory performances are spared.

However, there is much other work concerning which there is no consensus. In some instances the facts are too closely tied to particular theoretical positions to be usefully described without the theoretical context. These theoretical positions are remarkably diverse. Their range may be illustrated by a simple list of the main classes of hypotheses currently discussed concerning the organic amnesic syndrome: (i) amnesia is a defect of a process of 'consolidation', i.e. a process which gives durable status to information temporarily in store; (ii) amnesia results from inadequate encoding of information at the time it is entered into store; (iii) amnesia results from defective retrieval of information which is however encoded and stored normally. The second and third of these classes of hypothesis can be subdivided into a number of more specific and rather different hypotheses which receive attention later in this chapter. Associated with these theoretical disagreements are some disagreements as to the facts. Perhaps the most obtrusive of these is the question as to whether 'short-term memory' is impaired in organic amnesia.

SHORT-TERM MEMORY

Until recently there was fairly general agreement that, whereas 'long-term memory' (LTM) was severely impaired in organic amnesia, 'short-term memory' (STM) was unaffected. Today there is marked disagreement on this issue. As mentioned in the Introduction, there is by no means universal agreement that a two-process model adequately describes data concerning normal memory and, among those who adopt such a model, there is disagreement as to its precise characteristics. Because of suggestions, which are not reviewed here, that typical STM experiments in some degree tap the long-term component, an explicit distinction is sometimes made between the short- and long-term memory experimental paradigms and the hypothetical short-and long-term memory processes. The latter are often nowadays designated primary and secondary memory, respectively — the terms were first used by James (1890) — and this convention is adopted here.

Primary memory (PM) is usually regarded as a component of memory (typically verbal memory) showing rapid forgetting within seconds of item presentation or as a component characterized by a store of very limited capacity, or as both. Evidence mainly concerned with capacity and evidence mainly concerned with forgetting may be considered separately.

Capacity

A fairly direct test of the proposition that amnesic patients have unimpaired storage capacity in PM would be provided by a technique of the kind employed by Waugh and Norman (1965). They studied STM for digits varying not only the number of potentially interfering items but also the speed of presentation of items. A capacity constraint was inferred from the observation that forgetting was directly determined by number of items but negligibly affected by speed of presentation of items (faster speed of presentation involves a shorter retention interval for any given span of items). No attempt appears to have been made to apply this kind of test to amnesic patients. The nearest approach has been the simple digit-span test and, as mentioned earlier, there is no disagreement that this is typically within the normal range (Talland, 1965; Drachman and Arbit, 1966; Baddeley and Warrington, 1970). Although this task is commonly regarded as reflecting the capacity of PM, the fact that opportunity for passive decay is confounded with number of items cannot be wholly ignored. It is tempting to infer that, insofar as either reduced capacity or faster forgetting should result in a reduced span, amnesics must be free from either of these defects. However, the work on short-term forgetting reviewed below warns against immediate acceptance of such a conclusion. It does however seem reasonable to say that the performance of amnesic patients on digit span in quite consistent with unimpaired storage capacity in PM and that no evidence has been reported to suggest the contrary.

Forgetting

There is sharp disagreement as to the facts when amnesic and control subjects are examined on tests of short-term forgetting. There are two main studies which yield apparently contradictory results and these are considered in some detail because they exemplify a number of the methodological and theoretical difficulties of research into amnesia.

Baddeley and Warrington (1970) studied six amnesic and six control subjects using a technique introduced by Brown (1958) and by Peterson and Peterson (1959). Subjects were presented with sets of three 3-letter words and were then required to count backwards until recall was requested. The results are shown in *Figure 2* and there is obviously no difference between the forgetting curves of the amnesics and the normals, both groups reaching an asymptote at about 40 per cent correct after 60 seconds. At first sight this seems to endorse the suggestion that selective sparing of primary memory in amnesia provides critical additional evidence for the two-process theory of memory.

In startling contrast to this finding, Cermak, Butters and Goodglass (1971) observed six Korsakoff patients to be significantly inferior to controls on the same type of test (*Figure 3*). The performance of the groups is identical with zero delay but differs significantly even with retention intervals as brief as 3 seconds. Is the discrepancy between these two results attributable to differences between the patients who served as subjects or to small but critical differences in the technique of testing? No confident answer can be given but a number of considerations are relevant. The patients in the American study (Cermak, Butters

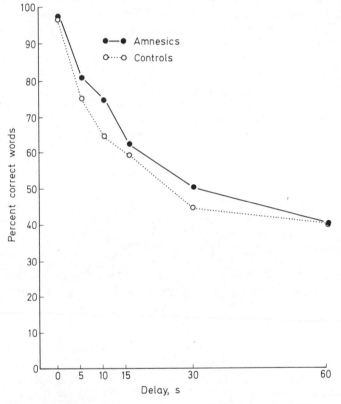

Figure 2. Short-term retention of word triads by amnesic and control subjects (Baddeley and Warrington, 1970. Reproduced by permission.)

and Goodglass, 1971) were all cases of the alcoholic Korsakoff syndrome whereas, of Baddeley and Warrington's six patients, four carried this diagnosis, one had undergone a right temporal lobectomy for epilepsy with no pre- or postoperative evidence of left hemisphere involvement, and one was thought to have had a vascular lesion. If Korsakoff patients have impaired PM and hippocampal patients do not, this would be insufficient to explain the discrepancy because the British results should be heavily weighted by the four Korsakoff patients.

Conceivably patients in the American sample had pronounced intellectual deficits additional to the amnesia but the authors specifically state that this possibility was excluded. Again, it is conceivable that the American patients were simply more amnesic than the British (studied

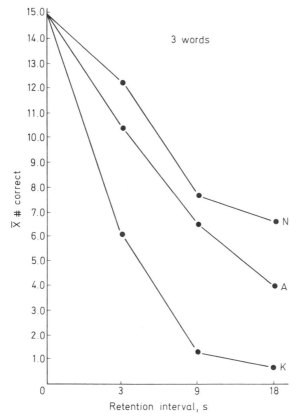

Figure 3. Short-term retention of word triads by Korsakoff (K), Alcoholic (A) and Normal (N) groups. (Cermak, Butters and Goodglass, 1971. Reproduced by permission.)

by Baddeley and Warrington) and that impairment of PM becomes apparent only when amnesia exceeds a certain threshold of severity. It is difficult to know how to exclude this possibility. There are no grounds for supposing that either group of investigators would include patients who were not on clinical examination severely amnesic. On the other hand, there are no empirical grounds for assuming that organic amnesia is an all or none state, or that an end-point of severity is identifiable, or that two severely but not equally amnesic patients are discriminable on clinical examination.

Whatever difficulties there may be between the patients serving as subjects in the two studies, Baddeley and Warrington's result poses important problems. The authors acknowledge that forgetting by normals was much slower in their experiment than is usual in the Brown–Peterson procedure. Why? Seeing that the performance of controls as well as amnesics was anomalous, the answer presumably concerns the technique used. If, despite the experimenters' pains to maintain verbal distraction, some rehearsal occurred throughout the retention interval, then much of the material may in consequence have been maintained in PM. This would be consistent with the fact that counting backwards was paced in the American study but not apparently in the British study (Baddeley and Warrington, 1970). But there is a more interesting and probable possibility. Unlike the American study and unlike the usual Brown–Peterson experiment, in the British study verbal distraction did not start until four seconds after stimulus presentation. If rehearsal occurred during this period then, at least among normals, material may have entered secondary memory (SM). In this case the controls' performance of 40 per cent correct responses after 60 seconds of verbal distraction would not be surprising. It would, however, be necessary to say that with this material and over this retention interval amnesics' SM is unimpaired compared with normal performance. It would no longer be necessary to assume remarkable differences between the patients studied in the two experiments but it would become necessary to reappraise the nature of the amnesics' defect of SM. Unimpaired verbal memory outside the STM paradigm would certainly be an exceptional observation in amnesia.

Serial position effects

One set of observations which has encouraged the 2-process theory of normal memory concerns the characteristics of the serial position curve for free recall (e.g. *see* Kintsch, 1970). This typically shows a marked but labile recency effect benefitting the last few items in a series (attributed to PM), and a smaller but stable primary effect benefitting the first few items in a series (attributed to SM). *Figure 4* shows the serial position curves obtained by Baddeley and Warrington (1970) for immediate free recall by their amnesic and control subjects.

The two groups perform equally well on the last items but the amnesic group is inferior on earlier items. Baddeley and Warrington argue that a normal recency effect suggests intact PM. However, it is difficult to be sure that the PM component in the recency effect is entirely normal because it is not entirely clear how early in the series the recency effect begins. Amnesics are unequivocally as good as controls only for the last two positions in the series of ten. Adopting a technique pre-

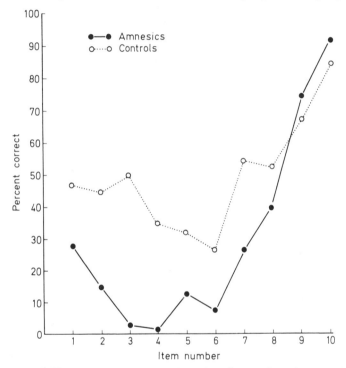

Figure 4. Mean percentage correct on immediate free recall as a function of order of presentation. (Baddeley and Warrington, 1970. Reproduced by permission.)

viously employed by Glanzer and Cunitz (1966), Baddeley and Warrington also tested free recall following a delay filled with verbal distraction. On the assumption that delayed recall is free from PM effects, they subtracted scores on delayed recall from scores on free recall and described this difference as an estimate of the number of items which, although represented in PM, fail to be represented in SM. They also computed a different estimate for the total content of PM. This estimate disregards the subsequent fate of these items in SM. They found no difference between amnesics and controls for either of these two estimates. The observations concerning the total content of PM are of course consistent with their hypothesis of intact PM in amnesia. However, the fact that there was no difference between the groups in the estimate of items represented in PM but not in SM is not consistent with their hypothesis. If the two groups differ markedly for SM but not at all for PM, a greater proportion of the content of amnesics' PM should fail subsequently to be recalled from SM. That is to say, the difference between immediate and delayed recall should be greater in amnesics than controls.

Neither of these estimates takes any account of serial position effects. Baddeley and Warrington's serial position curves for delayed recall, like those for immediate recall, are not easy to interpret. The amnesics appear to perform anomalously on the final item in the series, scoring nearly as well as the controls despite 30 seconds of interpolated verbal distraction. The various anomalies outlined above present some difficulties for Baddeley and Warrington's claim that their free recall data suggest intact PM but impaired SM in amnesia. These anomalies also raise again the possibility referred to in relation to the same authors' results concerning the Brown—Peterson task. The results of both experiments suggest that, even under conventional test conditions, some salient items of information may be retained by amnesics even after verbal distraction and — at least over the short retention intervals utilized in these experiments — may be recalled in a near-normal fashion.

Interference

The rapid forgetting which characterizes performance on the Brown—Peterson task represents the mean performance on numerous successive trials. However, Keppel and Underwood (1962) have shown that surprisingly little forgetting occurs on the first trial of such experiments although forgetting is very marked on second and subsequent trials. Inasmuch as forgetting is clearly increased by the occurrence of previous trials, Keppel and Underwood's suggestion that the effect is an instance of proactive interference (PI) may readily be accepted as a statement of the facts without accepting any particular theory. Both of the groups of investigators whose conflicting findings were described above have also examined the development of PI in amnesics and controls. Again their findings are grossly discrepant. Mean performance of amnesics and controls on successive trials using a 15-second retention interval is shown for Baddeley and Warrington's (1970) subjects in *Figure 5*.

There is a decrement in performance between the first and second items for both groups but no difference between the groups in amount of PI.

Cermak and Butters (1972) studied sensitivity to PI on STM tasks rather differently and obtained quite different results. In one experiment the Brown—Peterson technique was administered in blocks of

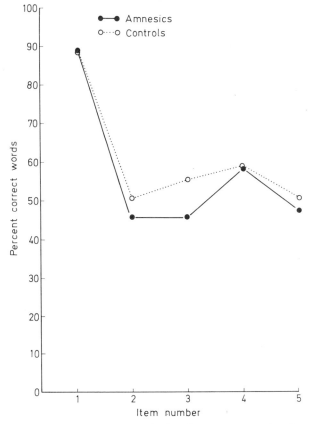

Figure 5. Development of proactive interference on successive short-term memory tasks. (Baddeley and Warrington, 1970. Reproduced by permission.)

two trials with a six-second inter-trial interval. In some blocks the same type of material was employed in both trials (words); in other blocks the material differed between the two trials (consonant trigrams in the first trial and words in the second). This procedure takes advantage of the demonstration by Wickens, Born and Allen (1963) that PI on successive trials of a STM task is maximized by similarity of materials to be remembered and minimized by dissimilarity. Table 1 shows Cermak and Butters' results for Korsakoff patients and alcoholic controls under conditions of high PI (similar materials) and low PI

TABLE 1

Effect of similarity of material between trials on proactive interference in STM performance.

	Korsakoff	Control
9 s	52%	23%
18 s	40%	14%

The percentages are recall decrements between high PI conditions and low PI conditions $(H-L)/(H+L)$ after 9- and 18-s retention intervals. (Cermak and Butters, 1972. Reproduced by permission.)

(dissimilar materials). The decrement between the low and high PI conditions is substantially greater in the Korsakoffs than the controls for each of the two retention intervals studied. In another experiment Cermak and Butters studied the effect of inter-trial intervals on STM performance. Loess and Waugh (1967) showed that in normals PI is greatest with short inter-trial intervals and becomes negligible with inter-trial intervals exceeding two minutes. Table 2 shows Cermak and Butters' results when the effect of inter-trial intervals of 6 seconds

TABLE 2

Effect of inter-trial interval on proactive interference in STM performance.

	Korsakoff	Control
CCC	30%	11%
WWW	76%	32%

The percentages are recall decrements between massed practice and distributed practice $(M-D)/(M+D)$ shown for consonant trigrams (CCC) and word triads (WWW). Inter-trial intervals: 6 s (massed practice); 60 s (distributed practice). (Cermak and Butters, 1972. Reproduced by permission.)

(massed practice) and 60 seconds (distributed practice) are compared. The decrement resulting from reducing the inter-trial interval is clearly much greater in the Korsakoffs than the controls for each of the two types of material used in the memory tests.

Possible explanations for the different results obtained by the two groups of investigators have already been considered and because each group used the same techniques and patient populations for both the short-term forgetting experiments and the PI experiments it is to be presumed that the same methodological considerations apply to both types of experiment. A curious theoretical ambiguity surrounds Cermak and Butters' observations. Although these authors appear to have demonstrated increased sensitivity to PI on STM tasks among amnesics, they do not regard this difficulty as primary. They consider that amnesic patients are more vulnerable to interference effects only as a consequence of the restricted coding operations which they believe to characterize amnesic memory. On the other hand, Warrington and Weiskrantz (1973) apparently do not accept that amnesics have difficulty on STM tasks (and hence presumably do not accept that they are particularly vulnerable to interference on these tasks). Nonetheless these authors suggest that amnesics' defective LTM performance results from abnormal sensitivity to PI! This confused state of affairs centres on the different ways in which interference is seen. Cermak and Butters have *demonstrated* increased sensitivity to interference in amnesics but interpret this observation in terms of defective coding in memory. In contrast, Warrington and Weiskrantz have *postulated* abnormal interference to explain other anomalies of amnesic performance, yet have not actually demonstrated that conventional methods of provoking interference produce greater effects in amnesics than controls.

One experiment may be suggested which conceivably could help decide whether abnormally high levels of PI in amnesia are the cause or the consequence of accelerated 'short-term' forgetting. The occurrence of PI provides undeniable evidence that the prior activity is still having an effect and is therefore, at least in some sense, still in store. In the Brown—Peterson paradigm when inter-trial intervals are progressively *increased*, up to what interval is STM performance of amnesics and controls facilitated? In normals this interval does not exceed two minutes (Loess and Waugh, 1967). If PI of this type lasts longer in amnesics than normals then it remains quite possible that PI is a prime cause of amnesics' STM defect. On the other hand, if PI in normals is detectable over an inter-trial interval which is greater than the maximum interval over which it can be detected in amnesics, a quite different interpretation is encouraged. It is improbable that amnesic forgetting is determined primarily by PI if this dissipates more rapidly in amnesics than in normals.

Although this experiment might throw light on the role of PI in amnesics' performance on STM tasks, it would not necessarily do the same for their performance on LTM tasks. Although in STM experiments PI decays within two minutes as a function of inter-trial interval, in LTM experiments PI *increases* as a function of retention interval over periods greatly in excess of two minutes. Although the term 'proactive interference' is used in connection with both effects, the relationship between them is obscure. It could in fact be argued that 'interference' is itself too much in need of explanation to be employed as an explanatory principle in amnesia.

To summarize the research into amnesic performance on STM tasks is to summarize a series of confusions. First, there is radical disagreement as to whether amnesic patients are impaired on standard short-term forgetting tasks. This conflict of evidence may result either from relatively small but crucial differences of experimental technique, or from major differences in the type of patients studied, or from both. Second, there has been no well controlled study of capacity constraints relating to immediate memory in amnesia but there is general agreement that digit span is essentially normal. This is *prima facie* evidence of a normal capacity constraint on amnesics' PM but whether the assumptions involved in describing their performance in terms of PM and SM are justified is quite unclear. Third, the only study of serial position effects in recall, although providing data broadly consistent with the intact digit span, does not yield a clear-cut picture of impaired SM and intact PM. Fourth, Butters and Cermak have demonstrated markedly increased susceptibility to interference on certain STM tasks among Korsakoff patients. A central theoretical issue is whether, as Butters and Cermak suggest for *all* amnesic memory, this is a consequence of defective encoding or whether, as Warrington and Weiskrantz suggest for amnesic *secondary* memory, abnormal interference is the central defect in amnesia. Finally, the theoretical significance of all this work on amnesic STM performance is clouded by uncertainties as to how normal STM performance should be specified and, in particular, by uncertainties as to the adequacy of the two-process model. Probably no general conclusion can be drawn which will not be disputed by one or other of the investigators already cited. The conclusions drawn here are : (1) that amnesic data shed no clear light on how normal STM performance should be specified, and (2) that, even if a two-process model of normal human memory is accepted, it remains unclear whether or not PM should be regarded as intact in amnesia.

ENCODING AND ORGANIZATIONAL FACTORS

Semantic encoding

It was mentioned in the Introduction that there is some dispute as to how, and even whether, PM may be distinguished from SM. Those who are convinced of the distinction will naturally be concerned as to whether

PM is intact or impaired in amnesia and the work of, for example, Baddeley and Warrington, and of Warrington and Weiskrantz, is formulated in terms of this distinction. For others, however, this distinction may appear largely irrelevant to the problems of amnesia. Thus Butters and Cermak do not endorse the conventional two-process view of memory but instead adopt a 'levels of processing' approach (e.g. Cermak, 1972; Craik and Lockhart, 1972) which assumes that memories may be sequentially processed up to varying levels, with amnesics being constrained as to the level to which processing can be carried. They consider that the primary defect in the Korsakoff syndrome concerns the encoding of information in memory. This encoding is naturally assumed to take place during or very soon after stimulus presentation, and it is for this reason that these investigators have made extensive use of the STM type of experiment.

Butters and Cermak point out that semantic features of such things as word lists and sentences are more durable in memory than acoustic

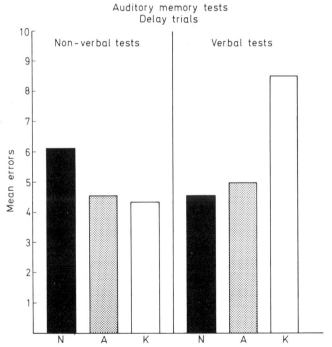

Figure 6. Errors on verbal and non-verbal auditory STM tasks compiled by Korsakoff (K), Alcoholic (A) and Normal (N) groups. (Butters et al. 1973. Reproduced by permission.)

features and suggest that semantic encoding is selectively impaired in amnesia. The abnormally rapid forgetting of three words shown in *Figure 3* has already been referred to. However, these authors point out that this only occurs for verbal material. *Figure 6* shows a comparison of verbal and non-verbal auditory memory in alcoholic Korsakoff patients and non-amnesic alcoholics (Butters, *et al.*, 1973). The verbal items were three unrelated consonants and the non-verbal items sequences of random piano notes. Retention was tested using a recognition technique. Verbal distraction during the retention intervals (9 to 18 seconds) was the same for all conditions. Korsakoffs are significantly impaired on the verbal task but not on the non-verbal. Similar results are reported for the visual and tactile modalities. It was assumed that 'semantic analysis' is not necessary for the storing of non-verbal material and that the material-specific defect observed in amnesics reflects impairment of semantic encoding in memory. 'Semantic' is not closely defined and it is not clear that the concept as used by these workers is distinguishable from 'verbal categorical'. More recent studies from this group (Butters and Cermak, 1975) appear to de-emphasize material-specificity of the defect. They have now shown that non-verbal material is spared in an STM experiment only when the distracting activity is verbal in character. When the distraction is non-verbal, Korsakoffs are impaired compared with controls on non-verbal STM tasks. This observation suggests that the amnesic defect is not confined to semantic encoding as originally defined by these investigators. If their concept of 'semantic' were broadened to include non-verbal codes, their hypothesis might lose some precision, but it would gain considerably in the range of data that it accommodated.

Perhaps the most persuasive evidence of an encoding defect in amnesia is provided by the results of an experiment by Cermak, Butters and Moreines (1974). They made use of an effect which has been discussed in detail by Wickens (1970). It has been shown in normals that PI in STM experiments may be highly specific to the material constituting successive trials. This is revealed when, after four trials on the Brown–Peterson task each using the same type of material (e.g. consonants), the material employed on the fifth trial is changed (e.g. to numerals). The decrement in performance with successive trials may be dramatically reversed when the material changes, and this effect is independent of whether the change is from consonants to numerals or from numerals to consonants. The effect is known as 'release from PI' and has been demonstrated not only with respect to obvious changes in material but also with respect to changes in semantic category when words are used (e.g. animals to plants) and more subtle semantic shifts of which the subject may be quite unaware

(Wickens and Clark, 1968). *Figure 7* shows the performance of Korsakoffs and alcoholic controls in five successive trials under two conditions. In the control condition, all five trials involve the same type of material, either consonant trigrams or three digits. In the experimental condition

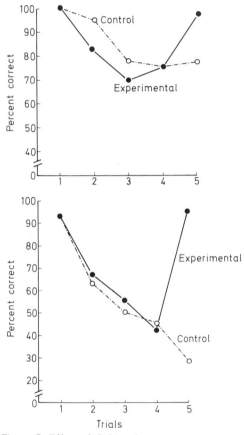

Figure 7. Effect of shifting from numbers to letters (and vice versa) on the STM performance of alcoholic control patients (top) and Korsakoff patients (bottom). (Cermak, Butters and Moreines, 1974. Reproduced by permission.)

the first four trials involve the same type of material (consonants or digits counterbalanced between subjects) but on the fifth trial there is a shift to the alternative material (digits or consonants). The release effect on the fifth trial is clearly evident in both amnesics and control patients. *Figure 8* shows the same experimental procedure except that all five trials involve words. Under both experimental and control conditions for each subject the words in the first four trials conform to the same taxonomic category (animals or vegetables) but on the fifth trial the experimental group shifts to the alternative taxonomic category (vegetables or animals), while the control group is exposed to further

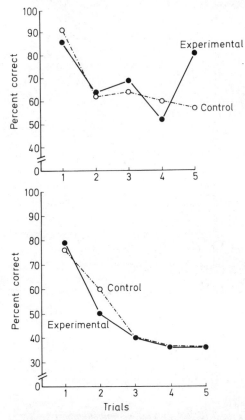

Figure 8. Effect of taxonomic shift on the STM for words of alcoholic control patients (top) and Korsakoff patients (bottom). (Cermak, Butters and Moreines, 1974. Reproduced by permission.)

words conforming to the original category. The non-amnesic patients show release from PI but the Korsakoff patients do not.

Why do Korsakoffs show the effect when the shift is between consonants and numerals but not when the shift is between taxonomic categories? Wickens' argument that release from PI reflects categorizing (or coding) operations is difficult to resist. May we therefore conclude that, at least in this type of experiment, Korsakoff patients do not encode words in memory according to their taxonomic category and accept the argument of Cermak *et al.* that this constitutes compelling evidence that semantic encoding in memory is defective in Korsakoff patients? This is certainly the most straightforward explanation but some account must be taken of the logical point that, although release from PI provides good evidence of categorization, it is possible that categorizing activity may take place without this being reflected in release from PI. Amnesics might be characterized by less concordance than normals between encoding in memory and parameters determining proactive interference. It would then be possible to argue that this experimental result does not reflect impaired semantic encoding. However, in the absence of independent evidence of a disturbed relationship between encoding and PI, the results argue for abnormal encoding in amnesia.

Cueing and recall

Organizational factors in memory have received much experimental attention recently and, influenced by this work, some investigators have examined the possibility that in the organic amnesic syndrome, information is inadequately organized. Some would argue that a defect of organization in memory is equivalent to a defect of encoding. However, it is possible to test amnesic patients for evidence of organization without prejudging this question.

Warrington and Weiskrantz (1971) compared amnesic patients and normal controls with respect to the influence of categorization on their memory for lists of words. In both amnesics and controls, when memory for words was cued by the category name, performance was superior to performance under conditions of free recall. Warrington and Weiskrantz suggested that this finding 'indicates that semantic categorization is as relevant to the performance of amnesic subjects as normal subjects'. Using the same retention interval (one minute) Cermak, Butters and Gerrein (1973) obtained essentially similar results but interpreted them quite differently. They suggest that although Korsakoff patients can encode words by category if encouraged to do so by the instructions or the conditions of the experiment, they nonetheless fail to categorize in this fashion when left to their own devices, e.g. under conditions of free recall. It is, however, noteworthy that the test for cued recall was differently administered by the two groups of workers. When the word list was presented to be remembered, Cermak, Butters and Gerrein drew the attention of their subjects to the fact that the list was categorized but Warrington and Weizkrantz apparently did not. So far as can be gathered from the description of their methods, lists for free recall and for cued recall were administered in an identical fashion. Accordingly, Warrington and Weiskrantz's result cannot readily be explained in terms of a special encoding strategy induced by the instructions, because they showed that, even when left to their own devices at the learning stage, amnesics were as much assisted by category cueing at retrieval as controls.

However, as well as comparing free and cued recall, Cermak, Butters and Gerrein (1973) also compared the effectiveness of different types of cue. In one experiment a list of words was read to Korsakoff patients and alcoholic controls who were then cued for the recall of specific words in the list. These cues were either a rhyme of the word or the category which the word exemplified. The effectiveness of these two types of cue was studied in relation to the number of items intervening between the test word and the relevant cue. No difference between amnesics and controls was observed for rhyming cues at any of the intervals studied but amnesics were significantly inferior to controls when responding to category cues after long delays. It was argued that category cues tapped more sophisticated levels of encoding than the rhyming cues and that these higher levels of encoding are normally more permanent than lower levels. A deficiency in this higher level encoding was held responsible for Korsakoff patients' defective memory. A further experiment by the same authors involved the presentation of paired associates and, in the case of target words which could not be retrieved following presentation of the stimulus words, cueing with a word which was closely associated with the target word (e.g. 'table' as a cue for 'chair'). Although alcoholic controls recalled more words than Korsakoff patients without cueing, the degree of facilitation by associative cueing did not differ significantly between the two groups. Associative cues, like rhyming cues, were regarded as related to levels of encoding which are less durable than categorical or semantic encoding. A third experiment analysed the incidence of different types of false recognitions. Words were presented visually at a regular rate and subjects were instructed to detect repetitions within the list. The list contained not only repetitions but also some words which were acoustically identical with previous items (homophones), some that were closely associated with previous words although distinct in meaning and others that were synonymous with previous words. Although the two groups did not differ significantly in the number of correctly identified repeats, the Korsakoffs, unlike the alcoholic controls, falsely recognized more homophones and associates than synonyms. Although this is interpreted in terms of a tendency among Korsakoffs not to encode spontaneously at the semantic level, the results of this particular experiment do not force this conclusion. Not only did the two groups not differ significantly in the number of repeats correctly identified, but the tendency to falsely recognize synonyms was no more marked in the controls than in the Korsakoff patients.

Imagery

Recent work concerned with semantic aspects of normal human memory has led to the postulation of two different but interacting systems underlying memory for meaningful material: one derived from language skills, the other associated with the use of imagery. The possible role of imagery in facilitating amnesic memory has received attention in three different experiments.

Baddeley and Warrington (1973) examined amnesics' and controls' memory for words when these were grouped according to (a) phonemic similarity, (b) membership of taxonomic category and (c) relevance to a composite visual image described by the experimenter. In the version involving visual imagery, four words were presented visually and linked together by a short spoken sentence describing a scene which the subject was instructed to visualize. On phonemic lists, both amnesic and control subjects did better on clustered lists than control lists and there was no difference in the extent to which amnesics and control subjects were helped by phonemic clustering. On taxonomic lists, amnesics and control subjects were again aided by clustering but amnesic subjects significantly less so than control subjects. Although the authors advise caution in interpreting this last result, it does appear consistent with the suggestion discussed earlier that amnesics are less efficient at taxonomic categorization in memory than phonemic categorization. In the experiment concerned with imagery, control subjects performed significantly better on the lists which were linked by a described scene which the subjects were instructed to visualize than on control lists. Amnesics however, were not significantly aided by the opportunity to form a linking visual image. On the basis of this result, Baddeley (1973) suggests that 'amnesics may be defective in their ability to utilize the imagery component of semantic memory'.

Two experiments have examined the usefulness of imagery in mediating amnesic memory for paired associates. Jones (1974) obtained essentially negative results. The two amnesic patients studied, in contrast to normal controls and patients with unilateral temporal lobectomies, obtained zero scores throughout the test, both with and without imagery. In contrast, Cermak (1975) showed that, compared with rote learning, the provision of a linking image significantly improved Korsakoff patients' performance both on initial learning of paired associates and on a savings measure 24 hours later. An important difference between Cermak's experiment and the other two experiments concerned with imagery is that he trained all subjects to the criterion of an errorless run (involving a mean of 13.5 runs for Korsakoffs in the imagery condition), whereas Jones used only three runs and Baddeley and Warrington only one. Furthermore, Cermak used only five paired associates in each list, (i.e. only 5 words had to be recalled), whereas Jones used ten and Baddeley and Warrington required recall of 16 words. Only Cermak and Baddeley and Warrington compared the effectiveness of imagery with other mnemonic aids. Baddeley and Warrington found imagery less effective for amnesics than either phonemic or semantic clustering but Cermak found imagery and a verbal mediating link equally helpful for amnesics. Only Cermak used strictly comparable training procedures for the imagery condition and other conditions. Baddeley and Warrington presented the imagery list once only but all other lists four times, although they say 'the total presentation time was the same' by virtue of allowing proportionately longer pauses between the items of the imagery list. On the basis of these studies, it would seem reasonable to conclude first that greater difficulty in utilizing imagery compared with other mnemonic aids is not conclusively proved in amnesic patients and second that, if there is such a defect in amnesia there is no reason to suppose that it amounts to complete incapacity to utilize imagery as an aid to memory.

Contextual memory

Although contextual memory in normal people has received relatively little experimental attention, there are grounds for supposing that contextual features may have an important organizing function in memory. Much information which is recalled or recognized tends to be associated in memory with the circumstances in which it was acquired (e.g. when, where and in whose company a new face became familiar). Norman and Rumelhart (1970) have suggested that the attributes of an item have attached to them information about the context in which the item occurred. In recall the contextual information is provided and the subject reconstructs the item from the attributes with the appropriate contextual markers. In recognition the attributes of the item are provided and the subject examines the contextual markers to determine whether the item occurred in the appropriate context.

Huppert and Piercy (1976) investigated the ability of amnesic patients to organize their memories with respect to temporal context, i.e. *when* an event occurred or an item was presented to be remembered. In one experiment they examined the ability of Korsakoff patients to discriminate between items seen ten minutes previously and items seen the previous day. Subjects were first familiarized with 80 pictures by repeated presentations and then, on the following day, were shown half of these together with an equal number of new pictures. The total shown on the second day comprised the list to be remembered. After a ten-minute retention interval, yes–no recognition was tested by showing subjects the items in the test list and an equal number of non-list pictures, half familiar, half new. The mean scores of Korsakoff patients and alcoholic controls are shown in Table 3. Although amnesics obtained

TABLE 3

Differential effect of familiarity of material on yes–no recognition performance by Korsakoff and control patients. (Huppert and Piercy, 1976. Reproduced by permission.)

	Familiar pictures			*Unfamiliar pictures*		
	TP	*FP*	*'Yes'*	*TP*	*FP*	*'Yes'*
Korsakoff	88.8	50.6	69.7	70.0	10.0	40.0
Control	97.5	3.1	50.3	89.4	1.3	45.4

TP – True positive responses as a percentage of all responses to stimulus items.
FP – False positive responses as a percentage of all responses to filler items.
'Yes' – Positive responses (true and false) as a percentage of all responses.

significantly lower scores than controls on both familiar and unfamiliar pictures, their performance was disproportionately poor on familiar pictures. This resulted almost entirely from a very marked tendency to make a positive identifying response to familiar pictures irrespective of whether they were in the list to be remembered. In effect, they were largely unable to discriminate between pictures seen ten minutes previously and those seen the previous day. In contrast, their performance on unfamiliar pictures was relatively efficient and not marked by the very high false positive rate which occurred in response to familiar pictures. The tendency to make a positive identifying response to familiar pictures irrespective of whether they were stimulus or filler items is not readily explained by a response bias constituting a low criterion of acceptance because familiar and unfamiliar items were in random sequence both when the list to be remembered was presented and during recognition testing. It is particularly notable that accurate performance on familiar pictures was possible only if subjects could discriminate between the items according to *when* they were previously seen. Accurate performance on unfamiliar pictures however, could have been achieved by a simple decision as to whether the item had *ever* been seen before. The performance of Korsakoff patients on both unfamiliar and familiar pictures was consistent with recognition judgements being largely determined by whether or not the item had been previously seen at any time.

Huppert and Piercy suggest that amnesics have comparatively little difficulty in judging the overall familiarity of an item but severe difficulty in assigning a temporal context to remembered items. They point out that if context has the role assigned to it in Norman and Rumelhart's model, then defective contextual memory in amnesia would explain not only grossly impaired recognition of pre-experimentally familiar material, but also the characteristically severe defect of recall in amnesia.

Considering the work described in this section as a whole, there would appear to be grounds for concluding that, at least in some respects, information is inadequately encoded or organized in the memory of amnesic patients. The strongest evidence for an encoding defect as such is the failure of Korsakoff patients to show release from PI following shifts between taxonomic categories of words despite showing normal release following shifts between letters and numerals (Cermak, Butters and Moreines, 1974). This evidence relating to verbal material may have a counterpart in non-verbal memory. Baddeley and Warrington's (1973) patients failed to show improved memory performance in association with a mnemonic aid involving imagery. There might therefore be a defect of both verbal and non-verbal semantic encoding in memory. At the same time, there is reason to believe that neither of these defects should be regarded as a complete incapacity. Warrington and Weiskrantz' findings (1971) relating to categorical organization of verbal material provide a reminder that semantic encoding in verbal memory can by no means be regarded as absent in amnesia, and Cermak's (1975) observation that imagery can improve paired associate learning by amnesics tempers the interpretation of Baddeley and Warrington's failure to find any facilitation of amnesic memory by this means. The suggestion of a defect of contextual memory (Huppert and Piercy, 1976) cuts across the verbal/non-verbal dichotomy and raises serious questions as to the ability of Korsakoff patients to organize remembered information with respect to time. Here again the defect is certainly not absolute because, despite severe impairment, they performed above chance in discriminating items seen 10 minutes previously from items seen 24 hours previously. If we provisionally accept that these various lines of evidence suggest some kind of defect or defects relating to the stage at which information is acquired, we should bear in mind that it does not necessarily follow that there are not other independent defects in organic amnesia. It is, however, the case that defects associated with later stages of the memory process could in principle be seen as secondary to defects of encoding or organization whereas, once an encoding defect is accepted, it cannot in principle be seen as secondary to a defect of storage or retrieval.

SPEED OF FORGETTING

It has become clear that, at least under some conditions, amnesic patients can retain information over considerable periods of time. There is also a large measure of agreement that, irrespective of the method of training employed, learning by amnesics, if it occurs at all, is very much slower than the normal. An important question arises as to the fate of those items of information which enter into the long-term memory of amnesic patients insofar as this is suggested by the occurrence of cumulative learning or correct retrieval after a retention interval of several minutes or more. Is the rate of forgetting of such items following further lapse of time comparable with the normal or is the rate of forgetting accelerated?

The answer to this question has important implications for the nature of the amnesic defect. Since it is universally found that, except for certain motor performances, amnesics are slow to learn material in excess of their immediate span, the only two possible types of performance requiring consideration are (i) abnormally slow learning and abnormally fast forgetting, (ii) abnormally slow learning but a normal rate of forgetting. The second possibility would suggest difficulty in getting information into store, but thereafter normal storage and normal retrieval — at least for the type of material with which such an effect is demonstrated. If this were found for most types of material it would be consistent with an encoding defect. It would also be consistent with a consolidation defect provided it was assumed that consolidation did not extend beyond the learning trials. Abnormally fast forgetting would be consistent with several different hypotheses concerning the nature of the amnesic defect. It would be consistent with a consolidation defect if consolidation were considered to have a relatively long time course; it would be consistent with an encoding defect if it was assumed that durability of memory was partly determined by richness of encoding over and above that necessary to reach a criterion of learning; it would be consistent with abnormal sensitivity to proactive interference because PI is known to increase with retention interval; it would also of course be consistent with a defect of the storage mechanism itself.

Investigations by five different groups are relevant to this question. Two studies by Weiskrantz and Warrington are of particular importance because they succeeded in training amnesics and normals on the same materials to the same criterion of learning. In both studies the material to be learnt was a short word-list, all subjects were brought to the criterion of two successive errorless trials and were retrained following a retention interval. Forgetting was measured by a savings score which compared performance on the first trial of relearning with performance on the first trial of original learning. In one study (Weiskrantz and Warrington, 1970a) subjects were trained by inspecting progressively less fragmented versions of the word until that word could be identified. An errorless trial was defined as identification of all words in the list on the basis of their most fragmented versions. Retention and relearning were tested using the same method after intervals of one hour, 24 hours and 72 hours. For the two shorter retention intervals, the control group showed significantly better savings than the amnesic group, but with the 72 hours retention interval the amnesic group did not show significantly less savings than the control group. In the second study (Weiskrantz and Warrington, 1970b) training was conducted by showing subjects the first two letters of each of the five-letter test words and asking them to guess the word. Following wrong guesses, the first three letters and then if necessary the complete word were shown. An errorless trial was a trial in which all words were correctly guessed on the basis of the first two letters. Following a retention interval of one hour, subjects were retrained to the same criterion and a savings score computed. This score was significantly higher in the controls than in the amnesics.

Although these two studies show that, for certain retention intervals, amnesics forget more than controls, the findings of the first study which examined forgetting at three different retention intervals call for discussion. If amnesics forget faster than normals, the difference in retention between the two groups should increase with increasing retention interval. In fact at the longest retention interval there is no significant difference between the groups. Inspection of the data makes it clear that this result cannot be attributed to a floor effect, i.e. virtually complete forgetting in both groups. Accordingly, it is not easy to accept the suggestion that, even when brought to the same criterion of learning, amnesics forget more rapidly than normals. It is possible that, at the shorter retention intervals, normals were aided by a strategy not available to amnesics, e.g. spontaneous unprompted recall of the material (*see* Milner, Corkin and Teuber, 1968). If, at the longest retention interval, this strategy were no longer available to the controls a more straightforward comparison might be available of the ability of normals and amnesics to remember on the basis of the cues provided. Certainly if performance at the longest retention interval is accepted as the most natural and least complicated measure of long-term retention, then the findings do not suggest more rapid forgetting of what has been learnt by amnesics than by controls.

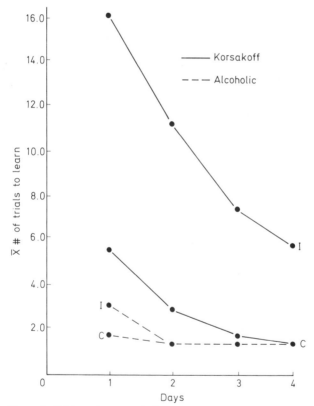

Figure 9. Trials to learn particular paired associates on successive days. For both groups, items learnt correctly by Korsakoff patients on Day 1 (C) and items not learnt correctly by Korsakoff patients on Day 1 (I) are plotted separately. (Cermak, Butters and Goodglass, 1971. Reproduced by permission.)

A normal rate of forgetting by amnesics is indeed claimed by Cermak, Butters and Goodglass (1971) on the basis of rather different evidence. They studied paired associate learning and training was provided on four successive days. Although the Korsakoff patients studied were far less efficient on this task than the non-amnesic alcoholic controls, the Korsakoffs displayed relatively rapid learning on the second and subsequent days of items which they succeeded in acquiring on the first day. The results are shown graphically in *Figure 9*. Although this effect is quite clear, it is not clear that relearning of initially correct items was as fast among the Korsakoffs as among the alcoholic controls. The suggestion by these authors that material which does get processed into the long-term memory of Korsakoff patients is retained in an almost normal fashion should perhaps be treated with caution. It is possible that items which were learnt on the first day were the easier items and would therefore more readily be relearnt after a delay and would be subject to more rapid cumulative learning between days. The authors attempted to control for this possibility by comparing controls' performance on items which Korsakoff patients did and did not learn on the first day. Unfortunately, although this difference was not significant, it was vitiated by a ceiling effect.

In the course of a larger investigation, Huppert and Piercy (1976) examined forgetting of verbal and non-verbal material over a period of seven weeks. Korsakoff patients and non-amnesic alcoholic controls were shown 80 complex pictures and 80 words, and tested for recognition of this material after intervals of ten minutes, one week and seven weeks. On each occasion of testing the same original stimulus items were presented but the filler items not previously seen by the subjects were different for each occasion of testing.

Figure 10 shows percentage of correct responses obtained by each group at the three retention intervals. For each of the three types of material, there is no significant interaction between subject group and retention interval. Decay rates do not therefore appear to differ between amnesics and controls in this experiment. Although forgetting was confounded with any cumulative learning which occurred as a consequence of the re-presentation of the stimulus items on the three occasions of testing, it is very unlikely that this could obscure any tendency of the amnesics to forget faster. For this to happen it would be necessary for amnesics to show more rapid cumulative learning than the controls.

The studies of forgetting so far described have either been confined to Korsakoff patients or else have included patients of this type. There are also two studies which raise the possibility of abnormal forgetting in individual patients with hippocampal lesions. Lhermitte and Signoret (1972) used a task requiring memory for the positions in a 3 X 3 matrix occupied by nine pictures of single objects. Only one of their three postencephalitic patients could be brought to a standard criterion of learning during the acquisition stage but when tested four minutes later, this patient showed defective memory for the positions compared

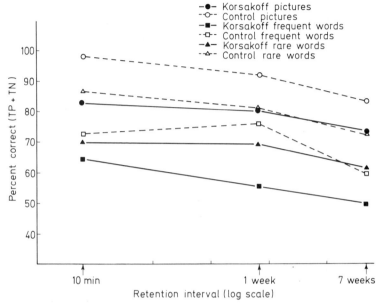

Figure 10. Mean percent correct responses by Korsakoff and control groups on yes—no recognition tests of pictures, high-frequency words and low-frequency words as a function of retention interval. (Huppert and Piercy, 1976. Reproduced by permission.)

with control subjects brought to the same criterion of learning. The same defect was apparent after retention intervals of one hour, 24 hours and four days. Unfortunately, the method of learning was quite different from either of the two methods of testing employed and it is not certain that the criterion performance had been forgotten rather than that it had failed to generalize to the test performance. It is, however, the case that the test performance could not have been correctly executed without memory of spatial position. Accordingly, the observation points at least to the possibility of abnormally rapid forgetting by patients of this type.

Somewhat similar results were obtained in Milner, Corkin and Teuber's (1968) study of maze learning in the patient H.M. While quite incapable of learning a 28-choice-point visual maze, this patient could be brought to the criterion of three successive errorless trials on a drastically shortened version. However, although he showed unmistakable savings when tested on subsequent days and was brought to criterion on three further occasions, he did not execute an errorless performance on any of the test days. Control subjects on the other hand 'show perfect or near-perfect retention of the 28-choice-point maze after 24 hours'. These results reveal undeniably defective learning ability and, at first sight, impaired retention as measured by amount of savings. However, some account must be taken of the fact that H.M. required 155 trials to reach criterion on the shortened maze whereas the 28-choice-point maze 'is mastered by control subjects of comparable age and intelligence in less than 25 trials' (Milner, Corkin and Teuber, 1968). Ettlinger (1962) has pointed out that when tasks are graded as easy or difficult on the basis of number of trials to reach a fixed criterion, training to criterion on an easy task involves more overtraining than training to criterion on a difficult task. He also reported that when tasks differ in difficulty, differences in speed of relearning following a retention interval may be reduced by making the number of trials constituting a criterial run on initial learning proportional to the number of trials the subject needs to reach the level of performance at which the criterial run begins (e.g. 90 per cent correct out of 20 consecutive trials if 200 trials needed, 90 per cent correct out of 40 if 400 trials needed, etc.) It is therefore quite possible that when a maze is learned to a fixed criterion in 155 trials, (as by H.M.), testing 24 hours later taxes relearning capacity much more severely than similar testing of a maze learned in 25 trials (as by controls).

There are in fact severe methodological difficulties in comparing rates of forgetting in groups which differ markedly in speed of learning, and satisfactory comparisons between amnesic and normal rates of forgetting are likely to require more sophisticated test methods than are currently used for this purpose. It appears necessary to conclude that none of the five studies described above has convincingly demonstrated faster forgetting by amnesics than normals in a long-term memory experiment. One of the studies which established comparable levels of initial learning showed no difference between the groups at the longest retention interval although significant differences were observed at the shorter intervals. It is therefore natural to speculate that in this experiment normals had some special advantage at the shorter intervals which was no longer available at the longest intervals. Another study which established criterial learning performance did not examine either savings or retention of the ability to execute the criterial performance. The third study which established criterial learning may have established greater overtraining in the controls than in the amnesic subject. Both of the other two studies were interpreted by their authors as providing no evidence that learnt material is forgotten more rapidly by amnesics than by normals and, in the one study where an interaction was sought between groups and retention interval, no such interaction was found.

It would therefore seem that nobody has yet fully succeeded in attempts to disconfirm the null hypothesis that amnesics do not forget more rapidly than normals information which successfully enters a comparatively long-term store. However, despite these serious reservations, it is of some interest that the two studies which are most suggestive of faster forgetting in amnesics are concerned with the performance of patients with lesions involving the hippocampus. The possibility that these patients have storage defects but that patients with mammillo-thalamic lesions do not, cannot be completely ignored. A prior question however is whether any patients with a selective 'global' amnesia have storage defects.

RETRIEVAL

The radical hypothesis

It has been suggested that retention failure can never conclusively be shown to result from an absence of stored information because some circumstance might always be found in which retention would be unimpaired (Weiskrantz, 1968). In practice however, we are not obliged to assume that amnesia is a defect of retrieval alone and this possibility can be compared with others in the light of available evidence. Indeed the logical difficulty implied by this suggestion is not as great as it seems. Where for example a temporary anterograde amnesia occurs — either naturally as transient global amnesia (*see* Chapter 2) or by injecting sodium amytal into the carotid artery contralateral to an existing hippocampal lesion (Milner, Branch and Rasmussen, 1962) — then, following return to a normal state, failure to remember any events during the amnesic episode is not readily understandable as a defect of retrieval alone.

The suggestion that the amnesic defect is located at the stage where retrieval is attempted has been repeatedly advocated recently, and this suggestion calls for critical attention. In its most radical form, this hypothesis suggests that information is encoded and entered into memory normally and survives normally in store, the defect being associated uniquely with the problem of access to the information in store, (e.g. in consequence of 'undue prominence of interference phenomena', (Warrington and Weiskrantz, 1973). According to this notion, events which occurred long before the onset of the amnesia should be just as vulnerable as events occurring since the onset; in other words the retrograde amnesia should be as severe as the anterograde amnesia. Most clinical descriptions do not accord with this view (*see* Chapter 2) but there is relevant experimental evidence. Sanders and Warrington (1971) tested five amnesic patients and a sample of healthy people on a questionnaire covering public events over several decades and on recognition of faces of people who had been famous. The patients performed worse than controls for all periods covered by the test and no better for remote than for recent events. Because the patients' performance was around the chance level, valid comparison of amnesic memory for different periods was precluded. However, the overall inferiority of the amnesic group to the healthy controls was dramatic for all periods as would be predicted by the hypothesis of a defect located at the stage of retrieval. There are, however, difficulties in basing far-reaching conclusions on these results. Four of the five amnesic patients were women and it is not clear that the test used was free from sex differences. A greater difficulty is the possibility that the amnesic patients did not receive normal exposure to the items constituting the test. Thus, three of the five patients were cases of the alcoholic Korsakoff syndrome and a fourth was a long-standing epileptic. It cannot readily be assumed that, for example, chronic alcoholics pay the same attention to current affairs and currently famous faces as other people.

A test of memory for famous faces has also been used by Marslen-Wilson and Teuber (1975) who studied the performance of the hippocampal patient H.M., Korsakoff patients and normal, head-injured and alcoholic controls. In this study amnesic memory was considerably more impaired for recent than for more remote events. This was particularly obvious in H.M. and, because the date of onset of his amnesia is known precisely, it is clear that memory for events prior to onset is far superior to memory for events which occurred subsequent to onset. Compared with controls, his performance was certainly unimpaired for the 1930s (20–30 years prior to onset), intermediate between head-injured and normal controls for the 1940s (10–20 years prior to onset) but grossly impaired for the years subsequent to onset. This result is frankly inconsistent with a thorough-going retrieval theory because such a theory predicts that memory for pre-onset and post-onset events will be equally impaired. It is not, however, the case that this experiment poses problems only for the retrieval theory. On a version of the test using graded prompts, there is evidence that both H.M. and Korsakoff patients perform well above chance levels (and well above their unprompted performance) in relation to items seen only subsequent to the onset of amnesia. This observation is inconsistent with any theory which postulates absence of new long-term storage.

The disinhibition hypothesis

This hypothesis (Warrington and Weiskrantz, 1970) proposes that amnesics are abnormally sensitive to interference from irrelevant competing memories as a consequence of 'a failure to inhibit or dissipate stored information' (Warrington and Weiskrantz, 1973). This is often referred to as a theory of defective retrieval, both by its authors and by others. As stated, however, the theory is ambiguous. If it is assumed that memories do not decay normally in store then something more than a retrieval defect is postulated. Indeed a failure of memories to decay normally carries no implication that there is any defect of the mechanisms of retrieval. Retrieval would be impaired as a direct consequence of failure to forget in a normal fashion. Such a theory would not entail any remarkable retrograde amnesia. If failure of inhibition is postulated, then this is a theory of retrieval failure only if the disinhibition is supposed to occur solely at the time of attempted retrieval. It is unclear whether Warrington and Weiskrantz are postulating such a retrieval defect or abnormal storage such as would be entailed by absence of normal decay processes. A true abnormal retrieval theory (but not an abnormal storage theory) would demand an across-the-board retrograde amnesia of the kind discussed above. However, both types of theory would find support in further lines of evidence discussed below.

Prior list intrusions

Evidence thought by some to favour the disinhibition hypothesis concerns the incidence of prior list intrusions in recall tests. When tested successively with word lists A and B, an amnesic patient may produce a word from list A when recall of list B is requested. It is pointed out that, although produced as an error, the word must have been stored throughout the period between the presentation of list A and attempted recall of list B. This is slightly misleading because high frequency words are normally used in these tests and such words were in store before the experiment began. Nonetheless it seems clear that production of the word was facilitated by its presentation in list A and that this facilitation was still apparent when list B was subsequently presented and tested. If it is accepted that the memory process impaired in amnesia is not necessarily completely absent, then prior list intrusions constitute evidence for a retrieval defect rather than some other disturbance of memory only if their incidence is higher among amnesics than controls. There seems to be no evidence that this is the case. Weiskrantz and Warrington draw attention to the fact that, in one of their recall experiments (1970b) 50 per cent of wrong responses were intrusions from previous lists. This intrusion rate is not numerically high, amounting to just over one per subject per list, and the rate for the controls is not given. Baddeley and Warrington (1970) also point to the occurrence of prior list intrusions in an experiment concerned with free recall and here both the amnesic and the normal rates can be computed. However, the data do not especially favour the retrieval theory of amnesia. The proportion of wrong responses which were prior list intrusions was 45 per cent among amnesics but 69 per cent among controls. If it is suggested that amnesics fail to recall correctly because they retrieve genuine but inappropriate memories, then the incidence of prior list intrusions should be higher in the amnesics than in the controls. Yet the reverse appears to be the case if the incidence is computed as a proportion of total wrong responses. It is inappropriate to compare prior list intrusions as a proportion of all responses (correct as well as incorrect) because controls will naturally make more correct responses than amnesics and so have less scope for producing prior list intrusions.

Effect of method of testing

1. *Partial cueing*

The authors of the disinhibition hypothesis have emphasized that clear evidence of long-term memory in amnesic patients may be observed if certain methods of testing are used. None would now disagree with this. However, in a later study (Weiskrantz and Warrington, 1970b) they provided evidence which, it was claimed, showed that amnesic memory was disproportionately facilitated by tests involving 'partial information'. It was argued that partial cueing had the effect of eliminating competing incorrect responses (false positives), which would otherwise severely impair the performance of amnesic subjects. Amnesic and control subjects were presented with a short word-list and after a retention interval of one minute were tested with one of four tests: free recall; yes—no recognition; a fragmented form of the words; the first three letters of each of the five-letter test words. The results are shown in Table 4 and analysis of these data revealed a significant interaction between groups and method of testing 'indicating that there was a differential effect of retention conditions in the two groups'. It was argued that responding to partial information was a particularly favourable retrieval method for amnesics but not for the controls. It was also suggested that the findings refuted the hypothesis

that partial information is a particularly favourable method of testing
memory for all subjects.

TABLE 4

Retention scores after 1 minute. (Weiskrantz and Warrington, 1970b. Reproduced
by permission.)

	Controls N = 8	Amnesics N = 4
Recall	13.0	8.0
Recognition	18.7	10.5
Fragmented words	11.1	11.5
Initial letters	16.0	14.5

This rather persuasive argument has recently been questioned on
the basis of a study of normal memory using similar techniques. Woods
and Piercy (1974) investigated the possibility of obtaining results
similar to Warrington and Weiskrantz without using any amnesic subjects
but substituting for them a group of normal subjects with a presumably
weak memory trace. Subjects were tested on half the material after
one minute and on the other half after one week with separate groups
for each method of testing. A recall group could not be included in the
experimental design but it may be seen from the comparisons presented
in Table 5 that, for the three test methods in common to the two

TABLE 5

Percentage of correct responses obtained by Woods and Piercy's (1974) normal
subjects.

	1-min test	1-week test
Yes–No recognition		
Total correct	83.0	63.7*
TP–FP	66.0 (77.9)	27.3*(43.8†)
Initial letters	43.0 (66.7)	28.4 (60.4)
Fragmented words	62.4 (46.3)	66.4 (48.0)

Figures in brackets are scores obtained by Weiskrantz and Warrington expressed
as percentages for amnesics (shown with Woods and Piercy's one-week test
scores) and for controls (shown with Woods and Piercy's one-minute test scores).

* Significantly inferior to score at 1 minute ($P < 0.025$)
† Significantly inferior to score of controls ($P < 0.02$)

experiments, differences on particular tests between controls' and amnesics' performance were closely paralleled by differences between normal performance after one minute and normal performance after one week.

In particular, only yes–no recognition showed a significant difference between groups, whereas the groups did not differ significantly on initial letters although in both experiments the difference was in the expected direction. Also in both experiments, on the fragmented words test, the theoretically inferior group actually performed insignificantly better. An analysis of variance carried out on Woods and Piercy's data revealed a significant interaction between method of testing and retention interval, analogous to the significant result obtained by Weiskrantz and Warrington. Although the two experiments are not identical in design and, in particular, the free recall condition was not accommodated in the more recent experiment, nonetheless the results are remarkably similar and it seems reasonable to conclude that it is unsafe to make inferences concerning the nature of amnesia simply on the basis of a profile of performance on a group of memory tests which departs from that of normals tested after the same retention interval. Given the results of both experiments it may be incautious to say more than that, when tested after one minute, the differential effect of test conditions on amnesic memory is more like that of normals tested after one week than of normals tested after one minute. Such a statement does not of course provide support for any particular hypothesis concerning the nature of the amnesic defect.

The disinhibition hypothesis assumes that methods of partial cueing specially benefit amnesic memory performance by preventing the occurrence of false positive responses. Studying normals, Woods and Piercy (1974) did indeed find that few false positives were produced in response to cues consisting of fragmented forms of test words. However, they also found that the incidence of false positives was high (35 per cent) when partial cueing took the form of the first two letters of the test words. In their experiment this incidence was higher than in yes–no recognition. Seeing that this method of cueing has been shown to facilitate amnesic memory, it becomes difficult to account for this facilitation in terms of forestalling false positives. Furthermore Huppert and Piercy (1976) have shown that when the number of alternative responses available to the subject is constrained in a quite different fashion, amnesics gain no special benefit from this procedure. They found that the advantage of two-choice recognition over yes–no recognition was no greater for amnesics than for normals. Warrington and Weiskrantz have argued that amnesics perform better on partial cueing than on yes–no recognition because 'the choice of possible responses is restricted by the partial information provided' (Warrington and Weiskrantz, 1973). However, two-choice recognition restricts this choice at least as much as cueing with initial letters of words, and should, according to the theory, specially facilitate amnesic memory. Since Huppert and Piercy found that recognition memory of amnesics and controls was equally facilitated by this method it seems reasonable to infer that partial cueing does not facilitate amnesic memory simply as a consequence of restricting the choice of possible responses.

2. Recognition vs. recall

A further point made by Warrington and Weiskrantz on the basis of two separate studies is that the normal relationship between recall and recognition is not found in the amnesic groups, recall being relatively more efficient and recognition less efficient than might be expected on the basis of normal performance. The evidence they cite however, is by no means unambiguous. In the first study (Warrington and Weiskrantz, 1968), deficit scores for amnesics are computed separately for yes—no recognition and recall by expressing the difference between amnesic and control performance as a percentage of control performance. The authors state that 'the amnesic group was more impaired than the control group on both methods of recognition as compared with recall (unadjusted score)'. They present recall scores adjusted and unadjusted for number of wrong responses but do not specify whether recognition scores are adjusted in any way when deficit scores are computed. However, inspection of their data makes it clear that, in computing deficit scores, recognition scores have been adjusted by subtracting 10 from the total correct (the total possible score being 20). Their conclusion in fact applies only to the comparison of unadjusted recall scores with adjusted recognition scores. When *unadjusted* recall is compared with *unadjusted* recognition and also when *adjusted* recall is compared with *adjusted* recognition, the amnesics' deficit scores are considerably greater on recall than on recognition (Table 6). Although this study has often been cited as demonstrating that amnesics are more impaired on recognition than recall (e.g. Weiskrantz, 1971; Weiskrantz and Warrington, 1970b; and Warrington and Weiskrantz, 1973) the results do not support this conclusion. Amnesics' deficit scores on recall are greater or less than those on recognition, depending on how recall and recognition are scored.

The other relevant study by these authors, Weiskrantz and Warrington, 1970b) comprised two experiments, the second being the one most often cited as suggesting special impairment of recognition in amnesia (e.g. by Weiskrantz, 1971; Gaffan, 1972; Warrington and Weiskrantz,

1973). Here total correct on recall was simply compared with true positives minus false positives on recognition, and it was found that for the 8 controls the difference was significant but for the 4 amnesics it was not. The effect of small sample size in the non-significant result for amnesics is suggested by the fact that the proportionality of the scores was closely similar for the two groups. Thus if, using the same data, deficit scores are calculated for the amnesics then these are

TABLE 6

Deficit scores as computed by Warrington and Weiskrantz (1968). All figures shown were obtained by expressing the differences between the control group and the amnesic group as a percentage of the control group score. The original adjusted recall scores were obtained by subtracting wrong responses from correct responses. The original adjusted recognition scores were obtained by subtracting 10 from the total correct, the total possible correct being 20. (Reproduced by permission.)

	Recall	Recognition
Unadjusted	48*	23†
Adjusted	93	58*

* Deficit scores compared by Warrington and Weiskrantz
† Deficit score obtained from inspection of Warrington and Weiskrantz's data.

39 per cent for recall and 44 per cent for recognition – not an impressive difference. But the first experiment in this study also permits comparison of recall and recognition although this is not usually cited in this context. Deficit scores calculated on those data are 78 per cent for recall (based on total correct) and 37 per cent for recognition (based on true positives minus false positives). It would seem therefore that the recurring statements in the recent literature on amnesia that these two studies by Warrington and Weiskrantz reveal a greater impairment of recognition than recall do not have a secure basis in evidence.

Examining memory for words and for pictures, Huppert and Piercy (1976) found amnesic performance to be markedly superior when tested on yes–no recognition after a 10-minute retention interval than when tested on free recall after a 1-minute interval (e.g. for words 29 per cent true positives minus false positives and 1.8 per cent correct recall. Corresponding figures for controls were 46 per cent and 11.2 per cent). It can be said in summary that no individual study provides clear evidence that, compared with controls, amnesics do relatively worse on tests of recognition than on tests of recall, and that the published evidence as a whole shows no overall tendency in this direction.

The evidence discussed above includes the principal findings which have been cited in support of the hypothesis that organic amnesia is primarily a defect in retrieving information which has been encoded and stored in a normal fashion. It may now tentatively be suggested that the evidence as a whole does not support such a radical theory and that, if there are defects of retrieval, there are very probably defects of another kind too. However, it must be remembered that, in the form in which it is most often presented nowadays, the retrieval theory postulates that defective retrieval is the consequence of excessive proactive interference (Warrington and Weiskrantz, 1973). This notion has an interesting parallel in theories of normal forgetting. Interference has long been regarded by many theorists as a primary and possibly sole cause of normal forgetting. A thorough-going interference theory of forgetting has however run into very considerable difficulties in recent years (Postman, 1969) and many consider that the role of interference in forgetting cannot now be formulated without careful reference to organizational factors. It is appropriate to bear this is mind when considering how to evaluate the role of interference in amnesia. It was mentioned earlier that Cermak and Butters (1972) showed markedly increased susceptibility to PI among amnesics but that they interpreted this as secondary to an encoding defect (i.e. to a defect of one aspect of organization). Their line of argument would suggest that Warrington and Weiskrantz are right to stress the importance of interference effects in amnesia but perhaps mistaken in regarding them as primary and independent of organizational factors. The difficulties encountered by the radical retrieval theory and by the disinhibition hypothesis, encourage a cautious approach to the problem of interference effects in amnesia and suggest that we may be on safer ground when we consider these effects as observations requiring explanation than when we consider interference as a theoretical construct which may be used to explain other amnesic phenomena.

AMNESIA OR AMNESIAS?

In the introduction to this chapter it was pointed out that different workers have used quite different criteria for the selection of amnesic patients to be studied and that this could be a source of apparently conflicting findings concerning what amnesic patients can and cannot do. It is possible that some disagreements of this kind arise from different kinds of memory impairment associated with different cerebral lesions. Although the organic amnesic syndrome is commonly understood as a unitary functional deficit which does not vary qualitatively with site of cerebral lesion, we nevertheless have no assurance that this assumption is correct. Indeed, given current disagreements concerning not only the nature of the defect but also the empirical facts, there seems little justification for making this assumption in advance of systematic comparison between different lesion groups. The problem is complicated by the fact that, when the results of psychological experiments are communicated, the site of the lesion is not usually known. Cases such as that of the patient H.M., where the defect arises as a direct consequence of well-defined surgical intervention, are quite exceptional. More commonly one knows little more than the aetiology of the illness. Although the alcoholic Korsakoff state and postencephalitic state are those most commonly studied, other patients included in experimental studies of amnesia have become amnesic as a consequence of vascular accident, unilateral temporal lobectomy, carbon monoxide poisoning and cardiac arrest. The difficulties involved in establishing the neuropathological basis of amnesia of varying aetiology is made clear in Chapter 7 and it would seem that it is unwise in advance of postmortem evidence to make assumptions as to the exact site and extent of cerebral lesions in patients who have become amnesic as a consequence of, for example, chronic alcoholism or encephalitis. Nevertheless some distinctions, albeit only approximate, can be made and would justify comparison of the performance of different types of amnesic patient. The alcoholic Korsakoff state typically involves the mammillary bodies and the thalamus but not the hippocampus, whereas certain cases of herpes encephalitis particularly affect various structures within the limbic system including the hippocampal formation. Although in nonfatal cases (the only ones in which amnesia can be studied) the type of encephalitis may be in serious doubt, nevertheless it does seem reasonable to suggest that Korsakoff patients and amnesic postencephalitic patients should be studied separately and systematically compared. Certainly experimental studies of amnesia which pool the performance of both types of patient in order to arrive at some theoretical conclusion, renounce any opportunity there may be to distinguish between the effects on memory of the two classes of lesion.

There is a related methodological point. The whole history of neuropsychology suggests that once some relatively circumscribed cognitive deficit is known to be associated with relatively focal neurological dysfunction, advance in understanding the deficit is likely to be most rapid if, in the case of human patients, selection for research purposes is by lesion rather than by symptom. In the case of animal research, when a lesion results in an inadequately understood cognitive deficit, it is standard research procedure to seek differential effects of more restricted lesions within the same cerebral region. A closely focused understanding of amnesic defects will not necessarily be yielded by functional analysis of the performance of supposedly 'pure' cases of amnesia selected regardless of aetiology.

Only very limited inferences can be made from comparisons of results obtained by workers studying different groups of patients. Korsakoff patients tend to be the most readily available and studies of aetiologically homogeneous groups of patients have mostly taken advantage of this fact. For the most part such studies can be compared only with intensive studies of individual patients with amnesia of different aetiology (such as that described in Chapter 5) or, much more rarely, with very small groups of other patients (such as the four postencephalitics described by Rose and Symonds (1960). But different investigators very commonly use different techniques of memory testing and, as the discussion of 'short-term memory' in this chapter suggests, relatively small differences in technique can sometimes exert powerful effects. However, Lhermitte and Signoret (1972) have compared the performance of 10 Korsakoff patients and 3 postencephalitic amnesic patients with specific reference to the possibility of differential impairment in the two groups. Their tests were specially designed for this experiment and unfortunately it is by no means clear what kind of disability is to be inferred from failure on a particular task. Four tasks were employed: learning a spatial array, learning a verbal sequence, learning a logical arrangement and learning a code. It appeared that the third and fourth tasks could be correctly executed without utilizing memory except for the instructions. The first task necessitated memory for spatial position and the second task necessitated memory for temporal sequence. Korsakoff patients were more impaired than postencephalitics on the second, third and fourth tasks and postencephalitics were more impaired than Korsakoffs on the first task. The authors interpret this result as showing that the postencephalitics have a more profound failure of retention than the Korsakoffs, whilst the Korsakoffs have greater difficulty with organization of material and with recall. This formulation may be questioned because, to take one specific point, it is by no means clear that remembering spatial position involves more as opposed to different powers of retention than remembering temporal sequence. Nevertheless, despite the difficulties of interpretation, and despite the fact that two patients showed generalized intellectual impairment, this work does constitute *prima facie* evidence for a qualitative difference between the amnesias associated with the Korsakoff state and the postencephalitic state. A careful search for and analysis of other such differences now appears to be called for. The unitary character of the organic amnesic syndrome was always a rather dubious assumption and it is now seriously in question.

CONCLUSIONS AND SUGGESTIONS

Theories of amnesia

Baddeley (1973) has undertaken an appraisal of a number of theories of amnesia and he has attempted to order these theories with respect to the number of different features of amnesic performance they are capable of explaining. A similar enterprise will not be undertaken here because the concern of this section is not a theoretical order of merit but the implications for future research of present theoretical inadequacies.

It does in fact seem to be the case that no current theory of amnesia is consistent with all the evidence available. This may be exemplified by a simple list of the main theories and the observations which they most obviously fail to accommodate.

(1) *The retrieval theory*   Any theory which maintains that the amnesic defect is located only at the stage where retrieval is attempted must predict that memory for events occurring prior to onset of amnesia will be as impaired as memory for events occurring subsequent to onset. Marslen-Wilson and Teuber's experiment (1975) showing that amnesics' pre-onset memory is superior to their post-onset memory disconfirms that prediction.

(2) *The disinhibition/interference theory*   It may be agreed that certain interference effects are more marked in amnesics than normals but the suggestion that amnesia results from failure to inhibit competing memories encounters two main classes of difficulty. First, insofar as it is a retrieval theory, it is subject to the objection just cited. Second, a number of the consequences deduced from the theory have not been confirmed. Thus, (a) prior list instrusions as a percentage of wrong responses in free recall do not appear to be higher in amnesics than controls, (b) the relative effect of different test conditions does not appear to differ between amnesics and controls except in consequence of a generally lower level of memory performance, (c) one of the methods of testing (cueing with initial letters of test words) which is supposed to benefit amnesic performance by preventing the occurrence of false positives, does not in fact prevent false positives in normals. The version of the disinhibition theory which postulates that stored information fails to *dissipate* in a normal fashion is a storage theory not a retrieval theory and as such is subject to the second class of difficulty just described but not to the first.

(3) *The semantic encoding hypothesis (verbal)* This fails principally because, in the form in which its authors described it, it is tied to verbal coding. The same authors have subsequently reported evidence that, under suitable conditions, Korsakoff patients are impaired on tasks of non-verbal short-term memory. This is inconsistent with their original theory.

(4) *The imagery coding hypothesis* Baddeley's suggestion that amnesics cannot utilize the imagery component in long-term semantic memory is directly contradicted by the results of Cermak (1975) who found that Korsakoff patients showed significantly improved learning and retention of paired associates when these were linked by imagery, and that imagery mediation was as effective as verbal mediation.

(5) *The consolidation hypothesis* Other authors (Warrington and Weiskrantz, 1973; Baddeley, 1973) have listed numerous observations which they regard as inconsistent with the consolidation hypothesis. Some of their strictures may be questioned, especially if failure of consolidation is not assumed to be absolute. However the observation that Korsakoffs are inferior to controls on verbal STM tasks even after retention intervals as short as three seconds is not explained by a defect of consolidation, if consolidation is defined as the means of transfer from primary memory to secondary memory.

(6) *The contextual memory hypothesis* The suggestion that in amnesia, there is severe impairment of memory for the context in which items were presented (e.g. when and where), but little impairment of memory for items as such, provides no explanation of the failure of amnesic patients to recognize new faces (Milner, 1968; Warrington and Taylor, 1973).

What has been described above is simply a list of theories and obvious instances which they fail to explain. It may however, be noted that there are two classes of these unexplained instances. There is the instance which suggests that the defect as postulated does not occur (at least among the patients studied in the disconfirming experiment); and there is the instance which suggests that the defect as postulated does not explain everything that is observed and that therefore, if there is a defect of the kind postulated, there must in addition be another kind of defect. The distinction is vital to any systematic appraisal of theories of amnesia but it is not pursued here because this discussion has the limited aim of suggesting that no one current theory provides a satisfactory account of the experimental observations as a whole. Some of these theories would explain more of the available data if they were less narrowly conceived. For example, the notion that consolidation is directly tied to the transfer of information from primary to secondary memory is not the only, or even necessarily the most plausible, formulation of a theoretical construct of this type. To define consolidation in this way and to postulate a defect of consolidation in amnesia was appropriately parsimonious at the time that it was thought that severely amnesic patients retained virtually no new information once they were distracted from rehearsing it. But once it was demonstrated that amnesics could retain certain kinds of information over appreciable periods, this hypothesis encountered difficulties and a systematic attempt to modify the original hypothesis might have been profitable. It has been suggested that memories may consolidate (i.e. become more durable) over minutes or hours rather than seconds (Huppert and Deutsch, 1969; McGaugh, 1966). If consolidation is defined in this way, it is very doubtful whether there are any established findings concerning amnesia which are frankly inconsistent with a consolidation defect. The hypothesis would not explain some of the observations which have encouraged the postulation of an encoding defect but the only obvious way of directly disconfirming the hypothesis of a defect of 'long-term consolidation' would be the demonstration of normal rates of forgetting in amnesics brought rapidly to the same criterion of learning as normals. As suggested in an earlier section, the facts of this matter have not been established.

In a similar fashion, the notion that amnesia results from a defect of semantic encoding would appear ripe for reformulation rather than rejection. If semantic encoding is construed as applying only to certain aspects of verbal memory, then it certainly does not explain all of the observations now available. It might however explain very much more if the term 'semantic' were broadened to encompass highly organized non-verbal information.

Assumptions and questions

The mis-match between fact and theory outlined above does not of course mean that the defect in amnesia must be of a character which has so far been completely unsuspected. Much of the difficulty seems to arise from possibly unjustified assumptions which are made either in proposing theories or in evaluating them. One of these assumptions (that there is only one type of organic amnesia) has been mentioned in the previous section. It is possible that amnesias associated with different aetiology are functionally different. If this were the case, no envelope theory of the type considered above could accommodate all of the evidence concerning amnesia, although it might adequately describe a particular kind of amnesia.

Another assumption which is certainly widespread although often tacit is that, if patients are carefully selected, and end-state of amnesia can be identified in which the defect is maximal and presumably absolute. In fact we have no agreed means of measuring the severity of amnesia and no reason whatsoever for claiming that whatever is lacking in amnesia is lacking absolutely. It is for example entirely reasonable to postulate a defect of consolidation without claiming that *no* consolidation occurs. But once this possibility is fully accepted (and on present evidence a relative defect is *at least* as probable as an absolute defect), the task of mediating between competing theories becomes very much more difficult and a much higher degree of ingenuity is demanded of research workers who seek to devise crucial experimental tests of particular theories. Theories of defective organization in memory or of defective storage are no longer disconfirmed by demonstrations that amnesics are assisted by organizational cues or that some information can be retained by amnesics over considerable periods. Furthermore, we cannot, in advance of empirical studies, assume that variations in severity of amnesia are reflected only in quantitative differences in performance. There may also be qualitative variations in performance which, if not recognized as being associated with variations in severity, could be a potent source of disagreements both as to the facts and as to the nature of the amnesic defect. An awareness that amnesia, however severe, may not reflect the absolute loss of a function, does not of course preclude the testing of appropriately formulated theories; it should, however, provide warning that we may not be as close to an answer as we have recently been tempted to believe.

One further assumption is made by most current theories. This is the assumption that organic amnesia is the impairment of one and only one subfunction of the memory process. The postulation of a single defect rather than multiple defects is encouraged by the habit of parsimonious inference. However, in this area there are good reasons for considering more complex possibilities. First, as stated above, it has been repeatedly observed that more refined neuropsychological analysis may result in considerable fractionation both of an observed deficit into component deficits and of the relevant cerebral region into more than one functional unit. Second, the hypothesis that in amnesia memory functions are impaired 'across the board' is, in some sense, as parsimonious and perhaps as probable as the various hypotheses concerning impairment of postulated component memory processes. The 'across the board' hypothesis may indeed sometimes directly suggest means of submitting narrower hypotheses to experimental test. These hypotheses often imply some qualitative difference between normal and amnesic performance. One example is the claim by Cermak, Butters and Moreines (1974) that, in Korsakoff patients but not in controls, release from proactive interference is dependent on the semantic level of the shift in stimulus material and that this constitutes evidence of an encoding defect. Another example is the claim by Warrington and Weiskrantz (1970) that amnesic memory is *selectively* benefitted by test techniques which rely on partial cueing and that this is evidence that amnesia is a defect of retrieval. If, instead of one or other of these theories being correct, amnesic memory were impaired in an undifferentiated fashion, it should in principle be possible to demonstrate in normals any anomalies of performance which seemed to distinguish amnesia from normal forgetting, provided appropriate test conditions were used (e.g. by attenuating normal memory in some way). Indeed Woods and Piercy (1974) claim to have done just this in relation to the example cited above concerning Warrington and Weiskrantz's disinhibition retrieval theory. As described earlier, they appear to have shown that the test technique which benefits amnesic performance more than normal performance also benefits normal memory after a long retention interval as compared with normal memory after a short retention interval. They claim that in consequence of the demonstration in normals of an effect previously considered to be uniquely characteristic of amnesics, Warrington and Weiskrantz's original observation no longer provides convincing support for their theory. This type of test may have some general usefulness. A strenuous attempt to demonstrate amnesic anomalies in normal people could, at least in some instances, provide a useful test of theories of amnesia which entail the postulation of a qualitative difference in the performance of normal and amnesic subjects.

The conceptual confusion associated with the three common assumptions which have been discussed can be resolved only by further empirical studies. We are largely ignorant as to whether there is a difference between the type of amnesia provoked by medial temporal lesions and the type associated with mammillothalamic lesions because the problem has not been systematically tackled. Similarly, doubts as to variations in the severity of amnesia complicate the theoretical interpretation of available evidence largely because we have paid little or no attention to the problem of what if any qualitative changes in performance are associated with variations in severity of amnesia. There is no serious doubt that milder forms of amnesia than those conventionally studied do in fact occur and, equally, we are entitled to be seriously doubtful as to whether there may not be similar variations in the severity of those apparently maximally amnesic patients who are at present studied. Possibly a study of milder forms of amnesia would be instructive. Certainly little is to be gained by assuming either that we do not need a detailed understanding of how memory performance varies with severity of amnesia or that the severely amnesic patients at present studied do not vary in the severity of their defects.

These doubts concerning the homogeneity of the syndrome raise the possibility that our theories of amnesia have so far taken too little account of the complexity of the issues involved. This possibility is also suggested by the fact that, despite the exclusive character of most theories of amnesia, when the published evidence is considered as a whole, there are remarkably few aspects of memory which have not been implicated in organic amnesia and these are not such as to enable us to choose between competing theories. This combination of difficulties might profitably be tackled from a position of theoretical modesty. Perhaps current theoretical positions make too many unverified assumptions concerning the unitary character of the syndrome. Possibly we should first attempt to answer more restricted questions concerning variation in the type of disabilities and in the severity of disabilities shown by different cases of the organic amnesic syndrome. Given answers to these questions, we might then be better placed to submit to experimental test the more far-reaching hypotheses concerning the nature of the defect or defects, perhaps in respect of particular, narrowly defined groups of patients.

It would however be misleading to overemphasize present theoretical difficulties and underemphasize the successful research which gave rise to them. If existing hypotheses seem inadequate, this is not because they were misconceived or obviously inappropriate to the data they sought to explain, but rather because the research which they subsequently provoked has introduced further complexities. The failure of early theories is a normal price for empirical advance.

Acknowledgement

The author is indebted to Dr Felicia Huppert for criticism of the original manuscript and much valuable discussion.

2 Amnesia in Cerebral Disease

C.W. M. Whitty, G. Stores, and W. A. Lishman

INTRODUCTION

The study of amnesia in cerebral disease has yielded increasing information both about memory itself and its cerebral correlates. Beginning as a rather amorphous and pervasive symptom in many varieties of brain disease, amnesia is now emerging as a psychologically well defined condition with a sure footing in cerebral pathology.

The recognition of memory defects as a presenting feature in certain disease, the detailed description of such defects and the observation of their clinical accompaniments, provided some of the striking pictures of amnesic states given a century ago. The syndrome associated with the name of Korsakoff, discussed in detail in Chapter 4, remains a classic example of such early clinical observations. Autopsy material at first occasionally allowed some correlation of clinical state with site of brain lesion. Since then, technical advances in investigating structural and functional changes in the living brain have extended the range of these correlations and allowed them to be attempted in transient, as well as permanent, disturbances of memory. Air-encephalography, angiography, and more recently, computerized axial tomography (the E.M.I. scan), echo-encephalography and scanning with radioactive isotopes, have given increasingly accurate localization of brain damage, while electroencephalography can provide information about changes in at least one aspect of cerebral function, and indicate something of their location. Neurosurgery now permits direct inspection of parts of the brain and allows study of the effects of electrical stimulation or ablation of certain areas.

These techniques have been combined with new and more discriminative psychological analysis of amnesia itself. Inability to give a clear account of past events has been shown to depend on many factors: on primary perception and the factors affecting its accuracy, on registration, on retention for a variable time and on recall. Tests have been devised with which to study each of these aspects as particularly as possible. Armed with all these methods, the clinician has been able to re-examine amnesia in its clinical setting. His interest has been directed chiefly to the site and type of brain lesion which may produce changes in memory, but inevitably, and increasingly as knowledge grows, such studies have given incidental information about the forms which amnesia may take and the mechanisms of memory itself.

From the clinical point of view, it is necessary to distinguish clearly between circumscribed periods of amnesia and continuing defects of the active process of memorizing by which memories are laid down for future recall. In the former, it must often remain uncertain whether the mechanisms of recall or of memorizing have been principally at fault: but where there is a persisting partial or total amnesic state, a lesion in those parts of the brain concerned with memorizing must be postulated. Such cases are likely to be most rewarding in trying to elucidate the anatomical basis of memory. It is therefore convenient to consider separately examples of transient amnesic states, which constitute by far the greater proportion of clinical examples, and persisting defects in memorizing in which causative brain lesions may be expected to be still present when death occurs.

In addition to these disturbances of memory in its usually accepted sense, there are also localized syndromes of cerebral dysfunction which may be considered to represent 'limited amnesias'. Some forms of dysphasia may be regarded as an amnesia for words. Dyspraxia, where requested or voluntary performance of a well-known motor task is impossible, may also be considered as a loss of memory in the sense of voluntary recall for this particular piece of behaviour. Visual object agnosia involves loss of recognition of the general meaning of an object, and a limited form is very occasionally seen in which the defect applies largely to people's faces — so-called prosopagnosia. In its milder forms, the clinical impression here is simply of an extreme forgetfulness and lack of recognition of friends and family, and it may readily be mistaken initially for a simple failure of memory. These conditions are known to be due to lesions of particular parts of the brain, mainly of the dominant hemisphere. They are of importance in formulating any coherent theory of memory and its neurological basis, but their relation to general amnesia is both complex and, as yet, ill understood and they will not be further considered here.

It will become evident that, in the material considered in this and the following three chapters, the theoretical difficulties and differences discussed in Chapter 1 are not resolved. The material presented is, so far as the clinical situation allows, factual. The interpretations and inferences derived from it remain, in many cases, tentative. What does emerge as a main theme in the conditions discussed, whether they are transient or permanent, is a defect of ongoing memorizing by which a store of experience and events is not laid down for future recall, so that a permanent memory gap exists for the period of defective memorizing. In addition, while the defect persists, there is a variable difficulty in recalling past experiences known to have been previously recorded and capable of recall, i.e. a retrograde amnesia; and this also may persist, but usually only for a brief space of past time. These two features give some unity to the amnesic states discussed.

TRANSIENT AMNESIC STATES

Toxic and metabolic factors

The examples of apparent causative agents for both transient and persistent amnesic states cited here seem multitudinous. While it is important clinically that they be recognized, they are of less value to our understanding of the mechanisms of amnesia and represent our present ignorance of the immediate and primary cytochemical changes involved. As knowledge grows, these discursive lists may give place to a more coherent classification of those agents known, or likely, to influence the primary cytochemical milieu of relevant neurones.

Any severe toxaemia may produce amnesia as part of a more general impairment of cerebral function. This was often seen in the so-called toxic confusional states of lobar pneumonia or typhoid fever, but may occur in any overwhelming systemic infection. Upon recovery, memory for events during the illness may be absent or greatly reduced, and the period covered by such amnesias may be quite sharp-edged in onset and ending. Typically, they cover periods during which consciousness was obviously impaired, or in which the patient was frankly delirious. Sometimes, however, the patient will have appeared superficially to be normal throughout, responding to his environment and even answering simple questions accurately. The persistent amnesic gap on recovery will then provide the only evidence that transient impairment of cerebral function had in fact occurred. Careful testing at the time would almost certainly have revealed minor degrees of inattention and disorientation.

In liver failure, before coma ensues, disorders of memory may be prominent and may fluctuate with the progress of the disease (Summerskill *et al.*, 1956). In kidney failure also, amnesic states may precede full uraemic coma.

In the early stages of hypoglycaemia, bizarre and inappropriate behaviour may occur and be followed by complete amnesia for the period in question. Very occasionally, memory may be selectively affected, and amnesia will then cover periods in which behaviour was seemingly normal (Romano and Coon, 1942). The following case provides an example of amnesic episodes with abnormal behaviour, in which hypoglycaemia was ultimately found to be the cause. The relative contributions of the hypoglycaemia itself and of the epileptic activity which it engendered are hard to separate clearly.

A man aged 32 was referred for neurological opinion because of episodes of abnormal behaviour, sometimes accompanied by complete loss of consciousness, and on a few occasions also by a grand-mal fit. He was a trained physicist working on problems of atomic energy, and a clear and accurate witness. His attacks consisted of the abrupt onset of inappropriate and often aggressive behaviour, sometimes involving attacks on people or destruction of his own belongings. He had no memory for this afterwards. Attacks might last for 30 minutes to one hour, and if they did not end in a fit or simple unconsciousness they would lead on to a period of emotional disturbance and confusion, for which memory would subsequently be incomplete and fragmentary.

No abnormalities were found on neurological examination. An electro-encephalogram showed some inconstant bilateral theta activity arising mainly in the temporal leads. Cerebrospinal fluid and air-encephalograms were normal. A 12-hour-fasting blood sugar was 84 mg per cent: and his electroencephalogram at this time showed no specific changes. He was regarded as having a cryptogenic temporal lobe epilepsy, but anticonvulsant treatment was quite ineffective. Subsequent and more thorough blood-sugar studies suggested the presence of an islet tumour. This was confirmed and removed at operation. Following this his attacks ceased.

Confusional states with subsequent amnesia may occur in a wide variety of other metabolic and endocrine disorders, although often in association with other psychiatric disturbance of varying degrees of severity (Granville-Grossman, 1971). They have been described in Cushing's syndrome (Ross, Marshall-Jones and Friedman, 1966), hyperthyroid crisis (Nelson and Becker, 1969) and less severe forms of hyperthyroidism where memorizing may be impaired because of the disruptive effect of anxiety on registration (Whybrow, Prange and Treadway, 1969), hypothyroidism (Tonks, 1964), hyperparathyroidism (Petersen, 1968) and other causes of hypercalcaemia (Strickland, Bold and Medd, 1967; Clunie, Gunn and Robson, 1967) as well as hypoparathyroidism (Hossain, 1970). Acute intermittent porphyria can also give rise to such changes (Stein and Tschudy, 1970). The physiological mechanism for these disturbances is not certain. Disorders of fluid and electrolyte balance may play a part. The occasional amnesic confusional state with the use of ion-exchange resins, or steroids, appears to operate in this way: and acute porphyria is also accompanied by striking changes in osmolality. However, with steroids, affective disorders and psychosis are more common reactions.

Some inorganic substances such as arsenic, lead, manganese or mercury are reported to affect memory selectively: and magnesium deficiency following massive intestinal resection has also been implicated (Fletcher *et al.*, 1960). Of organic compounds, carbon disulphide has been implicated in patchy amnesias and chronic difficulty in memorizing (Braceland, 1942).

Drug effects

The now extensive literature on behavioural effects of drugs used in general medicine, includes reports on adverse effects on memory, usually in a setting of toxic confusion from overdosage or hypersensitivity. The defect appears to be one of registration, with persisting amnesia for the period of confusion. Occasionally however the memory disorder is the main feature. Many drugs have been implicated. Of those used in cardiovascular disease, digitalis and potassium-depleting diuretics have been incriminated, especially in the elderly, as well as some antihypersensitive agents such as methyldopa and mecamylamine: although in general the usual psychiatric complication of this last group is depression (Granville-Grossman, 1971).

The stimulant effects of aminophylline and sympathomimetic drugs may sometimes give rise to confusional states. Anti-inflammatory drugs (De Nosaquo, 1969; Prescott, 1972) have also been indicted.

Toxic confusional states and, rarely, a clear-cut toxic encephalopathy are recorded in isoniazid treatment, but a more selective impairment of memory, which is reversible when the drug is stopped, is described by Olsen and Torning (1968). The psychiatric effects of this drug, unlike its neuropathy, do not seem to be counteracted by pyridoxine (Ross, 1958).

Amongst drugs used in neurology and psychiatry, anti-Parkinson remedies, benzhexol and similar compounds, as well as the newer L-dopa preparations, may produce behavioural changes of which impaired memory is a feature. A syndrome of acute delirium with hallucinations has been described, and amnesia for the episode, with retrograde spread, is recorded (Granville-Grossman, 1971).

Anti-epileptic drugs can have adverse effects on various aspects of behaviour including the learning process (Stores, 1975). A small amount of experimental work on this topic makes it difficult to know whether memorizing or some other phase of learning is primarily affected. Although enthusiastically proclaimed a few years ago, the role of anticonvulsant-induced folate deficiency in these behavioural disturbances remains controversial (Reynolds, 1975).

Impairment of concentration and memory occurs in chronic intoxication with barbiturates and other hypnotics, sedatives and minor tranquillizers: the elderly being more readily affected even with small dosage. Chronic bromide intoxication was an early example (Curran, 1944) and continues to occur (Carney, 1971).

The major tranquillizers such as the phenothiazines or haloperidol and the mono-oxidase inhibitors rarely produce impairment of memory. Tricyclic antidepressants on the other hand, may produce, especially in elderly patients, an hallucinatory confusional state for which there is a persisting memory gap.

The effect on memory of these agents represents a wide range from minor forgetfulness and difficulty in recall to a gross failure of current registration and ultimately disorientation. Confabulation may sometimes be added to this picture. Though the defect of memorizing is usually reversible, some permanent changes may occur when the toxin has acted for long periods or in heavy dosage. In the latter case, it may produce more profound effects than just amnesia, proceeding to stupor or coma, which may leave in its wake a permanent sequel of memory difficulty. In contrast to the defect in the ability to memorize, the periods of amnesia which may occur during the intoxication will usually remain complete and permanent. The mode of action of these agents is not clearly known, but it is likely that they act at cellular level by interfering with enzyme systems. In general, these conditions do not at present add anything to our knowledge of which parts of the brain are concerned in the memory disorder.

Cerebral anoxia and carbon monoxide poisoning

These two conditions almost certainly produce their effects on the brain by the same mechanism, carbon monoxide producing cerebral anoxia by the inactivation of the oxygen-carrying function of the haemoglobin molecule. Since carboxyhaemoglobin is relatively stable, the effects of exposure to carbon monoxide may be longer lasting and more profound than that of a transient reduction in oxygen supply *per se*.

Although these are usually transient disorders — unless so prolonged or so severe as to cause death — there may be some permanent sequelae. Amongst these, defects of memorizing are prominent, along with permanent amnesia for the period of the acute condition. In the majority of cases, especially of carbon monoxide poisoning, complete loss of consciousness is rapid, and amnesic abnormalities are seen only during the recovery phase.

Allison (1961) describes a woman of 70 admitted in coma as a result of accidental coal-gas poisoning. Only several weeks later had she recovered sufficiently to respond to simple commands and reply to questions. For the next two weeks she was grossly disorientated in time, giving the year variously as 1888 or 1918, and being equally wide of the mark for her age. Another week was to pass before she realized she was in hospital, yet insisted that it was in Armagh, the place of her childhood, though in fact she was in Belfast. At this stage she was able to repeat the months of the year correctly, could repeat four digits, but could retain nothing of a name and address after a three-minute interval. She could remember the names of her brothers and sisters and recall some episodes of her childhood. Two weeks later she had improved remarkably. She was then consistently orientated in time and place, had good general insight and was able to recall the circumstances leading right up to her accident.

Not all patients recover so completely, though the incidence of permanent severe disabilities varies in different series. Shillito, Drinker and Shaughnessy (1936) reported that of 21 000 victims of carbon monoxide poisoning in New York City, two-thirds were resuscitated, and of these, only 39 were found to show persistent psychiatric sequelae. The average time for complete recovery was three months, and memory defects were often the last to clear. Ajuriaguerra and Rouault de la Vigne (1946) found that a severe amnesic state could persist, in striking contrast to the absence of other intellectual impairment. In other cases there was profound inertia, indifference and slowing of cerebration, so that memory appeared more defective than it was in reality ('une sorte d'indifference amnestique'). On full recovery, there remained of course an amnesic gap for the period of coma, to which might be added a variable degree of retrograde amnesia and a patchy amnesia for part of the period of recovery. A strange feature, noted by both authors, is the occurrence of a latent period between exposure to the toxin and the onset of pronounced mental disorder in up to one-third of cases. This may average a fortnight, and a progressive vascular pathology has been postulated as its basis.

The importance of long-term follow-up of cases of carbon monoxide poisoning, because of the relapsing course or delayed onset of neuro-psychiatric complications, is emphasized in a recent survey by Smith and Brandon (1973). 74 survivors of acute carbon monoxide poisoning were followed up for a period of approximately three years. Three patients had committed suicide, eight had died from other causes and eight more had gross neuropsychiatric damage attributable to the poisoning. Of the 63 patients alive at follow-up, 27 reported an impairment of memory which was usually confirmed by psychological testing. Memory impairment was closely associated with deterioration of personality. In view of the close relationship between the development of gross neuropsychiatric complications and the patients' level of consciousness at the time of initial admission to hospital, these authors also rightly stress the necessity of prompt and effective treatment of carbon monoxide poisoning.

Similar amnesic symptoms are seen following periods of cerebral anoxia or hypoxia, especially in the elderly. Bedford (1955) has stressed the importance of anoxia as a cause of chronic amnesia in the elderly, and found 29 severely demented cases amongst a large population of patients who had had operations with general anaesthesia over the age of 50. Amongst 45 elderly patients in whom memory loss was a chief complaint, Allison (1961) ascribed six to anoxia; two due to temporary cardiac arrest (*see also* McNeill, Tidmarsh and Rastall, 1965); one due to defective aeration during anaesthesia, one to severe haematemesis, one to carbon monoxide poisoning and one to electrocution. Survival from attempted hanging has also been implicated (Berlyne and Strachan, 1968).

Anoxia *per se* has indeed been extensively studied in relation to its mental effects, both experimentally and in the course of mountaineering expeditions. Under conditions of slow acclimatization to lowered oxygen concentration in inspired air, memory is found to be impaired, along with other higher mental processes, when the concentration of oxygen falls below 9 per cent, corresponding to an altitude of 24 000 feet. Commonly this stage is preceded by a host of other minor psychological abnormalities; laziness, fatigue, irritability, slowness of reasoning, distractibility and by a varying degree of neuromuscular inco-ordination. The impairment of memory may, however, outlast the other symptoms on return to normal conditions. Kossmann (1947) reported a pilot who experienced severe hypoxia during a bombing mission, and showed impairment of memory even three weeks after the event. Pugh and Ward (1956) reported eight mountaineers who climbed 28 000 feet without additional oxygen. Only one showed residual mental difficulties and this took the form of impaired ability to memorize.

Acute alcoholic intoxication

Apart from the effects of chronic alcoholism resulting in brain damage, in which memory defects are often profound and which are considered later, one of the more familiar examples of toxic amnesia is the acute alcoholic 'blackout', which despite its name is not associated with loss of consciousness. Amnesia 'for the night before' may, of course, follow any bout of drinking which is carried to the point of severe impairment of consciousness or coma, and may be found to extend backwards in time for a considerable period. But the alcoholic 'blackout' appears to be a different kind of phenomenon. Here, there is a dense amnesia for a circumscribed period of time during which drinking was occurring. During this period, outward behaviour may have seemed scarcely disordered. There may have been no obvious signs of intoxication, the patient may have carried on a reasonable conversation and gone through quite elaborate activities, for all of which there is no trace of memory the next day. Spouses and close friends sometimes claim to know by subtle changes of behaviour when one has started. Occasionally, grossly abnormal and even criminal conduct may occur during the episode. The detailed evidence about such blackouts is, however, unsatisfactory as it has come largely from the subjects themselves.

The onset, as judged by subjective recall, is usually abrupt, and it may end equally sharply with the recovery of some highlight of experience, after which memory is resumed. The density and permanence of the amnesia suggests that it is brought about by a transient disturbance of the process of memorizing. Occasionally, however, isolated details may later be recalled. A further interesting point is the claim made by some subjects that events during such amnesias may sometimes be recalled under subsequent alcoholic intoxication. This evidence is even more difficult to assess, but, if accepted, would suggest that recall rather than memorizing is principally at fault. An additional difficulty is the emotional setting and possible psychogenesis of some such attacks. Nevertheless, the majority must be accepted as organically determined.

Alcoholic blackouts appear to be quite common. Goodwin and his colleagues (1969a) elicited a history of them in 64 out of 100 alcoholic patients without other psychiatric or neurological disorder. In fact, these authors described two types of amnesia in their patients: a complete and permanent 'en bloc' form of abrupt onset and termination, and a more fragmentary type which tended to improve in time, sometimes with the help of further drinking (Goodwin *et al.*, 1969b).

The pathogenesis of blackouts remains uncertain. They are commoner, apparently, after the ingestion of spirits than after wine or beer (WHO Technical Report, 1955). The sharpness of the rise and fall of the alcohol level in the blood would appear to be of more importance than the height to which it may rise, and the episodes may follow the drinking of medium or quite small amounts. On the other hand, in the series described by Goodwin, amnesic episodes were significantly associated with heavy drinking, especially in bouts, as well as a past history of head injury leading to unconsciousness. In these patients amnesias first appeared late in the course of the illness well after symptoms of physical dependence had been noted, although Jellinek (1952) has noted their frequency in the histories of established alcoholics, dating from a time before the drinking had gone out of control. He has suggested that repeated experience of the phenomenon is a prodromal sign of alcoholic addiction, and that its occurrence after only medium alcohol intake represents heightened susceptibility or sensitivity to the effects of alcohol in the prospective addict.

Deficiency diseases

Some well recognized clinical syndromes, in which disorders of memory figure prominently, are associated with deficiency of the vitamin B group, especially of thiamine (vitamin B_1). Provided death does not occur in the acute stage, these conditions, certainly in their florid forms, are in general reversible and transient, though slight sequelae may be permanent; and when the deficiency has been prolonged, it may give rise to structural brain changes with more severe permanent memory defects. A striking example of such a syndrome is Wernicke's encephalopathy. This has traditionally been assigned an alcoholic aetiology, but is now known to occur in a number of clinical conditions, all connected more or less closely with vitamin B deficiency. In Campbell and Russell's (1941) series of 21 cases, there was a definite history of alcoholism in only five.

Spillane (1947) lists the following precipitating factors in his review of reported cases at that time: alcoholism, carcinoma of the stomach, pregnancy, toxaemia, pernicious anaemia, vomiting, diarrhoea and dietary deficiency. Lopez and Collins (1968) give the same list with the addition of chronic dialysis. The importance of thiamine deficiency in the aetiology of the syndrome emerged clearly in the last war. In 1947 de Wardener and Lennox were able to report 52 cases occurring in British prisoners kept on a rice diet in Singapore, and they suggested the name cerebral beriberi to emphasize its cause.

The syndrome itself is characterized by ophthalmoplegias in conjunction with disturbance of consciousness, often acute in onset. Headache, vomiting, ataxia and polyneuritis may also be prominent features. Amongst the mental phenomena of the acute stage clouding of consciousness is foremost, progressing frequently to disorientation, delirium or coma. Impairment of recent memory is, however, an outstanding sign in those cases sufficiently accessible for testing. It was noted in 61 per cent of the de Wardener and Lennox cases, and a good example is provided by Spillane (1947).

A man aged 23 had been a prisoner of war for about 18 months. When first seen, he had neurological signs suggesting a Wernicke's encephalopathy, and some beriberi oedema. On mental examination, he was disorientated for time and place. He did not confabulate, but had almost complete loss of memory for recent events; by contrast, his memory for events before his illness was intact. When examined after two weeks of a liberal diet, and ten days of thiamine 20 mg daily by intramuscular injection, he was alert and co-operative and had no amnesia for the period of treatment, recalling accurately details of his examinations and treatment.

All cases are not so fortunate in the resolution of the memory defect, and indeed, the fully developed syndrome proves to be closely bound up with the development of a subsequent Korsakoff syndrome, which will be discussed in more detail elsewhere (*see* Chapters 4 and 8). This would appear to be particularly true of the cases with an alcoholic background, and therefore presumably a persisting aetiological agent. Victor and Adams (1953) reported that 75 per cent of their 86 cases progressed to a permanent amnesic confabulatory syndrome, while conversely, all but three of 69 cases with such a syndrome due to alcoholism had had previous episodes of Wernicke's encephalopathy. Before its aetiology was known, this encephalopathy was not uncommonly fatal in its acute form, and its pathology has therefore been extensively studied. It consists of foci of congestion and haemorrhage, largely confined to the periaqueductal grey matter, hypothalamus, brainstem and areas around the walls of the third ventricle; the mammillary bodies are nearly always markedly affected. It should be noticed, however, that this represents an acute pathology which may be modified by time and treatment.

Thiamine deficiency, in relation to the demands of carbohydrate metabolism, is now generally accepted as its cause. The production of lesions in the central nervous system of thiamine-deficient pigeons, similar in distribution and type to those of Wernicke's encephalopathy, was first clearly shown by Alexander in 1940.

Subsequently, the clinical response to treatment with thiamine has added confirmatory evidence. Within 48 hours of intravenous thiamine, provided treatment is started within days of the onset of acute symptoms, improvement occurs in the ophthalmoplegia and the gross disturbances of consciousness. The recovery of memory defects is less certain. When the condition has been caused by some short-lived but severe deficiency — a situation not uncommonly precipitated by a sudden increase in carbohydrate intake and consequent metabolic demand in someone chronically depleted of thiamine — the improvement in memory and other symptoms is rapid and complete. When the causative factor has been present for longer, and particularly when recurrent attacks of acute or subacute Wernicke's encephalopathy have occurred, and where permanent structural pathology is therefore likely, the recovery of memory function remains incomplete, even with continued and heavy thiamine dosage. Thus, Jolliffe, Wortis and Fein's (1941) conclusion that thiamine had little effect on memory disorders must be viewed in the context of their cases, which were mostly chronic alcoholics. In such a setting, permanent pathology and permanent functional defects would be expected. But it is interesting to note that the more widespread confusion and delirium of some of the patients *did* respond to thiamine – uncovering an amnesic state in the process. In de Wardener and Lennox's (1947) cases, permanent structural changes are likely to have been less, and the results of treatment are therefore seen to be better. Their cases represented more pure deficiency states, and although chronic, it is likely that a generally reduced diet lessened their metabolic demands for thiamine. These authors noted that, in mild cases, memory defects would recover within 48 hours of treatment. When symptoms of disorientation and impairment of consciousness were more severe or more long-standing, recovery might take weeks or months, defects of memorizing and recall of events recovering last.

Experimental thiamine deficiency in human subjects has certainly produced defective memory as a prominent complaint, among other minor mental abnormalities (Elsom, Lewy and Heublein, 1940; Williams and his colleagues, 1943). Defective memory has also figured largely amongst the incidental changes observed in beriberi (Cruickshank, 1961), and on treatment with thiamine, improvement has often been striking.

Nicotinic acid, a second member of the vitamin B group, has similarly been implicated in the memory process; though here the corresponding cerebral pathology has not so far been elucidated. Impairment of memory may figure prominently in the acute phase of pellagra, and where the disorder is allowed to progress to dementia a clinical picture resembling Korsakoff's syndrome has occasionally been recorded. In England, pellagra is now mostly seen in the feeble-minded and in chronic mental patients, and it is of course hard to exclude concomitant thiamine deficiency in such a setting. Nonetheless, nicotinic acid proves to be effective in reversing the disorder, and in some cases it may prove effective treatment when thiamine alone has failed. This has also been shown strikingly in a group of elderly patients rather commonly encountered in general hospitals (Sydenstricker, 1943; Gottlieb, 1944). Such patients have usually been living alone on an inadequate diet, and are admitted to hospital in a stuporose or delirious state. Memory defects may be prominent, simulating a Korsakoff syndrome. Empirical treatment with nicotinic acid gave dramatic relief to their symptoms.

A woman of 62 living on a very inadequate diet developed general somatic evidence of vitamin deficiency. Two weeks before she was seen her memory had become very unreliable. When examined, she was confused and disorientated and her memory for recent events was grossly defective. Her physical condition suggested a pellagra and she was given 150 mg of nicotinic acid and 90 mg of thiamine by mouth daily for ten days. There was no obvious improvement in her condition. She was then given nicotinic acid in large doses by intramuscular injection and showed a rapid, marked and permanent improvement in her mental state. Her physical condition improved more slowly.

Cytamen deficiency may also occasionally produce a dementia with early memory defects rather than the usual signs of subacute combined degeneration, or anaemia (Strachan and Henderson, 1965). Finally, folic acid deficiency of dietary origin (Strachan and Henderson, 1967) and due to long-term anticonvulsant treatment (Reynolds, 1971) has been similarly implicated. However, evidence on the relationship between neuropsychiatric disorder and folate deficiency, including the possibility of reversal by administration of folic acid, remains conflicting (Reynolds, 1975).

A number of vitamins must therefore be accepted as playing a potential role in the maintenance of memory. Of these, the claims of thiamine are most clearly established. However, multiple deficiencies are likely to be most common in clinical practice and may account for the frequency with which memory impairment figures in the mental disorders associated with long-continued semi-starvation (Helweg-Larsen and his colleagues, 1952). The implication for treatment is that vitamin supplements must be of the whole water-soluble group rather than of one or other member.

The conditions so far considered in the causation of amnesic states have been generalized, acting only indirectly on the brain, though they may at times produce localized structural changes there. A number of diseases producing striking memory defects are, however, primarily or entirely intracranial.

Intracranial infections

The classification of encephalitis, on both clinical and pathological grounds, remains incomplete. It is not uncommon, however, for memory defects to figure prominently in some reported series. In epidemic encephalitis lethargica a state of amnesia with confabulation has been recorded in the acute phase of the disease (Kirby and Davis, 1921), but usually the mental clouding and delirium will obscure the more specific disorder of memory. On recovery, memory disorder does not figure prominently amongst well-known mental sequelae. It is among the more sporadic and less completely understood forms of encephalitis that memory disorder may occasionally be striking. In a series of four cases reported by Rose and Symonds (1960), an acute illness, presumed on clinical grounds to be encephalitic in origin, resulted in permanent intellectual deficit characterized by gross impairment of memorizing. The defect of memory was out of all proportion to the other intellectual deficits, which in some cases were virtually non-existent. Immediate recall and grasp were good, along with preservation of remote memory and motor skills; but retention of new information was grossly reduced. In addition, there was a fixed amnesia for the period of the illness, and a striking feature was a period of retrograde amnesia for months or even years before. Other isolated cases have been reported, in which transient failure of recent memory was prominent during the acute phase of the illness. Conrad (1953b) described a case of encephalitis in a woman of 24, who against a background of general intellectual impairment, could not retain any experience for more than 40 to 60 seconds. She improved rapidly on recovering from the acute illness and the registration defect disappeared. No information about site of lesion was available in these cases.

The following case was clinically similar:

A woman of 34 began to show disturbances of behaviour while on a cycling holiday with her husband. She lost her way on familiar routes, would stop and wander off the road for no reason, and on two occasions temporarily lost her bicycle. However, it was not until three weeks later that she developed headache, slight fever and a gross confusional state, at one time with hallucinations. On examination at this time, she had some swelling of her optic discs and a marked lymphocytic pleocytosis in her cerebrospinal fluid, but no localized signs in the central nervous system. As the general confusion and hallucinations subsided, mental examination showed a gross fixation amnesia with florid confabulation. She recovered slowly, but it was over two months before she was fit to resume her household duties. When seen nine months after her illness, she had a permanent retrograde amnesia which involved some six weeks of her stay in hospital and the preceding three weeks, with a sharp end-point at one particular incident of her cycling holiday. Her memorizing was also persistently defective. She would lose things easily, forget household details and had difficulty in remembering acquaintances. However, these defects were minor ones and she was able to lead a normal life and look after her home satisfactorily. She died some two years later of an unrelated condition. At autopsy the brain was macroscopically normal. Histological examination showed evidence of localized perivascular cuffing in the floor of the third ventricle and extending a little into the periaqueductal region. No other abnormalities were found.

In acute encephalitis due to the virus of herpes simplex, the site of the cerebral lesion is often established, and amnesia may be an important symptom (Fields and Blattner, 1958). There is confusion, disorientation and sometimes frank delirium, but a defect of memory, particularly for recent events, can at times be clearly defined within this setting. The autopsy findings are of interest as they show lesions particularly in the hippocampal formation, the insula and the cingulate gyri, such that the term 'limbic encephalitis' has been used for the condition (Glaser and Pincus, 1969).

The evidence from cases of acute encephalitis is, however, in the main unsatisfactory, because general impairment of consciousness obscures the specific memory defect. Even when the latter can be clearly brought out, it is still difficult to be certain that it is a primary feature, and equally difficult to be sure that any cerebral lesion that can be defined is directly related to the memory defect. These arguments apply also to most cases of subacute encephalitis as described by Brierley and his colleagues (1961). In these, the pathological findings were clearly established and related to the limbic system, but the extent and specificity of memory defects was much less clear. However, cases have been reported in which severe impairment of recent memory was a relatively selective deficit, either recovering in the course of time (Himmelhoch *et al.*, 1970) or possibly not at all (Gascon and Gilles, 1973). The variability of both neurological and psychological long-term sequelae of herpes simplex encephalitis is evident from the recent follow-up study by Rennick and his colleagues (Rennick *et al.*, 1973) and from studies in which different aspects of memory have been carefully compared in the individual case (Starr and Phillips, 1970). Disordered memory may also be the first sign of encephalitis affecting limbic structure in carcinoma especially of the bronchus (Corsellis *et al.*, 1968).

In meningitis, apart from periods of acute toxic delirium which may accompany its severe forms, memory disorders do not usually appear. Tuberculous meningitis, however, now that treatment permits survival, has proved an exception, and this is of particular interest because the site and nature of its intracranial pathology has been extensively studied and correlated with the memory defects that may occur. Williams and Smith (1954) have fully documented the typical disorder of memory seen in the course of this disease. In the prodromal phases, subjective difficulty with memory may appear, and in one of their cases it was a presenting complaint. In the fully established disease the picture varies in degree but in kind it is remarkably constant. The authors described three characteristic stages in its evolution. In the early 'confusional' stage the patient is apathetic, drowsy, disorientated in time and place and unable to sustain a rational conversation. During treatment, this evolves to the 'amnesic' stage which may last many weeks and presents a highly characteristic picture. The patient may appear reasonably alert and intellectually intact, but proves to have a grave defect in retaining any new information for more than a few minutes. Confabulation may be much in evidence, and memory for temporal sequences is early disorganized. Memory for remote personal events is usually intact, but is hazy and poorly integrated for events of the illness and for those preceding it, sometimes for several months. With increasing recovery in the meningitis, retention of current events improves, often with dramatic suddenness, and the period of retrograde amnesia steadily contracts towards the time of onset of the illness. With cure of the infection, as judged particularly by the return of cerebrospinal fluid to normal, there is usually complete restitution of normal memory function, though a persistent memory gap remains for the period of the acute illness, proportional to the duration of the period of overt confusion. Nineteen cases were followed up for periods of up to four years; none showed measurable defect of intellect, personality or memorizing ability, although four did complain of some subjective forgetfulness for minor day-to-day events. All, however, had a dense amnesia for the early weeks or months of the illness, and this was so even for those who had seemed alert and rational throughout. Six had some additional retrograde amnesia. This amnesia was seldom uniform or global, but in some cases it extended for months, even up to four years, as an inability to organize past events in correct temporal sequence, with some complete gaps and a general haziness for details.

These features are well illustrated by Case 2 in their series.

After an unusually good scholastic career, this patient developed severe tuberculous meningitis at the age of 22. He had a long and difficult illness with a typical amnesic phase. However, after some nine months of treatment he was discharged as cured. Some three years later he was seen again and at this time was well, doing full-time clerical work and had recently been promoted. His memorizing of current experience was normal. However, he still had a substantial retrograde amnesia for events some six months before the clinical onset of his illness, and had entirely lost some specific skills such as typing, acquired during this period; the amnesia extended also to the first four months of the illness itself.

The value of these careful memory studies lies particularly in the equally accurate observations on the intracranial pathology of the condition. The characteristic feature of the pathology of these cases in the amnesic phase is an inflammatory process with massive organized exudate, largely limited to the more anterior basal cisterns of the brain. The inflammation also directly involves the floor of the third ventricle. The evidence linking these changes with the memory defects is circumstantial but convincing. Variations in the intensity of the pathological process during life can be correlated with similar changes in the memory defect; moreover, the occasional case in which the memory defect is absent is found to be free of involvement of the anterior basal cisterns and third ventricle, the exudate blocking instead the more posterior cisterna magna.

Where pyogenic infection leads to cerebral abscess formation, the localization of the site of lesion is often precise. This is especially so when antibiotic treatment is successful in preventing dissemination of the infection to neighbouring parts of the brain. In this respect, such cases should be especially useful in attempting to correlate site of lesion and defects of cerebral function. Unfortunately, however, specific memory defects are usually obscured by the more diffuse impairment of psychological functions which occurs. The occasional example is, however, seen in which amnesia is a presenting feature. The following case illustrates this:

> A child of 11 was seen because of increasing behaviour disorder and a gross loss of memorizing. A large abscess in the middle third of the dominant temporal lobe was finally diagnosed and successfully treated. In addition to much emotional disorder and some dysphasia, the child was left with a permanent dense amnesia for the period of her illness and for some weeks preceding its clinical onset. In the absence of autopsy studies, the causal relation between this local lesion and the memory defect must remain presumptive. The area involved is likely to include the hippocampus and some of its connections.

Transient vascular occlusions

In a number of cases, sudden attacks of amnesia without warning may last for a few minutes or a few hours and then there is complete recovery. Such attacks may be recurrent and be accompanied by focal neurological signs and severe headache. Occasionally these cases terminate in a cerebrovascular accident, and this has led to the supposition that they represent brief periods of local cerebral ischaemia.

> A case observed personally was that of a right-handed woman of 64, apparently healthy except for a moderate hypertension, who, while sitting in a chair one day, suddenly lost her memory. She walked into her kitchen and the garden and complained to her sister that she did not know where she was. The sister described her as 'confused'. Half an hour later, her memory returned suddenly and she complained of severe left-sided headache. These attacks recurred four or five times in the next eight years. She then had a massive right-sided stroke and died two weeks later. Autopsy showed a large haemorrhagic infarction of the left hemisphere.

Poser and Ziegler (1960) have reported examples of similar episodic transient amnesias, sometimes with motor and sensory signs in the limbs of one side, but none of their cases had permanent strokes, nor was autopsy information available. One 74-year-old man had had four episodes of temporary amnesia before the observed attack, which lasted for about eight hours. Upon return of his memory, he had severe generalized headache for some 12 hours.

Amnesia has been described also in migraine by Moersch (1924) and by Nielsen (1958), both during attacks of visual disturbance and headache and as a variant of classical attacks. The latter author describes the amnesic symptoms as highly characteristic, lasting from one to four hours and clearing more gradually than they appear. During attacks 'isolated thoughts and ideas come to mind unbidden, and those that are wanted cannot be recalled. Memory is thus patchy and these islands of thought cannot be associated'. Typical automatism is also said to occur at times. The attacks are more frequent in the 20s and 30s and tend to disappear with age, even though more typical migraine persists.

Here again, a vascular mechanism must be involved, and ischaemia from vasoconstriction is the generally accepted basis for cerebral symptoms in migraine. Nielsen has suggested that the posterior cerebral artery is at fault in such cases. If this is so, then the amnesia might represent vertebral-basilar artery spasm, with consequent ischaemia, either in the brainstem reticular formation or in the mammillary bodies and hippocampal formation.

Memory disorder may also be seen in diffuse cerebrovascular disorders. It may figure prominently in attacks of 'hypertensive encephalopathy', and may occur amongst the diverse and transient focal symptoms of cerebral thrombo-angiitis obliterans (Cloake, 1951). In addition, memory defects comprise one of the many neuropsychiatric manifestations of systemic lupus erythematosus (Bennett *et al.*, 1972) and may sometimes be responsive to steroids or immunosuppressive agents (Brook, 1969). In these cases also, transient local cerebral ischaemia, whether by occlusion of vessels or reduced blood flow, is assumed to be the causative mechanism.

Some of these cases, such as those of Poser and Ziegler, may be examples of the transient global amnesia syndrome which is considered in Chapter 3 in more detail.

Epilepsy

Epilepsy presents one of the commonest examples of transient amnesic states, and these form an integral part of many epileptic attacks. Indeed, subsequent amnesia for events during an attack may be a symptom of some value in arriving at a diagnosis of epilepsy, especially in some of its more bizarre forms. In most grand-mal attacks, as would be expected, memory recording ceases when consciousness is lost, and the subject is left with a fairly well demarcated memory gap for what transpires, up to the point where full consciousness is regained. Immediately after the attack, memory may be hazy for an extensive period antedating the attack, but clears rapidly and progressively thereafter. On some occasions, a variable degree of retrograde amnesia may persist, obscuring much of the warning aura and premonitory signs, even where evidence has been clear that such were experienced at the time. Amnesia also usually persists for any period of marked confusion which may follow the regaining of consciousness after a fit. In this phase, an outburst of wild, pointless, aggressive and destructive behaviour may rarely occur – the so-called epileptic furor. For this also, amnesia will be complete. However, loss of consciousness and amnesia are not essential to the diagnosis of epilepsy and very occasionally, memory persists even during the attack itself.

Thus, in ordinary grand-mal epilepsy, amnesia occurs merely as part of the acute confusional state with impairment of consciousness, or as the necessary accompaniment of complete loss of consciousness. By contrast, there are some forms of epileptic attack in which amnesia may present as the essential symptom. The outward abnormality consists not of a convulsion, but of altered confused behaviour or the automatic repetition of some motor sequence which becomes inappropriate and irrelevant. Subjectively, the constant content of these attacks is an amnesia for the period of the seizure. These are the epileptic conditions variously described as automatisms, epileptic equivalents, psychic variants, psychomotor attacks, twilight states or fugues. Automatisms have been fully reviewed by Fenton (1972).

Such conditions may vary greatly in duration, and in the extent to which consciousness appears outwardly to be impaired during the time that the seizure is in progress. They also show a great variety of content. The patient may simply appear to be dazed for a few moments and perform some regular stereotyped manoeuvre, or he may perform a whole sequence of related actions over a considerable period of time, sometimes involving aggressive or seemingly purposeful behaviour. Usually, the patient is clearly out of touch with his surroundings, movements are clumsy and intentions poorly conceived and executed, but sometimes chance observers may notice little abnormality or may simply consider that the patient is somewhat dazed or intoxicated.

Hughlings Jackson (1932) was one of the earliest to describe and analyse such cases. One of his patients, a physician, continued to write a prescription during an attack, though the details of dosage etc. were incorrect. On another occasion, he examined and correctly diagnosed a case of pneumonia during an amnesic episode.

In a case of our own, a boy of 20 while giving his history suddenly paused for a moment, got up, unbuttoned his coat, fumbled in his pockets and then sat down again and continued his story, first repeating the last thing he had said. He was entirely unaware of his actions. Another, a man of 48, set out for his work in Oxford at the normal time one morning and remembered nothing more until he found himself on the sea-front at Bournemouth. This was some ten hours later. He had apparently travelled by train, changing twice, and had eaten a meal and paid for it normally. During the period he had lost his hat and coat. This patient was known to have had occasional grand-mal epilepsy. Further investigation showed that he had an epileptic focus in the left temporal region; his wife recalled previous episodes of brief confused behaviour of which he had himself been unaware.

In cases of this sort, especially when a fugue state is prolonged and purposeful activity of antisocial type occurs, the possibility of a psychogenic hysterical fugue has to be considered. Spratling (1902) reported a case of a travelling salesman who for 28 days undertook his usual circuit of work, recording events in his diary, including convulsive seizures from which he was known to suffer, but had no recollection of anything that happened during this time. The epileptic nature of such a case must remain very doubtful in the absence of electrophysiological or other confirmation. In general, the occurrence of unequivocal grand-mal attacks in someone who also had fugues, rightly biases the diagnosis in favour of epilepsy; but epileptic and hysterical attacks can occur in the same individual, and this is not very uncommon especially where intelligence is low. However, modern diagnostic aids, such as continuous long-term EEG monitoring, leave no doubt, in many cases of amnesia with abrupt onset and ending, that they are in fact epileptic. Wilson, Rupp and Wilson (1950) reported 59 cases which presented in the neurological and psychiatric departments of a general hospital, with loss of personal identity. Fifteen were associated with proven organic cerebral disease, and three had followed upon an undoubted epileptic seizure.

The amnesic states that follow a grand-mal attack, although organically determined, have not the same value for localizing the site of cerebral dysfunction as have those which appear to be the intrinsic and initial content of the seizure, since these latter may logically be assigned to dysfunction of the area of brain in which the attack may be shown to arise. Increasing evidence combines to show that the type of attacks described above are due to epileptic discharges, which arise in the medial temporal lobe. This evidence comes from neurosurgical exploration, from the study of traumatic epilepsy after brain wounds of known location, and from the electroencephalogram. The evidence of Feindel and Penfield (1954) is particularly convincing – 78 per cent of 155 patients undergoing partial temporal lobectomies for epilepsy had a history of automatism as part of the attacks. Attacks themselves were usually accompanied by spontaneous epileptic discharges in the medial and inferior temporal regions, and in such cases, electrical stimulation within a fairly discrete area centring around the amygdaloid nucleus and deep in the uncus, could reproduce the automatism and subsequent amnesia. In a very much smaller group, automatism was found to depend on discharges originating in the frontal grey matter, anterior to the motor cortex. The discharge then spread to involve subcortical structures. However, such frontally determined automatisms differed from the temporal in that they *followed upon* generalized grand-mal seizures. In all these cases, spread of discharge from cortical to subcortical structures formed the necessary prelude to automatism with subsequent amnesia. From such observations, Penfield has argued that a portion of the subcortical 'centrencephalic system' must play an important part in laying down memories, and that this portion must be, to some extent, functionally distinct from that subserving the mechanisms of consciousness.

In temporal lobe epilepsy, certain characteristic and well-defined auras may immediately precede the automatism and thus aid diagnosis. Feindel and Penfield (1954) have studied this question in both spontaneous epilepsy and in that induced by electrical stimulation of the cortex. Commonly observed auras were epigastric sensations, 'butterflies in the stomach', or sensations which seemed to rise up from the epigastrium to the throat, awareness of confusion and difficulty with thinking, feelings of strangeness, dreaminess and unreality, and a variety of autonomic effects.

Epileptic auras may, of course, themselves include disturbances of memory, even when the fit proceeds ultimately to a typical grand-mal convulsion. Here again, the temporal lobe has proved to be chiefly responsible. In the hands of Penfield and his associates, stimulation of the temporal lobe in the unanaesthetized subject has provided valuable information about such auras. In those attacks induced from the medial aspect of the lobe, the auras may include feelings of strangeness in relationship to the present surroundings, intensified familiarity, or *déjà vu*. Although emotional factors are clearly important in the auras, these also imply some falsification and distortion of the memory process. The patient may also experience difficulty with recall of words or names, or may become aware that his thinking is clouded and obstinately refusing to function normally. With stimulation of the lateral surface of the lobe, false recollections of certain events of the

past may form a recurrent feature. The recalled events are often stereotyped and relatively banal, though sometimes relating to emotionally
charged experiences and circumstances. Such 'experimental' hallucinations have proved to be characteristic of epileptic discharges arising
in this area. They occurred in 53 (10 per cent) of 520 cases of temporal
lobe epilepsy reviewed by Penfield and Perot (1963). In 16 of the 53
patients, the typical memory experience of the habitual seizure pattern
could be artificially induced by electrical stimulation. In a further
eight cases, other experiential responses were obtained, not directly
related to the content of the spontaneous seizure.

It is noteworthy that such a response to electrical stimulation of
the brain has been found to occur only from stimulation of the lateral
aspects of the temporal lobes, and only where the temporal lobe is
already the site of spontaneous epileptic discharges. Penfield argues
that the phenomenon represents reactivation of previous fragments of
experience — some previous episode from the patient's past which is
suddenly thrust into the field of awareness. Both auditory and visual
material may be involved, along with the appropriate emotional tone
which appertained to the original experience. Nonetheless, the phenomenon would seem to differ from that of normal recollection, in the
vividness, the wealth of detail and the sense of immediacy which seems
at times to interfere with current experiencing and approaches that
of a true hallucination. Where responses are obtained from several
adjacent points, there is similarity in content amongst the successive
experiences evoked. When stimulation is long continued, re-enactment
seems to be at the speed of the original experience — again in some
ways unlike normal memory.

Bickford and his colleagues (1958) have produced similar results
using implanted electrodes, thus allowing for repeated testing under
the conditions of the ordinary interview situation. Recall of the same
'stereotyped memory' was achieved, and could be repeated on several
occasions, provided the parameters of stimulation were held constant.
However, one is obliged to consider carefully, when reading accounts
of these phenomena, whether they truly represent reactivation of
segments of past experience, rather than the production of complex
hallucinations together with 'identifying paramnesia' as Piercy (1964)
has suggested.

These findings are only indirectly relevant to amnesia. They show
the obverse of the coin, and demonstrate something of the neurological
mechanism of remembering, whose function must be in some way
impaired in amnesia. Some additional results of Bickford are, however,
of more direct relevance. In two of his patients, stimulation in the
posterior part of the middle temporal gyrus, 1.5 to 2 cm below the surface,

produced a short-lived syndrome of amnesia for recent events – those for several days before the experiment – with normal recall of events preceding the amnesic gap. In these examples of an isolated and transient interference with recall from electrical stimulation of a limited area of the brain, the precise point of stimulation is unfortunately not known. However, it would be approaching the lateral border of the hippocampus.

Psychological assessment of patients with temporal lobe epilepsies sometimes reveals impairment of verbal or non-verbal learning, depending on the side of lesion, similar to those associated with structural hemisphere lesions (Milner, 1975). In seizures originating in the hemisphere dominant for speech, there is some indication that the memorizing defect is largely confined to meaningful material (Glowinski, 1973).

True petit-mal attacks, originating subcortically and showing characteristic three per second spike and waves on the electroencephalogram, are also characterized at times by a memory gap, no matter how brief and insignificant the outward appearance of the attack may have seemed. The transient 'absence' may lead only to a discontinuity in the appreciation of current activity, sometimes barely apparent to the subject himself. Mild, but repeated, attacks may in this way have an adverse effect on learning in young children and may sometimes go unrecognized. Such attacks are also associated with retrograde amnesias. Jus and Jus (1962) carried out continuous electroencephalograph recordings, accompanied by tests of continuous registration, in children suffering from repeated attacks of petit mal. A retrograde amnesia of 4 to 15 seconds was found in many attacks, to some extent varying with the active involvement and interest of the subjects during the period under observation: though the results indicated a disturbance of recall, not of registration. Such memorizing difficulties however are not confined to attacks with an EEG pattern of classic petit mal. Bursts of generalized atypical spike and wave may be accompanied by psychological changes of such subtlety that they go undetected except by sensitive laboratory measures. Depending on the time of their occurrence, such subclinical paroxysms have been shown experimentally to upset the memorizing process in children at the registration, storage and retrieval phases (Hutt, 1967).

Occasionally continuous generalized seizure discharge may produce dramatic cognitive change without gross motor manifestations: the condition of minor or petit mal epileptic status. This has been described in both children (Brett, 1966) and adults (Schwartz and Scott, 1971) and without electrographic evidence may be mistaken for subnormality, dementia, or psychosis. During bouts, registration of events is absent or variable so that there is no subsequent memory for the period or only patchy fragmentary recall.

A potential anatomical link exists between temporal lobe epilepsy and the so-called centrencephalic epilepsies, such as classic petit mal, which may account for the amnesia occurring in both. Present evidence suggests that, although they are probably not the actual source of the activity, thalamic structures are closely involved in the propagation of seizure discharge in electrographically generalized epilepsy (Williams, 1953); while in the amnesic temporal lobe seizure, the hippocampal formation and its connections are implicated. Both thalamus and hippocampus are part of the limbic system and interconnected via the fornix system, mammillothalamic tract and septal pathways.

The complex relationship between abnormal electrical activity and memorizing is illustrated by Mirsky and Van Buren's (1965) demonstration that the occurrence of spike-wave bursts is not necessarily accompanied by inattention. Where inattention does occur, its onset may precede the appearance of spike-wave activity, or inattention may occur after the onset of a burst but not persist throughout it. In addition, some children with centrencephalic epilepsy may show attention or registration defects between overt attacks in the absence of EEG abnormalities, possibly because of a persistent disturbance of subcortical mechanisms. These and other behavioural effects of recurrent generalized seizure activity, including that accompanied by clinical absences, have been reviewed by Penry (1973). While disruptive effects on memorizing and other aspects of learning have been repeatedly demonstrated in the laboratory setting, recent findings suggest that children with this type of EEG abnormality are not in general at an educational disadvantage, and, indeed, there is no simple relationship between the number of reported clinical absences and school attainments (Stores and Hart, 1976).

PERSISTENT ABNORMALITIES OF MEMORY

As seen above, transient or episodic amnesic states have yielded some information about likely sites of causative lesions. They also provide the most satisfactory direct information that we are likely to obtain about the form and content of *partial* amnesias, for when normal memory returns detailed subjective descriptions of the preceding state are often possible. When defects of memory are permanent, the patient's description of his disability is usually severely limited even when other intellectual functions are intact, and the condition has to be largely assessed by changes in outward behaviour which imply memory loss. However, permanent defects have some advantages for the objective study of amnesia. In such cases, tests can be planned and carried out at leisure and repeated at intervals. Moreover, the causative lesion is also permanent and likely sooner or later to be structural and accessible to autopsy study. It is, in fact, from cases of persistent abnormalities of memory that information as to their anatomical background was first obtained, and they remain our most valuable source.

The division into transient and permanent changes is not a rigid one. As we have already indicated, some of the conditions causing transient amnesia may occasionally lead on to permanent memory changes. In fact, since memory is seldom stretched to its full capacity either in formal testing or in everyday life, it is possible that slight defects persist after the apparent recovery of many gross amnesias of the type considered so far. In practice, this is seen especially in toxic and deficiency states, where the causative factor has been operating for so long a time that structural brain changes have occurred.

It remains to consider those cerebral disorders in which irreversible structural damage regularly occurs, and in which permanent amnesic defects may result — chronic alcoholism, cerebrovascular disease, neoplasms and degenerative disease. The results of lobectomy and other brain operations will be briefly considered here, and in more detail in Chapter 6.

Chronic alcoholism

A number of the patients which Korsakoff used in his original description of the amnesic confabulatory syndrome now associated with his name were chronic alcoholics. Although the Korsakoff syndrome has since been recognized as occurring in a number of different clinical settings, with nutritional deficiency or specific vitamin lack as a common denominator, it is still most commonly seen in alcoholism. The psychological abnormalities in this condition are usually more widespread than a simple defect of memory alone; nevertheless, a fixation amnesia with a facile and expansive confabulation is a common feature. The vagaries of the memory defects and other behavioural, personality and intellectual changes have been very fully recorded by Talland (1965). Clinically, episodes of Wernicke's encephalopathy and delirium tremens may temporarily obscure the amnesic confabulatory syndrome in such cases; but in many this emerges, sooner or later, as a clear and constant background disability. The value of such cases for the study of amnesia is that their confinement to institutions for the chronic sick allows lengthy examination of mental function, and that treatment and supervision maintain relatively static cerebral lesions which can be fully defined at autopsy. They have thus provided much of the classical evidence for clinico-anatomical correlations in amnesia. Since diffuse and widespread cerebral degenerative changes may be found in some cases, information has to be gleaned especially from a study of those sites which are constantly affected in patients who showed a well-defined and persistent Korsakoff syndrome during life. In the past, evidence from this source has implicated the mammillary bodies and nearby fornix system in the hypothalamus, as most markedly and consistently affected. However Victor (1964) suggests that the medial dorsal nucleus of the thalamus, the pulvinar and the anteroventral nuclei are equally constant sites of lesion and that even severe and chronic involvement of mammillary bodies need not of itself produce a Korsakoff state. Some cases with this damage were known to have no memory defect to adequate psychometric testing during life: moreover, in the cases examined by this author where amnesic states were present, all had involvement of the medial dorsal nucleus of the thalamus in addition to any lesions present in mammillary bodies and terminal portions of the fornices. If this evidence is confirmed, it will implicate the medial dorsal nucleus of the thalamus as a crucial site. However a more recent clinicopathological study by Victor and his colleagues (1971) illustrates the difficulty of assigning an exclusive role in the production of the amnesic syndrome to a particular part of the mesencephalic, diencephalic and limbic structures.

On the psychological side, attempts to define the exact nature of the defect have been made. Weiskrantz and his colleagues (Warrington and Weizkrantz, 1974; Winocur and Weiskrantz, 1976) have shown that in some cases indiscriminate and inappropriate retrieval, rather than a failure of storage, may be part of the disability; and that a reduction in factors interfering with retrieval may improve performance. Very long retrograde amnesias, involving memories long before any likely start of the causative disease, may sometimes be found: so that to view it as solely affecting recent memories, for which a defect of registration or storage might account, may be misleading (Sanders and Warrington, 1971). Further studies suggest (Sanders and Warrington, 1975) that here too a failure of appropriate retrieval rather than a true loss of memory material may be an important factor. It is accepted that some retention of new memories, albeit reduced and erratic, can occur in the Korsakoff syndrome (Talland, 1965): and a loss of the normal temporal orientation of memory has been invoked as one explanation. The above findings might lend this theory some support.

Vascular disorders

Infarction or haemorrhage can give rise to discrete cerebral pathology, and the resulting clinical picture may include diverse forms of intellectual deficit, including disorders of memory. The latter is said to be particularly prominent in lesions of the posterior choroidal artery which supplies part of the hippocampus (Ajuriaguerra and Hecaen, 1960). Certainly, striking cases have been reported in which apoplexy, followed by profound disturbances of memory, has proved at necropsy to have implicated the hippocampal formation of the brain.

> Glees and Griffith (1952) reported a woman of 58 who was admitted to hospital agitated, confused, disorientated and with grossly defective memory. She remained severely demented until her death 15 years later, and memory defect figured prominently throughout. She retained little of current impressions, and could not even remember which was her own bed in the ward, though it had remained the same for many years. At necropsy, the medial parts of both temporal lobes were found to be largely replaced by cystic degeneration. On each side the hippocampi were severely damaged, the hippocampal and fusiform gyri completely destroyed, and the fornix fibres depleted to some 25 per cent of their expected amount. The mammillary bodies appeared normal, as did the remainder of the brain. The pathological picture suggested a vascular catastrophe, probably haemorrhagic, at the outset of the illness.

Victor and his colleagues (1961) reported a case caused by bilateral occlusion of both posterior cerebral arteries. Two years intervened between the two strokes responsible, each producing loss of peripheral vision in the opposite field. It was only after the second episode that memory disorder declared itself, and persisted until death three years later. The patient showed a striking defect in immediate recall and in the ability to learn and retain new facts and skills. Instructions were completely forgotten in a few minutes. Memory for events in the distant past was virtually unaffected, though there was an incomplete retrograde amnesia for some two and a half years preceding the second stroke. There was also some mild but definite behavioural change, with apathy and loss of initiative. Otherwise, on examination he was alert and responsive, showed no apraxia, agnosia or dysphasia, and his general intelligence on the Wechsler scale was 'bright normal'. At postmortem three years later, lesions were found in the inferomedial portions of both temporal lobes involving the hippocampal formation and fornix, and in the mammillary bodies.

A striking case was early described by Mabille and Pitres (1913).

> A 34-year-old man was admitted to a mental hospital following an apoplectic seizure, and was initially diagnosed as dementia. On detailed examination, however, he proved to have a remarkable memory defect as the principal

psychological symptom. Memory for events preceding the stroke was said to be well preserved, but he was incapable of fixing any new memory for more than a few seconds, even though care was taken not to distract him in the interval. Throughout his 23 years in the hospital he would always give his age as 30, and never learned his place at table nor his bed. He lived amongst men whom he always seemed to be meeting for the first time. He was obliged to follow fellow patients around or he would lose his way, and he could work only in a group. By contrast, he answered promptly, consistently and without hesitation when questioned about his life before the stroke. He could dress and feed himself and read and write. At autopsy, a syphilitic arteriopathy, suspected during life, was confirmed. However, the striking macroscopic lesions of the brain were symmetrically placed areas of infarction in the frontal white matter, immediately in front of the head of each caudate nucleus. Detailed histological examination was not reported. The authors point out that these lesions must have interrupted long association fibres from the frontal to the temporal and occipital lobes, though the relevance of this to the amnesia would now be considered doubtful.

Brindley and Janota (1975) have recently described two long-surviving cases of cortical blindness of vascular origin associated with severe defects of recent memory which were of short duration in one patient but lasted six years until the time of death in the other. Only one case came to autopsy and this showed extensive changes in both hippocampi and other limbic structures in addition to calcarine lesions.

Some mention must also be made of subarachnoid haemorrhage and subdural haematoma. The amnesias associated with these conditions may be prolonged and in part permanent, and are considered in the persistent group because opportunity for repeated examination is often possible. However, in most cases substantial recovery finally occurs. The incidence of memory disorder is variable. When it occurs, it may be striking and amount to a full and definite Korsakoff syndrome with fixation amnesia and florid confabulation. Three cases of this sort were reported by Tarachow (1939) from a series of 105 examples of subarachnoid haemorrhage. A latent interval ranging from days to months was seen between the onset of the haemorrhage and the emergence of the memory disorder, and complete recovery was the rule. This interval calls for an explanation. It may sometimes be due to a more general confusion, at first masking the memory defect; in other cases, the secondary changes in an organizing clot in the region of the third ventricle may be responsible.

Indeed, the site of the aneurysm is very important. Impairment of memory of varying severity and duration was quite common in a series of patients with anterior cerebral aneurysms described by Logue and his colleagues (1968) and it was suggested that this was because of the close proximity of the aneurysm to the base of the third ventricle. Storey (1967) considered neuropsychiatric disturbance in relation to both the site of aneurysm and management, whether conservative or operative. Overall mental morbidity was reported in 55 per cent of his 261 patients and consisted of depressive and anxiety symptoms, intellectual loss (including memory disorders the details of which, however, were not given) and personality change. Patients most affected were those with a demonstrable aneurysm. Patients with middle cerebral artery aneurysms, especially those with left-sided lesions, had a higher morbidity with operative treatment, whereas in the other aneurysm group, operative treatment was followed by a slightly lower overall mental morbidity. Improvement of personality was reported in 13 cases.

Chronic subdural haematoma is characterized by an insidious onset and fluctuating course to its mental symptoms. Along with headache and motor and sensory abnormalities, a deterioration of memory may be noticed early by the patient or his relatives. Episodes of mental aberration, difficulty in concentration and frank amnesia are also seen. As the clot enlarges, mental abnormalities increase, along with neurological defects, and progressive retardation, disorientation, confusion and somnolence appear. In general, inefficient and defective memory is more common than a picture of total amnesia. When the clot is evacuated improvement occurs, but because this condition is common in the elderly, some slight permanent brain damage may remain, with persistent mental symptoms.

Cerebral tumours

Memory disorders of one sort or another are a common accompaniment of cerebral tumours. Most frequently they form part of a generalized impairment of intellectual function, with loss of concentration, apathy and drowsiness. In this setting, it is not easy to establish that they are primarily changes in the essential memory processes, rather than a reflection of altered attention, alertness or ability to co-operate. Occasionally, however, the early and prominent symptom of a tumour is an amnesic syndrome, which may occur in a setting of general alertness and clarity of consciousness. Sometimes the picture is of a florid Korsakoff syndrome. Even in such cases, there is still controversy as to whether the memory defect is of localizing diagnostic value and related to tumours involving certain specific areas of the brain, or whether it simply reflects one aspect, which happens to be prominent in that individual, of a general disturbance of cerebral function. On the whole, the evidence is steadily growing in favour of amnesia, and particularly of any marked amnesic confabulatory syndrome, being a symptom of tumours located in specific cerebral areas.

The difficulty in reaching firm conclusions has arisen largely from the fact that a cerebral tumour, in any situation, may produce widespread physiological changes indirectly by a rise in intracranial pressure or interference with blood supply, and that these effects are probably present to some degree in most tumours. Such mechanisms may produce general confusional syndromes in which memory defects can figure prominently, and it is hard to disentangle the specific from the general contribution to the final clinical picture. Thus, if valid evidence is to be obtained, cases must be chosen in which the tumour is well localized, and in which there are no signs of these general intracranial changes, nor of widespread psychological changes at the time of memory-testing.

In 1940, Busch considered the problem of mental changes and memory defect in cerebral tumours and concluded, after viewing some hundreds of cases, that general intracranial changes could be dismissed as an adequate explanation for many cases, and that when memory changes did occur, they would be the more serious the more widespread the actual cerebral lesion was. He did not produce clear evidence as to the siting of the tumours causing memory changes. However, Bleuler (1951) examined 600 unselected cases of cerebral tumours in a wide variety of sites, and investigated especially the psychological changes present. He concluded that amnesia is not associated with any particular site of lesion and that cases showed a wide uniformity in their psychopathological picture. As many as 83 per cent of his whole group showed some mental changes, and all tended to have similar syndromes: general clouding of consciousness in the acute stage, and a 'chronic amnesic syndrome' in the chronic stage. The latter syndrome, in fact, embraces for him much more than a memory defect alone. In addition to impairment of retention and recall of new experiences, there was confusion, increased fatigability and emotional instability or apathy. However, these features of general cerebral deterioration occur in variously sited cerebral tumours, if of infiltrating type or producing the general changes mentioned above. Some support is given to Bleuler's view that amnesia is not associated with any particular site of lesion, by the findings of McFie and Piercy (1952). In a study of 58 patients with localized cerebral lesions, they showed that several intellectual abilities were selectively impaired by specifically-sited lesions, but impairment of retention and learning was related to size rather than locus of lesion.

Against this must be set the evidence for a characteristic and marked amnesic confabulatory syndrome, in association with localized tumours and in the absence of more general psychological or intracranial changes. This constitutes an increasingly impressive argument for associating the site of the tumour with the symptoms produced. Sprofkin and Sciarra (1952) report three such cases in which the clinical picture was that of a Korsakoff syndrome, but alcoholic and other likely causes had been fully excluded. All three had tumours limited to the midline structures in the region of the hypothalamus and third ventricle. Williams and Pennybacker (1954) supplied evidence from a more thorough and widespread study of 180 patients with verified intracranial tumours. All were given specific psychological tests for memory function. In 26, impairment of memory was the outstanding psychological defect; the main changes were inability to fixate current events, impairment of new learning, distortion of the recent past and general difficulty with recall. Fifteen of these 26 patients had deep midline tumours. Four cases had a classic amnesic confabulatory syndrome, and all four had localized lesions involving the floor and walls of the third ventricle. Pursuing the question of localization, these authors further reviewed 32 cases of craniopharyngiomas involving the diencephalon and third ventricular structures. In 21 of these, the more posterior hypothalamus and third ventricle were involved by tumour, and some 75 per cent of them showed characteristic memory defects; while in the other 11 cases the lesion was more anteriorly placed, and memory in these was substantially normal. A group of 24 posterior fossa tumours was used as a control for the effects of raised intracranial pressure *per se*; less then half had memory disturbances and none had a florid amnesic syndrome. The distinction which can at times be made between the general mental changes of raised intracranial pressure and specific memory changes related to a focal lesion, is well illustrated in one of their cases.

A young man of 22 was found to have a craniopharyngioma involving the floor of the third ventricle. It had interrupted the cerebrospinal fluid circulation and caused a marked rise in intracranial pressure, giving rise to some local brainstem signs and severe confusion, drowsiness and, at times, coma. Ventricular tapping relieved these symptoms and he became alert and cooperative. However, a marked memory defect for recent events, with elaborate and detailed confabulation, then emerged. Part of the local tumour was cystic and was directly tapped, thus reducing local pressure on hypothalamic nuclei. Following this, he became fully orientated and his confabulation ceased. As the cyst again filled up, the amnesic confabulatory syndrome reappeared. As cerebrospinal fluid circulation was again interrupted and general intracranial tension rose, so drowsiness and confusion supervened. This sequence was repeated on several occasions.

Such observations, which continue to be made in neurosurgical practice (Kohn and Crosby, 1972), serve to point out the importance of quite limited areas of brain in the occurrence of amnesia. Hécaen and Ajuriaguerra (1956) added further evidence. A consideration of 450 cases of cerebral tumour of widely varying sites, and an extensive review of the literature, led them to conclude that certain sites are particularly associated with memory disturbance. A number of their cases had the fully developed amnesic confabulatory syndrome. The diencephalon and deep midline region was most clearly involved and must be regarded as being of practical diagnostic value in the clinical localization of lesions causing such symptoms. A second area, less implicated, was the frontal region. The latter finding may reflect the previously noted tendency for corpus callosum tumours to present with mental changes and especially memory defects. Amongst tumours involving the posterior part of the corpus callosum, Schlesinger (1950) found disturbances of memory to be common, and again, in some they took the form of a mild Korsakoff syndrome. In the more anterior part of the corpus callosum, memory changes also occurred, though here, tumours had usually spread to involve both frontal lobes. However, one clear-cut case with histological evidence of a lesion limited to the anterior two-thirds of the corpus callosum and with no frontal involvement, was reported by Hécaen and Ajuriaguerra. Here, memory disturbance was a prominent early symptom and there later developed a gross defect of fixation and of recent memory.

That frontal lesions, especially when bilateral, may be accompanied by memory changes is widely accepted. Sachs (1927) included loss of memory for recent events as a characteristic feature of such lesions. Hécaen and Ajuriaguerra also noted that intermittent memory defects were mentioned frequently in the literature of frontal lobe tumours. In their own 80 cases, ten presented with mental disturbances in which *amnésie de fixation* was prominent. However, the more characteristic change in these lesions is a defect of motivation and attention, and it is difficult at times to evaluate the effect of these on the tests used for assessing memory. Failure to remember or recall, in the patient with a frontal tumour, is often seen in a setting of gross fatuousness, apathy or indifference, which raises the question of whether the patient is trying to remember or give the right answer, even if he knows it. This difficulty has to be constantly recognized when assessing such evidence.

Temporal lobe tumours are sometimes associated with selective impairments of memory depending on the side of the lesion. As in other types of temporal lobe pathology such as vascular lesions (Barbizet and Cary, 1970) and possibly seizure sources (Blakemore, Ettlinger and Falconer, 1966), tumours are sometimes associated with memory impairment for verbal material if on the left (Barbizet and Cary, 1970) and non-verbal material if on the right (Benton and Van Allen, 1968). However they do not seem to be especially associated with permanent memory defects (Kolodny, 1928; Hécaen and Ajuriaguerra, 1956), despite the occurrence of episodic amnesia as a characteristic feature of temporal lobe epilepsy. This may well be due to the bilateral functional representation of memory mechanisms in the temporal lobe, so that damage to one side only is not enough to produce any marked defect. As we shall see later when considering temporal lobectomy, bilateral injury to medial temporal lobe structures certainly produces a severe and characteristic amnesic syndrome.

Occipital tumours have at times been thought to be especially liable to cause memory disturbance. This was suggested by the early work of Frazier and Waggoner (1929) and Allen (1930). However, it is difficult to exclude the effects of raised intracranial pressure in these posteriorly situated tumours. This applies equally to subtentorial tumours of the posterior fossa where, however, the frequency of memory disorder is surprisingly low despite the prevalence of raised intracranial pressure (Hécaen and Ajuriaguerra, 1956).

The nature of the memory impairment may be very circumscribed. Lesions in different regions of the same hemisphere may affect different aspects of memory (Luria, 1971). Patients with left hemisphere lesions may encounter difficulty with auditorily presented material, but be able to cope with the same material presented visually (Warrington and Shallice, 1969; Warrington, Logue and Pratt, 1971). Lesions in the posterior part of the right hemisphere may cause difficulties in visual perception and visual retention tests (Warrington and James, 1967): while in the left hemisphere visual short-term memory may be defective as a background to simultanagnosia (Warrington, 1971). Moreover, memories for motor skills can be functionally separate from verbal and non-verbal memories and impaired selectively by lesions of the right parietal area.

In general, it may be said that no site of tumour is so convincingly related to memory changes as that of the hypothalamus and periventricular area. It may be relevant that in this region a number of bilateral structures are closely related topographically, so that both sides are likely to be injured by a single lesion.

Finally, it is of considerable practical importance that cerebral tumours may be a common cause of failing memory and seeming dementia in the elderly. Among 45 elderly patients in whom memory disorder was the chief if not the only complaint, six proved to be due to cerebral tumour (Allison, 1961). Since the tumours were mostly benign and accessible to surgical treatment, their early diagnosis was all the more important.

Lobectomy and other brain operations

The amnesias associated with accidental injuries of the brain, and the information about memory mechanisms revealed by surgical operations, are both considered in detail in other chapters. However, some of the evidence obtained from brain operations is so germane to the problems arising from study of local disease of the brain that it will be referred to briefly here.

Surgical procedures are undertaken for the removal of tumours, the relief of epilepsy or the alteration of the course of chronic psychiatric illnesses. They therefore suffer from the disadvantage of dealing with a brain already in part diseased or abnormal. Nevertheless, the memory defects produced are sometimes clear-cut and unequivocally related to the lesion incurred. Some of the most impressive confirmatory evidence for the importance of medial temporal lobe structures in normal memory formation is provided from this source. Scoville in 1954, and later Scoville and Milner (1957) reported a gross loss of retention of current experiences with some variable retrograde amnesia for periods immediately prior to operation, in patients who had undergone bilateral removal of the anterior two-thirds of the hippocampus and hippocampal gyrus, and with removal of the uncus and amygdala. So severe was the defect of registration and so brief the memory for new experiences, that these patients seemed to live in a state of almost continuous anterograde amnesia following the operation. The defect was largely limited to this particular aspect of memory. There was no general deterioration in personality, intelligence or perceptual ability. Earlier learned skills were preserved and the patient's behaviour might appear superficially normal. Remote events were well recalled, but a variable and usually partly recovered retrograde amnesia occurred for events before operation. The syndrome appeared only with bilateral removal of the structures discussed. The findings were in general similar in cases reported by Milner and Penfield (1955). In their cases, although the surgical lesion was only unilateral, they considered that there was some evidence of pre-existing damage to the other side. Although some of these cases showed slight improvement in the memory defect, in general the changes appeared to be permanent (*see also* Chapter 6). On the other hand, defects of recent memory have been described in patients with unilateral surgical lesions and without evidence of disturbance on the other side (Walker, 1958; Luria and Karraseva, 1968).

We have to conclude that the areas damaged are an essential part of the cerebral mechanisms of memory and specifically for the registration of new memories. It is clear that parts of the temporal lobe, particularly the medial part, must be counted with the hypothalamus and periventricular areas as essential anatomical substrata for memory.

Less consistent and less clearly defined losses of memory have been recorded after surgical lesions of other parts of the brain — of the frontal lobes, including quite limited ablations of the anterior cingulate areas, and possibly also after damage to the fornix fibres and anterior thalamic nuclei.

Operations on the frontal lobes rarely produce enduring memory disorder, though Rylander (1939) did note that after frontal lobectomy for tumour, patients were significantly more forgetful of test material than controls. However, no marked memory changes have been noted as a permanent sequel in the now very large number of frontal leucotomy and similar operations. In the early postoperative period, however, striking evidence of memory disorder may be seen. Klein (1952) found a marked defect of retention during the first few days after operation. This defect was closely associated with distractability: immediate recall was good, but if attention was distracted by another task, retention was at once reduced. With this there was also some retrograde amnesia of a patchy kind, sometimes including events of high emotional significance such as the preparation for operation. Denial of operation was common, though this of course may often include something more than amnesia, and many patients could not recall the first dressing on the fourth postoperative day when bandages were replaced by plaster. The examiners' daily visits were often not recalled from one day to the next for the first four to seven days, yet at the time of examination patients were alert, attentive, and without impairment of other intellectual functions. A marked aspect of this temporary amnesic state was a disorganization of the temporal sequence of events.

Kral and Durost (1953) confirmed these findings, but added, in some of their cases, some permanent partial defect of retaining new experiences, even two to three years after operation. A memory disorder involving especially the temporal sequence of events, was also noted as a transient phenomenon following limited ablations of the anterior cingulate cortex (Whitty and Lewin, 1960). There was apparent confabulation, because events accurately recalled were misplaced in time. Lesions designed to disconnect anterior cingulate and other frontal areas from the limbic system have also been reported (Kelly *et al.*, 1973). However they are tract-cutting rather than discrete cortical excisions. Detailed studies of early postoperative cognitive and memory functions were not recorded, though Wechsler Adult Intelligence Scale tests showed no significant change.

Stereotactic operations on the thalamus have been undertaken for the treatment of Parkinsonism and similar disorders of movement. The aim is to place a limited lesion in the dorsomedial nucleus, though the close juxtaposition of the anterior nuclei makes it probable that at times they also are involved. Spiegel and his colleagues (1956), reporting the results of a series of such operations, noted transient memory deficits in a high proportion of cases. These usually cleared in a few weeks. Hassler (1962) also reported an isolated case where bilateral coagulation of the anterior thalamic nuclei was specifically aimed at, in the treatment of severe schizophrenia with auditory and tactile hallucinations. These particular symptoms seemed to be completely abolished by the operation, but a severe amnesic syndrome appeared. There was some general confusion with disorientation in time and place, but memory also was grossly defective and the patient could not recognize familiar objects and people, even his own close relatives. The more florid disturbance cleared in three months or so, but defective recall and recognition persisted. In these cases, the exact site of lesion must remain suppositional. However, in a patient described by Watkins and Oppenheimer (1962), full autopsy examination was possible, since death occurred from unrelated causes nine months after an operation undertaken for Parkinsonism. Immediately after a left thalamolysis, using an injected alcohol technique, the patient had a marked confusional state with probable hallucination. This cleared in a few days to reveal a severe defect of fixation of new memories, accompanied by confabulation. Some months later, his memory for recent events had improved, but he still had a complete amnesia for a period of some three weeks following operation. By contrast, memory was clear for events right up to the infliction of the thalamic lesion. Detailed examination of the brain at autopsy showed that the main lesion centred in the ventrolateral thalamic nucleus, and extended downwards and forwards to involve the internal capsule and the medial tip of the globus pallidus. The exact extent of indirect damage was difficult to assess, but the medial and anterior nuclei appeared to be spared. The authors point out the possibility that the anterior choroidal artery may have been temporarily occluded. There was no evidence of involvement of the opposite hemisphere, so that this case represents the result of a unilateral lesion in the dominant hemisphere.

The results of surgical interference with the fornix bundle have produced conflicting evidence where memory disorder is concerned. Sweet, Talland and Ervin (1959) have reported a woman in whom a colloid cyst of the third ventricle was removed. This necessitated bilateral section of the anterior columns of the fornix, but the operation, in the opinion of the surgeons, did not involve any damage to the floor or walls of the ventricle. Postoperatively the patient showed a gross defect of recent memory and a markedly reduced memory span in formal testing. By contrast, her remote memory was well preserved. No autopsy examination was available. In this case, the possibility of incidental damage to periventricular structures must still be considered, especially because changes in memory have not been found in other reported instances of bilateral section of the fornix (Clark and his colleagues, 1938; Cairns, 1950); when such changes have been reported, coincidental periventricular damage has usually been demonstrated (Davison and Demuth, 1946; Ajuriaguerra, Hécaen and Sadoun, 1954).

The senile and pre-senile dementias

In dementia, impairment of function may invade all areas of mental life, and the pleomorphic symptomatology is marked by correspondingly widespread pathological changes in the brain. Nonetheless, disorder of memory plays a prominent and often a leading role in the condition.

In many respects, the clinical features of the early stages of dementia find a parallel in the so-called normal process of ageing. The parallel must not, however, be drawn too closely, since the pathology of the ageing brain commonly includes changes which are, in part, independent of the ageing process itself. Thus, cerebral arteriosclerosis with consequent ischaemia and cell loss is common, and the mental defects of ageing may in fact be the result of such incidental damage, rather than of old age *per se*. This is not of practical importance in trying to correlate the memory disturbance of old age with local or specific brain lesions.

The psychological symptoms of old age are well known. Along with narrowing of interests, impairment of reasoning and mental fatiguability, there is progressive loss of learning ability and memory. Individuals differ widely in this respect, and it has not yet proved possible to define the significant histological or physiological variables which might account for these changes (Lewis, 1954). Busse (1962) has reported a relatively high incidence of electroencephalographic abnormality in the region of the temporal lobes in elderly persons, and there is a tendency for this to be more marked when learning ability is clearly deficient.

Numerous studies of memory function with advancing years agree in showing that, in the average person, the ability to retain new material declines gradually from the third or fourth decade onwards. The decline is global, affecting all kinds of material, but as age advances there is special difficulty in learning and retaining novel associations or in changing well-established mental habits. The memory impairment in old age, and in other instances where widespread and diffuse cerebral changes are known to be present, is traditionally held to conform to Ribot's law; that is, to affect recent memory most severely and old memories progressively less as they recede in time. This common assumption would appear, however, to rest largely on the fact that old people are relatively uninterested in the present and tend to dwell much more on the past. In fact, recall of the remote, as well as the recent past, may often be shown to be impaired. The evidence rests heavily on the recall of striking personal events of special interest, and the experiences recalled are often repetitious and lacking in detail. Moreover, it is often difficult to check the accuracy of such remote events. Among elderly patients with known organic cerebral disease, Shapiro and his colleagues (1956) were able to demonstrate convincingly that, in fact, remote memory was often severely impaired. Nevertheless, it is clear that the learning of new material and the establishing of a durable record of *current* experience are especially vulnerable to the ageing process. Welford (1958) has shown that this is due not to impaired perception, but to defective short-term storage of immediate perceptions. Not only is the memory trace for new experiences of itself more short-lived, but it is more readily impaired by subsequent impressions (Inglis, 1962; Mackay and Inglis, 1963).

While a dementing process will tend to produce permanent defects, depression in the elderly may cause temporary impairments. A distinction between the two groups may be important in management. Some qualitative differences in the memory changes have recently been suggested (Whitehead, 1973). In formal memory tests, depressives make less random errors and fewer false positive answers but tend to make more errors of transposition in remembered material.

Whatever the psychological or neurological basis, the aged may in practice show marked impairments of memory. This may be seen as a diffuse and general forgetfulness, so that routine tasks are left unfinished, possessions mislaid, letters unanswered and past and present events muddled — a common example is to confuse children, grandchildren and their own brothers and sisters. In other cases, short periods of complete amnesia may occur unpredictably, while the general level of memory is reasonably well maintained. Such amnesias may include events of much emotional significance. Thus, the visits of near and dear relatives, some special celebration or the signing of important documents may pass completely and irretrievably from memory.

Kral (1958) has attempted to distinguish a 'benign' and 'malignant' form of memory defect in old age; the former being mainly a difficulty in the recall of names, dates and occasions, and affecting objective and impersonal more than personal data; the latter, a progressive amnesia with marked defects in registration and recall of recent events and merging into a confusional state. The segregation of the two groups for old age as such is artificial, and probably reflects the development of a progressive organic cerebral disease such as arteriosclerosis in the more severe group.

Arteriosclerotic dementia begins typically in the 60s and 70s. The dementing process is characterized by intermittent stepwise downward progression. There is some evidence from autopsy studies to suggest that multiple small cerebral infarcts form the pathological background to the clinical course. Intellectual impairment shows fluctuations, though each acute episode leaves further residual defect. Memory function rarely escapes; impairment of memory for recent events is often the earliest sign and may long remain a relatively isolated defect (Mayer-Gross, Slater and Roth, 1960). Later, short-lived episodes of clouding of consciousness and delirium may occur, and amnesia for new experiences with confabulation may form a permanent background to the final picture. Eventually, memory may be grossly impaired in all its aspects, or virtually untestable, owing to the inaccessibility of the patient. Although minor clinical features such as the serrated course and the physical signs of generalized arterial degeneration may aid the clinical diagnosis, the psychological picture does not differ greatly from that of other dementias of old age, and the definitive diagnosis has to be made postmortem.

If a purely senile psychosis exists, then it is represented by a very similar clinical picture to that of arteriosclerotic dementia, but without the diagnostic arterial changes or the histological features of presenile dementia being found at autopsy. It is sometimes claimed that memory disorder, and particularly a failure of retention of new experiences, is an early and striking feature of the purely senile cases. A further suggestion is that in this group, a hereditary factor can be defined in the family history. The evidence is by no means convincing that either of these factors distinguishes a special group. Arterial changes occur to a greater or lesser degree in all brains over the age of 50, and the precise siting of this pathology must determine the exact mental picture that results. Thus, any memory defect noted in the elderly may be due to *specifically sited* arterial changes rather than to their total quantity.

The group of presenile dementias occurs largely in the fifth and sixth decades, though cases have been reported as early as the third and fourth. These show histological changes in the brain which are clear-cut and often diagnostic, and their familial hereditary nature in many cases is convincing. While a substantial number remain at present unclassified, four types are more or less clearly delineated on clinical and pathological grounds: Alzheimer's disease, Pick's disease, Huntington's chorea and Jakob-Creutzfeld's disease. In the last three, memory defects are either not marked or are early submerged in a more diffuse intellectual loss; in Huntington's chorea choreic movements are associated with progressive general intellectual loss similar to that seen in normal ageing persons (Aminoff *et al.*, 1975); in Jakob-Creutzfeld's disease rapid deterioration in intellectual function is accompanied by equally rapidly increasing spasticity and cerebellar dysfunction; in Pick's disease early changes occur most often in the spheres of conation, attention and emotion. All three of these conditions have pathological changes which are characteristic, either in site or type. All may show marked memory defects as part of the picture, but these rarely emerge early or in isolation.

In Alzheimer's disease, however, memory defects are commonly a presenting feature. In the early states there is simple forgetfulness for everyday events, and especially for names and words, which may soon merge into an obvious amnesic dysphasia. This progresses to a severe fixation amnesia which may lead to abnormalities of behaviour, such as inappropriate repetition of some recently performed act or denial of recent occurrences. Sometimes for years a facade of social normality may be preserved, but ultimately generalized intellectual impairment and disorientation supervene. In the early stages, however, a capricious loss of memory, which includes limited periods of apparently complete amnesia, is usual. At this stage and later, though Miller (1973 and 1975) reports impairment of both short-term memory and long-term storage with faulty retrieval similar to the findings of Warrington and Weiskrantz (1974), there may be relative preservation of more distant memories, and if aphasia is not prominent, coherent and sensible conversation about long past events is possible. Such patients are often partially aware of their memory deficits and this gives a characteristic anxiety to their reactions.

The pathology of this condition is also characteristic. There is neuronal loss with glial reaction, and specific argentophil plaques and neurofibrillary whorls are distributed throughout the cortex. They are often most marked in certain areas, the frontal cortex and the hippocampus being especially involved (Corsellis, 1970). However a qualitative difference in the memory defects of such patients and those associated with other causes of bilateral hippocampal damage may be found (Miller, 1973). The pathological changes in this and other amnesic conditions are more fully considered in Chapter 8.

In the field of mental handicap a movement away from the idea of global intellectual disability towards more selective learning difficulties, has uncovered specific defects in the input or registration phase of memory. No anatomical basis has yet been defined, but successful design of remedial programmes gives it some importance (Clarke, 1969; O'Connor and Hermelin, 1971).

The neuropsychiatric approach attempts to identify cerebral mechanisms involved in behaviour. This chapter serves to illustrate it in the field of memory. Some of the earliest and still widely accepted evidence suggests the limbic system as a substrate for emotion and memory — two functions closely linked in mental life. Smythies (1970) has marshalled much detailed evidence in support of this system as a major channel for behavioural activity. The biochemical and pharmacological factors which influence the system are as yet little known. In mentioning them he indicates a field of enquiry which will have to be increasingly tilled if we are to understand memory mechanisms.

CONCLUSIONS

Defects of memory are a common symptom of cerebral disease. As a transient phenomenon they occur in a wide variety of diseases, both those intrinsically cerebral and those of a more generalized nature affecting the brain indirectly. They are often but one part of a more widespread cerebral dysfunction such as is manifested in diffuse intellectual impairment, delirium, stupor or coma. Sometimes they are the predominant, and occasionally the only recognizable, features of the dysfunction.

The range of memory defect is considerable. It may be a partial loss of registration, appearing simply as exaggerated forgetfulness; a severe inability to recall or record all current events, with preservation of more distant memories; a limited but complete amnesia for a sharply defined period; repeated episodes of such amnesia; or a period of partial amnesia with hazy and inaccurate recollection.

In these cases the defects of memorizing itself are transient, and as the causative disease recovers, so does the ability to lay down durable memories. The limited amnesic period, however, is usually permanent; the implication being that registration was defective at the time and so no memory was established for subsequent recall.

Permanent defects of memorizing also occur. Here, irreversible structural brain damage is responsible.

In both transient and permanent defects, consistent and convincing evidence points to lesions in certain limited areas of the brain as being responsible. The hypothalamic nuclei, the hippocampal structures, and parts of the anterior thalamus and frontal cortex seem to be most clearly implicated. The anatomical and pathological evidence for this is deployed more fully elsewhere in this book. The clinical study of amnesia in cerebral disease serves mainly to emphasize and illustrate the wide range, both in type and severity, of memory defects that may occur.

3 Transient Global Amnesia

C.W.M. Whitty

Isolated attacks of amnesia associated with known cerebrovascular disease and examples considered to be due to migraine, have been mentioned in Chapter 2. However in 1964, Fisher and Adams in a monograph entitled 'Transient Global Amnesia' reported 17 patients with a stereotyped syndrome of sudden attacks of amnesia and confusion, without headache or any other neurological or psychiatric abnormality. Although Bender (1956) and probably Guyotat and Courjon (1956) had published similar cases using other descriptive titles, Fisher and Adams's detailed report makes it a definitive monograph of the condition. With hindsight, as always, a number of previous cases are now regarded as examples: Bechterew's report (1900b) of a man who had ten brief attacks of amnesia following a stroke, being one of the earliest quoted; though Bechterew himself seems to have considered them epileptic attacks. Cases must have occurred over the centuries, their brief duration, infrequent recurrence and benign prognosis perhaps allowing them to pass unrecorded.

Reported cases now number over 200. Of the larger series Bender (1956 and 1960) and Jaffe and Bender (1966) mention a total of 51 examples. Shuttleworth and Morris (1966) cite seven, Godlewski (1968) lists 33 cases with 40 attacks, Mumenthaler and von Roll (1969) 14, Martin (1971) 10, and Heathfield, Croft and Swash (1973) 19. While Lou (1968) gave details of multiple attacks in two patients; and Bolwig (1968), Evans (1966) and Gilbert (1972) report particularly on possible aetiology.

THE CLINICAL PICTURE

Attacks occur mainly in the 50 to 70 age group, in males more than females, and usually in a setting of previous good health. The onset is sudden. Patients describe some subjective confusion in phrases such as 'I can't seem to think straight'. The main objective feature is a loss of memorizing so that events are no longer registered. While immediate memory as measured by digit retention is normal, memory span for current experience is reduced to minutes. During the attack, spontaneous remarks or enquiry will reveal some retrograde amnesia for events preceding it. There is a degree of confusion shown characteristically by a rather mechanical repetition of questions such as 'What am I doing here?', 'Why aren't I at work?', 'When did I arrive here?', etc. Awareness of the memory difficulty may cause apprehension. Otherwise there are no other psychiatric or neurological abnormalities. The attack lasts a few hours — very rarely more than one day. Recovery of memory function is rapid and complete, though there is a permanent memory gap for the duration of the attack. Resolution of retrograde amnesia is discussed below. In the earlier descriptions single attacks were the rule. However repeated attacks are now being more often reported (Lou, 1968; Godlewski, 1968; Heathfield, Croft and Swash, 1973).

This is the central core of the syndrome. There are some less constant aspects. Minimal neurological deficit, in particular visual field involvement, hemiparesis or dysphasia, have been noted as transient early accompaniments, very occasionally persisting after the amnesia. Attacks lasting several days have been recorded, though rarely. If their progress remains basically similar, such cases may be regarded as part of the syndrome, though involving pathologically more extensive cerebral areas. Occasionally hesitancy and confusion in initiating some familiar task which is then carried out accurately may be noted: and Godlewski (1968) mentions a single case in his series in which the signature on a cheque made out during the amnesia was questioned by the bank. In general, however, it is striking that no loss of learned motor skills occurs: simple acts such as dressing, preparing food, and eating, and more complex activities such as driving a car or typing are well executed. This applies to skills known to have been acquired during a period involved in a long transient retrograde amnesia. One further constantly noted feature of the attacks is the absence of any automatic, confused or purposeless motor behaviour such as is associated with some of the temporal lobe epilepsies.

Since the first cases were reported views on aetiology have been divided between epilepsy and cerebrovascular abnormality. Bender (1956) favoured a vascular mechanism. Fisher and Adams (1964) considered either epilepsy or vascular disease possible, but favoured epilepsy. Attacks have been ascribed to probable or certain cerebrovascular disease in an increasing number of cases (Heathfield, Croft and Swash, 1973; Bolwig, 1968; Martin, 1971; Dimsdale, 1971;

van Crewel, 1969). An association with hypertension has been noted. A few cases linked with migraine would also fall into the cerebrovascular category. Precipitation of attacks by neck movements suggest a vascular pathology, with either mechanical obstruction or precipitation of emboli as the immediate cause. It is also argued that sudden response to cold, as noted in some cases, may precipitate vascular changes. In general, opinion favouring a vascular origin is growing. The question is further discussed later.

In a typical case seen personally there was opportunity to observe the patient throughout the attack.

A woman of 62 while visiting Oxford from her home in London for her son's graduation suddenly became confused while at lunch. She arrived at my house by taxi a quarter of an hour later at about 1.30 p.m. She had not been able to recall the address which was familiar to her, but recognized me at once. She complained of feeling muddled and strange and suggested this was due to the hot weather and very stuffy atmosphere of the lunch room. She was able to carry on a normal conversation on general matters, recognized various relatives, was alert and responsive and showed no evidence of intellectual loss. Neurological examination was normal. Blood pressure was 150/90. Digit retention forwards and backwards was normal but new information about family and friends was retained only for minutes. She had no memory of why she was in Oxford, nor of her car journey there. Her conversation was punctuated by remarks such as 'How long have I been here?', 'I don't really know why I'm here', etc. She enquired about a niece who had been talking to her some 15 minutes before. When her son arrived she asked why he was wearing his academic dress. At one stage she suggested ringing her husband who had been dead for more than a year. During conversation it became clear that current events were retained for only two or three minutes. There was also a dense retrograde amnesia of at least two days. She recalled nothing of the previous day, or her preparations for the journey including a phone call to check the graduation timetable, nor of a local council meeting she had attended on the day before that. Some remarks about family events also suggested a much longer but patchy retrograde amnesia. About 9.30 p.m. she retired to bed, finding her way to the room she usually slept in and knowing the location of the lavatory and bathroom. At that time memory span was still limited to minutes. She forgot that night clothes had been laid out for her, and a conversation which had resulted in a particular Jane Austen novel being put out for bedside reading. When she awoke next morning at about 8 a.m. memorizing had returned and appeared normal. There was however a dense memory gap of some nine hours for events of the preceding afternoon and evening, including her lunch and the start of the attack. Memory for the earlier part of the day, including her journey, was hazy but recovered in 48 hours. However a permanent retrograde amnesia ranging from ½ to 1 hour remained.

She had a moderate hypertension diagnosed three years previously and adequately controlled by methyldopa and a thiazide diuretic. It is interesting that she remembered her night-time tablet, found it in her handbag and took it She had no further attacks and remained well, apart from a short period of congestive cardiac failure until she died of a stroke nine years later. No autopsy was obtained.

DISCUSSION

This syndrome has clinical value. It allows us to recognize a condition, which may be very alarming to patients and relatives, as transient and benign: and, since the clinical picture is now so clear cut, to do so usually without the use of 'invasive' diagnostic tests. Nevertheless it remains a syndrome without an established aetiology. At the level of pathophysiology also, vascular and epileptic mechanisms are each proposed. Of the former, reversible vascular spasm, which brings it into the category of migraine, microemboli, changes in blood pressure (both a drop in central pressure with consequent reduced cerebral perfusion and a sudden rise as in hypertensive encephalopathy) and mechanical obstruction of cerebral vessels have all been discussed. A variant of temporal lobe epilepsy akin to a temporal lobe fugue is an alternative. The discharge is envisaged as occupying only in those neuronal circuits subserving memory. Since it does not generalize to produce a grand-mal fit, it does not invoke the powerful inhibitory mechanisms that normally end such a discharge, and can thus be maintained for the hours of the attack. A model for such local discharge is contained in the observations of Bickford and colleagues (1958). In two patients being prepared for surgical treatment of focal epilepsy, stimulation of the hippocampal complex caused a transient retrograde amnesia whose duration varied with that of the stimulation, and a permanent antero-grade amnesia for a short period after stimulation. Both bilateral and unilateral after-discharge from stimulation were effective: though it is not stated whether dominant hemisphere stimulation was required. Less direct support is also provided by Kesner, whose work in rats he termed 'an experimental model of transient global amnesia' (Kesner, *et al.*, 1975). Hippocampal after-discharge produced temporary amnesia for a previously learned habit, with a permanent amnesia for experiences during the period of after-discharge. However these findings must be regarded as primarily anatomical rather than physiological evidence, since focal embolization and probably other forms of local ischaemia can produce such discharges (Patrick and Whitty, 1965).

In the majority of cases the EEG is within normal limits, even when recorded during or shortly after an attack (Jaffe and Bender, 1966). The duration of attacks range from hours to a maximum of some days. The only symptoms are those of defective memory, with confusion which could be derived solely from the memory defect. Single attacks in the older age groups are the rule. These features together with such apparent precipitating factors as neck movements, blood pressure changes and occasional association with migraine make a primary vascular mechanism most probable. If such ischaemia is to be transient and limited to those cerebral areas known to be concerned with memory, local spasm of vessels might operate as in migraine, but microemboli could equally account for the phenomenon; and this offers an easier explanation for the limited anatomical extent of the dysfunction and, with variable associated thrombosis, for the differing durations. It could be argued that such a mechanism requires either bilateral involvement of hypothalamic nuclei or hippocampal formations, or sufficient pre-existing damage to one side to render remaining function unilateral, or a degree of memory 'dominance' in one or other hemisphere. The difficulty applies also to permanent memory deficits due to known unilateral temporal lesions. However the physiological evidence for *bilateral* hippocampal after-discharge following unilateral stimulation may make the requirement of bilateral lesions unnecessary. Present evidence supports the view, expressed by a number of those reporting examples of T.G.A., that this is a symptom of transient hippocampal dysfunction (Fisher and Adams, 1964; Bolwig, 1968; van Crewel, 1969; Tharp, 1969; Mumenthaler and von Roll, 1969; Martin 1971).

For an understanding of amnesia, the syndrome is also valuable. Its essential content is a temporary loss of memorizing for which Delay (1942) coined the phrase 'amnesie de memoration' – an inability to lay down memory traces available for later recall. This is accompanied by some defect of recall of already implanted memories as shown by a variable duration of retrograde amnesia. The loss of ongoing memorizing, so that the time span of current experience is reduced to minutes or less, causes a variable amount of anxiety and confusion, but in general the picture presented is of an isolated defect of memory unalloyed by intellectual loss, apathy, lack of initiative and emotional disturbances such as Talland (1965) has described in the alcoholic Korsakoff syndrome, and which presumably represent the more widespread cerebral changes subsequently found in many such cases.

While recall of past events, sometimes long past, is transiently defective, the preservation of learned motor skills seems to be complete. They are not included in any retrograde amnesia whether temporary or permanent. The acquisition of novel motor skills during the actual attack and their subsequent retention has not been studied. Motor tasks not involving visual or auditory aspects of memory, and likely to be learned in the limited time of the attack, might be hard to devise. In patients with severe head injury and prolonged retrograde amnesia (R.A.), such skills may occasionally appear to be lost. In some instances this is clearly a part of a more general traumatic dementia; while in others the possibility of an associated hysterical amnesia arises. One case, not traumatic, has been reported however in which a colloid cyst of the third ventricle was removed with cutting of the anterior pillars of the fornix. Immediately after operation the patient did show a long retrograde amnesia with marked loss of motor skills. She was reported as being unable even to use a knife and fork. Recovery of motor habits was rapid over a period of two to three days, but a substantial retrograde amnesia persisted for the two years of the follow-up (Sweet, Talland and Ervin, 1959). This isolated observation needs careful assessment. Damage to this area of the brain is known to produce behavioural changes such as akinetic mutism involving much more than just amnesia. At present there seems no convincing evidence that motor skills form part of the general memory system. An observation which is more firmly established is the remembering of a learned skill, while the circumstances of acquiring it may be engulfed in a retrograde amnesia. This may occur when active memorizing has been restored in both traumatic amnesia and cases of tuberculous meningitis (Russell, 1971; Williams and Smith, 1954). The acquisition of new motor skills has been investigated more fully in some cases of persistent defective memorizing with associated permanent retrograde amnesias. These conditions are provided in Korsakoff's syndrome, but more general intellectual and conative changes also occur. They are also shown in some patients surviving herpes simplex encephalitis, where the main damage is known to be in the temporal lobes, including the hippocampal formation. In one such case where the memory difficulty was unassociated with any general intellectual impairment or loss of alertness, simple finger maze-learning was possible. The skill was shown not only to be registered, but also to be retained for periods of months; this is in contrast to the duration of memory for events which followed the usual pattern of minutes only (Cermak, 1976). Both these observations would support a segregation of the cerebral mechanisms serving registration and recall of past events and those for motor skills.

The loss of memorizing appears to be completely reversible, but for the period of the malfunction there remains a permanent complete memory gap – 'un trou de memoire' as Godlewski (1968) puts it.

The course of the R.A. once the attack has ended is less well charted. There appears to be some recovery in all cases: and in the majority it is substantially complete. However, recorded observations on duration of R.A. are fewer than the plentiful records of the attack itself. This point needs special consideration. It applies to descriptions of amnesic states in general, and to their interpretation. Some of what is here discussed has by intention a wider frame of reference than T.G.A. There is a general difficulty in establishing length and content of R.A. Recent events in a given biography are plentiful and known to numerous witnesses, while more distant happenings are less widely known and tend to be represented by the highlights of public events. What is retained personally however will be influenced by emotional associations. Moreover memories are subject to a continuous process of tidying up and adjustment, dictated largely by the need to establish and maintain personal identity and to mould it nearer to an ideal — a process which by no means ends with the passing of the 'identity crisis' of adolescence. This too adds to the difficulty of objective assessment of R.A. Thus both material examined and methods of doing so differ in the two cases. The evidence for short and long R.A. must therefore be viewed critically. The brief 'legal' details of personal identity cannot be regarded as exclusively older memories since they are almost daily reinforced. The ascription of a retrograde amnesia of some years solely to a mis-statement of age is hardly valid, but the forgetting of a single family event with wide repercussions will have greater evidential value. The renewed interest in normal forgetting as part of the problem of amnesia has certainly shown that the more carefully distant memory is examined, the larger the element of R.A. appears to be (Squire, 1974).

With these provisos, R.A. was specifically mentioned in 40 reported cases (Fisher and Adams, 1964; Godlewski, 1968; Evans, 1966; Martin, 1971). In 30 it was recorded as a transient finding during the attack and varies from years to 12 hours. Only four cases involved more than one year, the majority being of days or weeks. In all of these it rapidly shortened or cleared completely when the attack ceased. However, persisting R.A., rechecked months to years after the event, was noted in 18 cases: most, though including significant items, were incomplete. Durations varied from half an hour to one week, the majority being of one to three hours. In addition to these 40 cases, indirect evidence in a further 28 case histories suggested a transient R.A. varying from one month to one day, with a persisting R.A. varying from 12 hours to one hour in 16.

In general these findings support the view expressed by Fisher and Adams (1964), amongst others, that R.A. is linked to the defect of memorizing. These authors further suggest that there may be a mechanism common to the two. If this is so, then with complete loss of memorizing there should be complete loss of recall. On this point detailed observations made during the attack of R.A. for events known to be accessible to recall before the attack are usually lacking, and we can only say that in some cases, substantial loss of important memories is demonstrated. Moreover, the view fails to account for persisting R.A. when memorizing has returned; though here too the evidence for significant R.A. known not to be present *before* the attack may be difficult to substantiate.

A widely held view that R.A. changes tend to involve more recent rather than more distant memories, also needs critical assessment. It

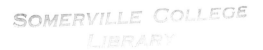

may for instance be an artifact of the greater accessibility to checking of recent memories: and of the converse, that the personal store of distant memories on which R.A. must operate is not likely to be well known to others before an attack. Thus the evidence must rely largely on the patient's personal statement made after the event. Assuming that persistent R.A. *is* of more recent material, one explanation proposed (Ritchie Russell, 1971) is that the hippocampal formation has a persisting activating function which re-enforces memories initially laid down via hippocampal circuits. If loss of memorizing represents loss of hippo-campal function, this will also involve loss of activating in recently acquired memories. On such an hypothesis, the *duration* of T.G.A. would be expected to have no influence on the length of R.A. which would depend solely on the time interval between an event to be remembered and the *onset* of T.G.A. This is, on the whole, supported by the evidence, though it may be noted that in traumatic amnesia, retrograde amnesias do appear linked to the length of post-traumatic amnesia (P.T.A.) – the equivalent in that situation to loss of memorizing, since a permanent memory gap exists for the P.T.A. period. This difficulty Symonds (1966) meets by postulating a time scale of normal decay for a memory, which if completed during a prolonged post-traumatic amnesia, will leave no trace for hippocampal activation to work on when its function is resumed. A major difficulty with this theory also remains the problem of a permanent R.A. for events known to be firmly registered and accessible to recall long before the attack.

Another neurological model for memorizing which has been proposed rather tentatively needs brief consideration.

Goddard, McIntyre and Leech (1969) observed that repeated electrical stimulation of one part of the brain could induce transynaptic changes in other areas, involving behavioural epileptic seizures. This process, referred to as 'kindling' has been extensively studied (Symposium on Kindling, 1975). It can arise from both electrical and chemical stimulation and is particularly readily elicited from the amygdala. The induced changes seem to be relatively permanent.

Goddard and Douglas (1975) has analysed the potential explanatory value of kindling as a model for the engram of memory. The general trend of physiological explanation for memory already assumes that an initial activity induced by perception in one part of the cerebrum results in permanent change in some other area. While it is of interest that kindling is readily fired from the amygdala, its value as an explanation, if it is to be more than tautologous, must lie in the physiological and biochemical changes that it represents. These so far have not been elucidated. Of itself it does not help to explain T.G.A. but it offers a possible mechanism by which the hippocampal formation subserves long-term memorizing.

It appears to have no direct relevance to the associated R.A.; but if kindling, from limbic structures at least, is a more general and possibly spontaneous physiological process than experimental observation yet shows, then its temporary abolition might be expected to interfere with engram reactivation. Further experimental study of the process in primates in which it is known to occur, may contribute to our understanding of the mechanism of transient amnesias.

It has been noted previously that in a number of amnesic states, particularly in alcoholic Korsakoff and other conditions of persisting memorizing defect which allow careful study, some recall of previous experience may be distorted and inaccurate, rather than abolished, but not a part of normal memory for which orientation of events in time is essential. Instances may also be seen in T.G.A. The process of transferring perception to memory includes the addition of a time label to perceptions. Lack of such labelling would account for a memory gap and for such briefly preceding R.A. as required the items of the memory gap to include it in a memory continuum. It could account for a more extensive *associated* R.A. if recall of already labelled material also required the use of the time-labelling mechanism. To account for persisting R.A. when memorizing is resumed, either *some* continuing abnormality of the mechanism must be postulated, or some change in the already established label — hence the importance of precise information about items of prolonged R.A. The analogy of a disordered filing system is obvious, but should not be pressed too far.

Can we assign the function of time-labelling and recall to the hippocampus and related formations of the limbic system which are implicated in amnesic syndromes? The view derives indirect support from the temporal disorientation seen occasionally as a presenting feature in temporal lobe lesions, the *deja arrivé* of some forms of temporal lobe epilepsy and the temporal sequence of induced memories in Penfield's stimulation experiments.

Symonds (1966) concluded his review of memory: 'we shall better understand disorders of memory when we know more about the physiology of time'. T.G.A., as a model of amnesic syndrome in general, deserves further study. In particular, the duration and content of R.A. during attacks, and the time relations of recalled events need detailed records. The nature of the 'mild confusion' so often mentioned also needs clarification. Is this simply a reflection of the memorizing defect or of a more general inability to maintain temporal orientation? Further analysis of time appreciation during the attack could be rewarding.

ADDENDUM

In the clinical field of amnesia, particularly in those problems which are potential material for solution by experimental psychology, definitions common to both disciplines are important. Psychology derives its models largely from the viewpoint of 'normal' memory; and in animal work it has to concentrate on the narrower problem of learning. Clinical studies rely primarily on the obverse — 'abnormal' failure of memory — and are largely restricted to man. In this latter context 'memory' has a meaning both wider and more narrowly defined than that used in experimental psychology. It embraces the retention and voluntary recall of events and experiences in relation, more or less, to an autobiographical time scale. Psychology's models of memory, especially those based on the concept of 'semantic' memory (Quillian, 1968) often have little reference to what is studied experimentally in man and particularly to the content of clinical studies. Tulving (1973) has made this point, and has proposed as a tentative guide in formulating theory, that we recognize two memory systems, 'semantic' and 'episodic'. Of the two, the episodic is more clearly delineated. It deals with information about episodes and events and their temporal and spatial relations in terms of individual experience. It has therefore an autobiographical reference. Reference for the semantic is cognitive. It has an input from perception and from thought; though perceptual input may be needed only to identify an entry and will not be recorded in the semantic system. Since the use of inference, generalization and formulae are considered part of the method of utilizing the semantic system, its validity as a memory system, rather than a congeries of cognitive function, is open to criticism.

Examples from the two systems may help to clarify the approach. 'I have booked my haircut for 12.30 tomorrow' and 'I remember my brother fell and broke his leg two years ago on that icebound road' are both essentially episodic. Whereas 'I know water and oil do not mix' or 'I remember that the circumference of a circle is $2\pi r$' belong to the semantic. It is evident that clinical amnesia is concerned almost wholly with the episodic system. This is true also of much of the material of experimental psychology on remembering and forgetting in man. While associative memory demonstrably contains semantic links in both clinical and experimental material, this does not necessarily place such material in the semantic. It simply illustrates a functional interaction between the two. For neurologists, the definition of a 'not semantic' system has advantages. It can provide a useful frame of reference in interpreting the kind of material they handle. It may also allow us to abandon the rather forced attempt to include aphasia, agnosia, constructional apraxia and loss of motor skills in amnesia. While their inclusion, with the possible exception of agnosia, in the semantic system is partial or dubious, they scarcely belong to the episodic. The functioning of this system is being increasingly assigned a clear cut cerebral substrate, involving parts of the limbic system. Since the known functions of the latter include the experience and expression of emotion, an anatomical background is offered for an association, which is obtrusive in both clinical and normal material, between memory and emotion. Such a link with semantic memory seems less necessary or direct.

4 The Amnesic Syndrome

O. L. Zangwill

In 1887, S. S. Korsakoff published the first of his several papers on the psychical symptoms, in particular, defect of memory, that so frequently accompany alcoholic neuropathy. He did not, however, lay claim to and special priority, observing that '. . . the psychical disorder that interests us here had already been noted a long time ago by M. Huss' (Korsakoff, 1889a). Indeed, his main object was to define what he believed to be a new disease entity ('cerebropathia toxaemia psychica'), having both peripheral and central nervous manifestations. If in this respect Korsakoff proved to be mistaken, the clinical descriptions which he gave of the syndrome which has come to bear his name, have seldom, if ever, been surpassed (*see particularly* Korsakoff, 1889b). Although there has been some dispute regarding the nosology of the syndrome (Angelergues, 1958; Talland, 1965), it is generally accepted today as a relatively well-demarcated psychiatric entity, distinguished from confusional states by clarity of consciousness and intact perception, and from the dementias by the relatively good preservation of intellectual capacity.

Korsakoff's observations aroused considerable interest, particularly in Germany, where comparable cases were soon described. The first to suggest that the psychiatric condition described by Korsakoff is not necessarily linked with peripheral neuritis, appears to have been Tiling (1890, 1892), who pointed out that it is more properly to be regarded as a general reaction of the brain to a wide variety of *noxa* (Körner, 1935).* It is to Bonhoeffer (1901, 1904), however, that our modern

* According to Talland (1965), the term *Korsakoff syndrome* was first used by Jolly (1897), though Barbizet (1964) attributes priority to Chaslin (1895).

conception of the Korsakoff syndrome as an exogenous reaction type is principally due. Bonhoeffer (1901) also gave the syndrome its definitive formulation in terms of the four 'cardinal elements', namely, memory defect for current events (*Merkunfähigkeit*), retrograde amnesia, disorientation and confabulation. Apart from some variation in emphasis (most authors stressing principally the first of these defects but some the last), this formulation has survived virtually without challenge to the present day.

Whereas the defect of memory has always been regarded as central, opinion has been somewhat divided as to the status of the other components of the syndrome, in particular, confabulation. As is well known, confabulation is by no means always in evidence (Williams and Rupp, 1938; Talland, 1961; Victor, 1964), and where it is present, bears no clear-cut relationship to the severity of the memory defect (Weinstein and Kahn, 1955). Further, defects in other spheres of psychological function are commonly in evidence. For example, lack of initiative is almost invariable (Meggendorfer, 1928), and though it may derive in part from the memory defect (intentions being forgotten before they can be acted upon), it probably reflects a more extensive disorganization of volitional activity (Krauss, 1930). A variety of cognitive defects, if relatively minor in comparison with the severity of the memory disorder, have also been disclosed in many cases by careful psychological examination. Thus, speed of perception is often reduced (Gregor and Römer, 1907), and careful study of perceptual activity may reveal appreciable defects in its adequacy and organization (Bürger, 1927; Bürger-Prinz and Kaila, 1930; Lidz, 1942). Perseverative and confabulatory features are not uncommon (Wyke and Warrington, 1960). Thinking, as Korsakoff (1889b) himself appreciated, is facile and stereotyped and confined as a rule to a narrow circle of ideas. A measure of conceptual weakness can also be demonstrated by the use of special tests (Talland, 1965). Although the significance of these relatively inconspicuous defects should not be exaggerated, it is plain that the Korsakoff state represents a relatively complex pattern of psychological deficit, which transcends uncomplicated amnesia.

In the view of the present writer, one of the most important features of the Korsakoff syndrome is the striking deficiency of insight, to which Korsakoff (1889b) himself drew attention. Few Korsakoff patients appreciate that they are ill, and in those that do, the gravity of the illness is invariably minimized. Insight into the memory defect is either lacking, or, at best, very partial, and when attention is drawn to obvious failures of memory, these are explained away by facile rationalization. Not uncommonly, this failure of insight extends to the appreciation of concomitant physical disability, for example, peripheral neuritis. Lack of insight also appears to underlie, and in part to explain, the curious anomalies in reasoning and judgement first described by Pick (1915), which are particularly marked when matters bearing on the patient's own conception of his circumstances (for example, his age or orientation) are discussed. In such cases, the patient may utterly reject evidence at variance with his own beliefs, or attempt to reconcile incompatible propositions in the most facile and implausible manner (Paterson and Zangwill, 1944; Zangwill, 1953). These phenomena have been held to reflect an active attempt on the part of the patient to maintain as consistent an attitude towards himself and his circumstances as his disabilities and attendant lack of insight into them permit; that is, as a defence against 'catastrophic reaction' (Zangwill, 1953).

At the same time, it has long been known that gross defect of memory may, on occasion, present without the more florid manifestations of the Korsakoff syndrome. Unusual cases of so-called 'continuous amnesia' without confabulation were reported many years ago in France (Chaslin and Portocalis, 1908; Mabille and Pitres, 1913), but attracted comparatively little interest at the time. More recently, sporadic attempts have been made, particularly in German psychiatry, to distinguish between the classic Korsakoff syndrome and cases in which memory defect, albeit severe, presents in relative isolation (the 'amnesic syndrome' of Ewald, 1940, and Conrad, 1953a, b). But it is only in the last twenty years, as evidence for the cerebral localization of memory defect has steadily grown stronger, that the importance of this earlier work has come to be appreciated (Milner and Penfield, 1955; Scoville and Milner, 1957; Rose and Symonds, 1960; Russell and Espir, 1961; Victor and his colleagues, 1961; Adams, Collins and Victor, 1962; Whitty, 1962; Dimsdale, Logue and Piercy, 1964; Victor, 1964). Although we shall not be directly concerned with the issue of localization in the present chapter (*see* Chapters 7 and 9), the extreme psychological interest of 'pure' amnesia would seem to justify its separate consideration.

The following case provides an excellent illustration of a well-circumscribed amnesic syndrome in a young adult of good intelligence and personality.

Case 1. A private soldier, aged 24, was admitted to the Brain Injuries Unit, Edinburgh, in 1942, with the complaint of marked and persistent defect of memory for the past two months. This had followed on an attack of meningitis, probably meningococcal, contracted while the patient was stationed in the Shetland Islands. Physical examination revealed paraesthesiae of the left arm and leg, continuously present but not interfering with sleep, and a bilateral right quadrantic homonymous hemianopia. Air encephalography gave evidence of a localized and considerable dilatation of the posterior horn of the left lateral ventricle, without displacement or excess of subarachnoid air.

This was thought to indicate a localized subependymal gliosis, according with the visual pathway lesion and suggesting a lesion of the radiation where it is disposed around the posterior horn of the left lateral ventricle.

The patient was closely studied from the psychological point of view over a period of two months. It was immediately apparent that he retained virtually no memory for events which had taken place since the onset of his illness, apart from one or two 'islands of memory' (for example, a visit from his relatives while in hospital in the Shetlands). These, however, were fragmentary and ill-localized in time. He had also a retrograde amnesia for events which had preceded the onset of the illness of at least several weeks, though its duration could not be established with any precision. The patient had considerable insight into his amnesia and attendant difficulties, and would spontaneously remark that his memory was 'desperate'. He showed no tendency to minimize or deny his handicap and was never observed to confabulate.

While in hospital, the patient was orientated for place but only vaguely orientated for time. He had marked difficulty in keeping track of the days of the week and to a lesser extent, of time of day. He gradually learned the names of members of the staff and of one or two fellow patients, but could hardly ever recall where or when he had last seen a particular individual, even after intervals as brief as five minutes. He reported great difficulty in 'placing' such few recent experiences as he could recall, especially with regard to time or date. He was very slow in learning his way around the hospital and, even after several weeks, the descriptions he gave of places he visited daily (for example, the Occupational Therapy Department) were fragmentary and often grossly inaccurate. He consistently underestimated the passage of time – interviews of up to an hour long being said to have lasted about ten minutes. Only slight improvement in memory was observed over the two months in hospital.

The patient performed well on psychological tests, apart, of course, from those involving recent memory. He achieved a score of 75 (high average) on the Terman Vocabulary, and 41 (above the 25th percentile point for his age group) on the Progressive Matrices. His 'immediate memory span' was eight or nine digits. Connected passages of up to about 25 words could be reproduced verbatim but were thereafter immediately forgotten. He produced an extremely condensed version of the 'Cowboy' story from immediate memory and was unable to reproduce anything of it two minutes later without a prompt. Ten minutes later, it was completely forgotten. On recognition tests, performance was a little better, though nonetheless, grossly impaired. Thus, on one occasion the patient was shown three pictures for ten seconds and then again five minutes later, together with three new pictures. Only one of the original three pictures was said to be familiar. He was, however, often able to recognize drawings that he had done himself, but was quite unable to recall when or where he had done them, even after intervals as short as three minutes.

Learning capacity was grossly impaired. The patient was quite unable to learn a passage of 82 words by heart after innumerable repetitions spread over several days. He also failed to master the exceedingly simple Rey-Davis peg-board test (Zangwill, 1946b). These results were entirely consistent with his poor learning in day to day life.

A Rorschach test gave evidence of mild organic impairment without evidence of psychoneurotic reaction.

Given Sodium Amytal intravenously (7½ gr), the patient became frankly confused and disorientated, believing himself to be still in hospital in the

Shetlands and misidentifying those present accordingly. No improvement of recent memory or shrinkage of retrograde amnesia could be demonstrated (Dr. A. Paterson).

This is a case of remarkably clear-cut and circumscribed defect of memory, indisputably organic in origin, which today would no doubt be related to the evidence of left temporal lobe pathology.

As several authors have pointed out (Scoville and Milner, 1957; Rose and Symonds, 1960), a memory defect of this kind may be extremely persistent and show little improvement over long periods of time. This is well borne out by the following case:

Case 2. A clerk, aged 53, was admitted with the complaint of long-standing difficulty with his memory, dating from an illness thought to have been mumps encephalitis, which he had contracted at the age of eighteen. In spite of his poor memory, the patient had secured employment as a clerk and had managed to retain one post for a number of years. Recently, however, he had experienced great difficulty at work, having held (and lost) ten jobs in the course of the past two years. In every case his dismissal was directly attributable to his defective memory. The patient had also had a number of 'blackouts' over the past six years, which were not, however, nearly as great a source of distress to him as his memory defect.

Neurological examination was negative. Electroencephalography gave evidence of a focus of slow waves in the left anterior temporal region, probably on the medial surface of the left temporal lobe.

On psychological examination, the patient had an IQ of 140 on the Wechsler-Bellevue Full Scale. His memory, on the other hand, was evidently much impaired. Although orientated in all spheres and able to recall his recent activities in broad outline, he could give no detail even of happenings earlier on in the same day. He stated that he relied heavily on his notebook, always entering his engagements and jobs that he had been instructed to perform. His knowledge of recent news events was very poor but he did not confabulate. His insight into his limitations of memory was remarkably adequate.

This patient could repeat nine digits forwards and gave the gist of the 'Cowboy' story fairly adequately from immediate memory. But he could reproduce nothing of the story a quarter of an hour later without a number of prompts. Visual test material was reproduced no better than verbal. Verbal learning was very slow and incomplete, and the patient failed to master the Rey-Davis peg-board test in spite of a large number of trials.

The patient was seen on three further occasions at yearly intervals. No significant change in the nature or severity of his memory defect could be ascertained.

These cases show clearly that gross defect of recent memory can co-exist with remarkably good preservation of general intellectual capacity. They also suggest that memory defect, in itself identical with that displayed in the Korsakoff syndrome, can present in the absence of disorientation, confabulation, disorders of judgement or denial of disability. For purposes of comparison, a very typical case of

Wernicke's encephalopathy with an alcoholic Korsakoff syndrome may be briefly described:

Case 3. A publican, aged 60, was admitted with a history of excessive alcoholic consumption for many years. Three months previously, he had had two major epileptic fits in one day, and in the past few weeks had become progressively more unsteady on his feet. His wife had noted some slurring of speech. One month previously he developed diplopia, which had, however, cleared by the time of his admission. His memory had deteriorated progressively and there had been episodes of confusion, disorientation and confabulation.

On admission, the patient was amnesic, disorientated and confabulatory. There was marked peripheral neuropathy and ataxia.

The patient was seen repeatedly in the Psychological Department, over a period of seven weeks. On the Wechsler-Bellevue Full Scale, he achieved an IQ of 105, without undue scatter or other evidence of appreciable recent deterioration. Weigl's Sorting Test, which calls for some measure of conceptual grasp and flexibility, was executed satisfactorily. On the other hand, the patient failed to learn the Babcock sentence or sequences of nine or ten digits in spite of innumerable trials. He was also unable to reproduce the gist of the 'Cowboy' story from immediate memory, but with the aid of prompts recalled one or two points, which he linked in a confabulatory way. When the story was repeated five minutes later, the patient denied that he had heard this particular story before, but thought he had heard a similar one. He gave a similar response on recognition tests with objects or pictures, thus exhibiting well-marked reduplicative paramnesia (Zangwill, 1941).

At first, the patient was completely disorientated, believing himself to be in a hospital in the vicinity of his own home. He gave the month (July) as January, the year (1963) as 1956, and his own age (60) as 52. He gave his present home address as one from which he had in fact moved five years previously, and when asked about his recent doings, described activities appropriate to a newsagent, though he had in fact sold up his newspaper business at about the time he moved to his present address. He betrayed no knowledge of his life as a licensed victualler, and completely denied his second marriage, which had taken place two years earlier. (Nonetheless, he recognized his present wife and accepted her as such when she visited him in hospital.) Although aware that he was in hospital (which he rationalized in a facile manner), the patient blandly denied that he was ill or that his memory was in any way affected.

There was little change in this patient's psychological state during the ensuing weeks. He continued to show dense retrograde amnesia for the four to five years prior to the onset of his illness, and appeared to retain practically nothing of his current experiences, whether tested by recall or recognition. Nonetheless, some degree of retention, at a quasi-automatic level, could be demonstrated. For example, while claiming not to recognize his examiners from day to day, the patient did not appear to react to them as total strangers. Again, although he denied that he knew the name of the hospital, he could select it correctly from a list containing the names of several hospitals, justifying his choice in an *ad hoc* manner. At this time, too, he showed a tendency to reduplication, stating that he had previously been in a hospital similar to the present one, though smaller and in the vicinity of his own home. Appreciation of his memory loss remained virtually non-existent.

Although this patient's defect of recent memory was little, if at all, more severe than in Case 1, the impression given is quite different. This patient was disorientated, confabulatory, totally lacking in insight and prone to reduplicative falsification. His disability clearly involved not only his memory, but his entire appreciation of his circumstances and his own relation to them. This is not an uncomplicated amnesic syndrome but the classic picture of Korsakoff's psychosis.

DISCUSSION

The exceptional 'purity' of the memory defect in Cases 1 and 2, as in others described in the literature, may well give rise to the suspicion — especially among psychiatrists — that its origin was not wholly organic. So far as our own two cases are concerned, this suspicion may be confidently allayed. In Case 1, an hysterical complication was considered very carefully at the time, but rejected on the following grounds. First, the pattern of memory defect, as exhibited both clinically and on psychological tests, accorded in all particulars with the organic type. Secondly, no change in the amnesia could be induced under barbiturate hypnosis; indeed, the patient became even more confused and disorientated. And thirdly, no evidence of hysterical personality or of motivation to maintain the disability was forthcoming on repeated psychiatric investigation. Although psychiatric inquiry was less exhaustive in Case 2, nothing whatsoever came to light to suggest a psychogenic element; in particular, no consideration of compensation or secondary gain could possibly have applied in a case such as this.

Very similar considerations arise in the four cases of severe and persisting memory defect following encephalitis, reported by Rose and Symonds (1960), three of which were seen by the present writer. Although one of their patients (Rose and Symonds, 1960, Case 1) is reported to have given indication of hysterical personality, the fact that intravenous amytal sedation led to no improvement in memory — indeed the difficulties became rather worse — was thought sufficient to exclude this as a significant factor. This patient certainly did not impress the present writer as in any sense hysterical, and the pattern of memory defect as displayed on psychological tests was wholly consistent with an organic substructure. Indeed, in cases such as these, it is almost impossible to believe that any part of the amnesia could have arisen on a psychogenic basis.

At the same time, it cannot be denied that an hysterical element has been implicated in certain cases of amnesia originally deemed to be wholly organic, as in the celebrated case of Grünthal and Störring (1930a, b); and conversely, that organic brain disease has subsequently been ascertained in certain cases of amnesia originally diagnosed as functional, as in the case of partially arrested G.P.I. (general paralysis of the insane) with severe superadded hysterical manifestations, reported by Lewis (1953). In the Grünthal–Störring case, a memory defect of unparalleled 'purity' supervened upon an episode of coal gas poisoning, not apparently of undue severity. When first seen in Reichardt's clinic at Würzburg a few months later, this patient was said to have presented a complete abolition of memory retention, his span of 'immediate memory' being apparently reduced to a second or two (*Sekundengedächtnis*), as was subsequently ascertained by extremely thorough clinical and psychological examination (Grünthal and Störring, 1930a, b,; Störring, 1931, 1936). The gross defect of recent memory has apparently persisted ever since.

In their original reports on this case, Grünthal and Störring had no doubt whatsoever that the basis of the memory disorder was wholly organic, a diagnosis with which Bumke (1931) and Kleist (1934) concurred, though the former was later to express certain reservations (Bumke, 1947). Doubts were also expressed, if tentatively, by Ewald (1930) and Syz (1937). Yet more recent investigation of the case, initiated by Scheller (1950, 1956) and carried further by Völkel and Stolze (1956), together with the careful critical studies of Lotmar (1954, 1958), have left little doubt that the amnesic state, whatever its original nature, has been maintained for many years on an hysterical basis. Indeed, this interpretation has now been accepted by the original authors themselves (Grünthal and Störring, 1950, 1956), at all events, in relation to the later stages of the illness. But they still maintain, in opposition to Lotmar (1954, 1958), that at the time of their original investigations this amazing disorder of memory was wholly organic.

Although it is always easy to be wise after the event, one may agree with Lotmar (1958) that even the early reports of the Grünthal–Störring case contain a number of features difficult to reconcile with the diagnosis of organic amnesia. In the first place, the initial period of hospitalization (one week) was surprisingly short, and the gross memory defect does not appear to have attracted the notice of the physicians at that time in charge of the case. In the second place, retrograde amnesia was limited to an hour only, which, bearing in mind the great severity of the retention defect for current events, must be regarded as exceptionally brief. In the third place, disorientation for both time and place was suspiciously fixed. And in the fourth place, there was the severe restriction of immediate memory, the patient being unable to reproduce more than a single digit from immediate memory, or to grasp the gist of a question or instruction unless it was repeated to him rapidly a number of times. A comparable reduction of memory span has not been seen in any other case of amnesic syndrome known to the writer, either from his own experience of from the literature. It may also be noted that an EEG examination conducted by Berger himself was reported as normal

(Berger, 1936), and that air-encephalography disclosed no abnormality (Störring, 1936). Although by no means conclusive from the standpoint of differential diagnosis, these negative findings might well cause a neurological eyebrow to be raised.

This case has been fully reviewed elsewhere by the present writer (Zangwill, 1967). In his opinion a strong case could be made out for regarding the amnesia in the Grünthal—Störring case as functional, if not from the outset, at all events from a relatively early stage. At the same time, no really convincing explanation for this prolonged and disabling illness has so far been adduced. The compensation issue was given much weight by Lotmar (1954) and is also regarded by Scheller (personal communication, 1957) as an important factor in perpetuation of the disability. If so, however, the loss would appear greatly to have outweighed the gain. Nor does the attempt by Völkel and Stolze (1956) to unearth deeper psychological motives for the amnesia appear altogether convincing. Rather than speculate upon an improbable psychogenesis, it might be more profitable to view the syndrome as a pseudodemential reaction secondary to mild brain damage, and no doubt maintained by various social pressures, to which both compensation and the attitude of the patient's wife contributed in no small measure. The relations between organic and functional amnesias, which may well be more complex than is often supposed (Lewis, 1953, 1961), are discussed more authoritatively elsewhere in this volume (*see* Chapter 11).

Let us now return to the circumscribed — and genuinely organic — amnesias described above, and consider their relation to the fully-fledged Korsakoff syndrome. As we have suggested, it is hardly possible to ascribe symptoms such as confabulation, disorientation and failure to reconcile conflicting propositions simply to the presence of memory defect. This is well borne out by the two cases we have described, in which, despite very appreciable memory defect, there was no confabulation and a measure of orientation remained possible. It is likewise apparent that in the four cases of severe postencephalitic amnesia reported by Rose and Symonds (1960), the picture was not strictly that of the Korsakoff syndrome. In the most severely affected of their patients (Rose and Symonds, 1960, Case 2), who was seen on several occasions by the present writer, the patient exhibited virtually complete loss of memory-retention, being quite unable to remember anything of his current experiences after the lapse of a few minutes. Yet this patient appreciated his memory defect, did not confabulate, and though unable to keep track of his whereabouts, seldom, if ever, positively misidentified his environment. His deficit was a surprisingly specific one, to which he reacted not without a certain dignity.

It might be thought that the level of intelligence plays some part in determining whether an amnesic state will evolve into a fully-fledged Korsakoff syndrome. Certainly our first two patients were a good deal more intelligent than the third, and had sustained little in the way of general intellectual deterioration. On the other hand, typical Korsakoff syndromes with florid confabulation have been described in many patients of good intelligence and education who still perform above the average on the standard intelligence tests. Further, the four patients described by Rose and Symonds (1960), who differed markedly in intelligence, showed much the same kind of memory disorder. While intelligence may well play some part in governing reaction to memory deficit, it would seem that other and more extensive psychological dysfunction must co-exist with amnesia for the classic picture of Korsakoff's syndrome to emerge.

What is the nature of this additional dysfunction? Weinstein and Kahn (1955) drew attention to a characteristic psychopathological reaction in patients with acute lesions in the region of the third and lateral ventricles, the diencephalon and the midbrain, as well as in some patients with rapidly growing neoplasms in various parts of the forebrain. This reaction, the so-called 'denial of illness' syndrome, is marked by unawareness or denial of disability (anosognosia), disorientation and confabulation, and may also display elements of reduplication and paraphasia. These features have been more fully considered by the authors in separate publications (Weinstein and Kahn, 1950, 1951, 1952, 1953; Weinstein, Kahn and Sugarman, 1952). Although gross memory defect was obviously present in the majority of their cases, the authors claim that the 'denial' syndrome bears no direct relation to the severity of the amnesia and may, on occasion, present when the latter is relatively mild. In their view, 'denial of illness' is to be regarded as a general form of reaction to acute cerebral dysfunction and as in no sense peculiar to the amnesic state.

While the present writer would not necessarily wish to derive features such as confabulation, disorientation or paraphasia exclusively from the element of anosognosia, he finds it plausible to regard the more florid features of the Korsakoff syndrome as due to the association of an amnesic syndrome with a more generalized psychopathological reaction of the kind described by Weinstein and Kahn (1955). Lack of insight, often amounting to outright denial of disability, is extremely common in the Korsakoff syndrome and is not, as we have seen, intrinsic to the amnesic state. Disorientation, too, is almost constant, and reduplication, when looked for, far from rare. Confabulation is notorious and even paraphasia, though relatively uncommon in Korsakoff states, is by no means unknown (Clarke, Wyke and Zangwill, 1958). It is these features which, when conjoined with memory defect, endow the Korsakoff syndrome with its characteristic complexion.

This interpretation of the Korsakoff syndrome finds some support from neuroanatomical considerations. While it might appear that 'pure' amnesic syndromes owe their origin to lesions involving the hippocampal region (Scoville and Milner, 1957; Victor and his colleagues, 1961; *see also* Chapter 7), the Korsakoff syndrome commonly involves more widespread brain damage, in particular to the subcortical structures implicated by Weinstein and Kahn (1955) in the origin of the 'denial' syndrome (*see* Chapter 9). Ultimately, therefore, the special features of the Korsakoff syndrome may well turn out to depend on the nature and localization of the underlying pathology.

POSTSCRIPT

This short account of the amnesic syndrome originally appeared as a chapter in *Amnesia* (1966), edited by C. W. M. Whitty and O. L. Zangwill. In the past ten years, a number of books and papers have been published which throw further light on its clinical and neuropathological aspects (Benson and Geschwind, 1967; Milner, Corkin and Teuber, 1968; Teuber, Milner and Vaughan, 1968; Adams, 1969; Brion, 1969; Delay and Brion, 1969; Victor, Adams and Collins, 1971; Kohn and Crosby, 1972; Jarho, 1973; Barbizet, 1970; McEntee, Biber, Perl and Benson, 1976). Although inevitably selective, the following short appendix directs attention to some more recent contributions of particular clinical and psychological interest.

A famous case of severe amnesic syndrome following bilateral temporal lobectomy (Scoville and Milner, 1957) has been followed up 14 years after surgery by Milner, Corkin and Teuber (1968). It was found that this patient (known as H.M.), showed little change in the severity of his recent memory defect but was none the less able to acquire simple motor skills, if relatively slowly. He was quite unable, however, to recall when or where he had learned these skills (*see* Corkin (1965b), for details of procedure). In the same way, a degree of perceptual learning could also be demonstrated, using the method of 'partial information' described by Warrington and Weiskrantz (1968). (*See also* Warrington, 1971). More recently, the capacity to acquire novel motor skills in spite of severe recent memory defect has been studied by Starr and Phillips (1970) in a case of postencephalitic amnesic syndrome. This patient successfully learned to play a hitherto unfamiliar melody on the piano though, as with H.M., having no recollection whatsoever of having learned it on the previous day. These findings are of special interest in view of the early observations of Claparède (1911) and MacCurdy (1928) that even severe cases of Korsakoff psychosis may on occasion learn to recognize or recall persons or places in spite of gross amnesia and disorientation. (This phenomenon is also shown in Case 3 above.) As Milner, Corkin and Teuber (1968) point out with reference to H.M., however, this emphasis on residual learning capacities should not detract from the gravity of the patient's amnesic state, or minimize the extent to which he is handicapped in daily life.

Korsakoff-like amnesic states following penetrating brain injury have been described by Teuber, Milner and Vaughan (1968), and by Jarho (1973). Teuber, Milner and Vaughan (1968) communicate a single case of severe and persistent anterograde amnesia following a stab wound involving principally the rostral midbrain. This patient improved to some extent but remained severely disabled from the standpoint of memory. In a follow-up of Finnish war veterans, Jarho (1973) describes an amnesic syndrome in seven cases, in six of which there was evidence of a bilateral diencephalic lesion and in the seventh evidence of bilateral involvement of the medial portions of the temporal lobes. This study is considered in greater detail in Chapter 5. Jarho (1973) comments on the paucity of confabulation in these cases and on the frequency of denial of disability, at all events in the early stages. On the other hand, in spite of persistence of amnesia some insight was commonly regained.

Extensive and persistent retrograde amnesia has long been described as a characteristic feature of the Korsakoff syndrome (Bonhoeffer, 1901). It may also occur, if transitorily, in the course of recovery from severe head injury (Symonds, 1960). Benson and Geschwind (1967) have studied the 'shrinkage' of retrograde amnesia in a case of post-traumatic encephalopathy and have stressed its association with denial of illness (Weinstein and Kahn, 1955). They suggest that a patient with 'shrinking amnesia' represents a transitional form between those with chronic defect of recent memory and prolonged retrograde amnesia (as in the classic Korsakoff syndrome) and those with the much more common type of brief permanent retrograde amnesia after recovery from concussional head injuries. In this patient (as in Case 1 above), certain features of the acute amnesic state, viz. disorientation and denial of illness, were caused to reappear in the course of an amytal interview shortly before the patient's discharge.

In the course of retrogressive amnesia in patients with progressive diffuse cerebral disease and in the restitution of memory ('shrinkage' of amnesia) in recovery from severe head injury, it has traditionally been supposed that memories more remote in time from the onset of the illness are lost later (or recovered earlier) than those which are more recent. This is Ribot's so-called 'law of regression' which is usually stated in the form that the resistance of any given engram (or memory trace) to dissolution consequent upon cerebral injury or disease varies inversely with its age (Ribot, 1882). Although, as has been pointed out elsewhere (Zangwill, 1961), this law admits of many exceptions, it is commonly accepted by clinicians as a reliable guide to the scope or duration of retrograde amnesia and, in traumatic cases, as an index of the severity of head injury (Russell, 1971).

In the last few years attempts have been made to test the validity of Ribot's law, using questionnaire methods and recognition tests to assess memory for events which had occurred in the preceding decades of the patient's life. Inevitably, these methods are somewhat crude and can have relevance only to public events which can be assumed to have been generally known at the time of their occurrence. Using a questionnaire method to test for recall of public events and a recognition test of photographs of faces of formerly well-known public figures, Sanders and Warrington (1971) report that in both normal and amnesic subjects memory for relatively remote events is no better than for those relatively more recent. This they consider to cast doubt on Ribot's assumption that memory traces undergo progressive consolidation as a function of time. Seltzer and Benson (1974), on the other hand, using a somewhat similar questionnaire method, obtained results much more closely in line with traditional expectations: every Korsakoff patient showed a better score on his more remote memories (*see also* Marslen-Wilson and Teuber, 1975). It would seem desirable to extend these inquiries to the study of personal as well as impersonal memory and to supplement questionnaire methods by carefully designed clinical inquiry.

In conclusion, the distinction drawn in this chapter between 'pure' cases of amnesic syndrome and the classical Korsakoff picture has continued to attract some interest (Liebaldt and Scheller, 1971; Jarho, 1973). It remains, however, somewhat controversial. Jarho's work might suggest that localization of the lesion is not necessarily the critical factor, for although his patients with amnesic states associated with diencephalic lesions did not confabulate, some degree of insight was commonly regained. At the same time, his work confirms the link suggested in this chapter between lack of insight into memory defect on the one hand and disorientation and denial of illness on the other. It is hoped that further studies of amnesic states associated with diencephalic and bitemporal lesions, respectively, will clarify this issue.

Acknowledgements

I am greatly indebted to the late Professor Norman M. Dott, formerly Director of the Brain Injuries Unit, Edinburgh, for his kindness in granting me access to the notes of Case 1 and for permission to publish this report. Cases 2 and 3 were studied at the National Hospital, Queen Square, London, and are communicated by kind permission of Dr. J. Purdon Martin and Dr Denis Williams, respectively.

5 Traumatic Amnesia

C.W.M. Whitty and O.L. Zangwill

Apart from the hazards of transferring animal work to man, the experimental study of amnesia, which has rightly been increasingly attempted in the past few years, contends with two obstacles. Many amnesic states are transitory and this applies especially to those which may be regarded as most purely amnesic and unaccompanied by more general mental changes such as confusion, inattention and lack of initiative. Opportunity for planned experiment is therefore limited. Moreover those facets of memory which are most readily measured may be only partially relevant to 'clinical' amnesia. Tests may define defects of memory which may include both more and less than what is understood as amnesia. Many much used tests include elements of attention, logical analysis, recognition, general orientation, rote learning and assumptions of previous stored information which may not be an intrinsic part of amnesia, either as loss of active memorizing or as persisting memory gap. The difficulty, though mitigated by segregating immediate, short-term and long-term memory, remains. Both obstacles occur in the interpretation of traumatic amnesia. Nevertheless some useful attempts by appropriate special tests are now being made to analyse the content of traumatic amnesia while it is present, and to recognize residual long-term defects.

Some of the commonest amnesias met with in clinical practice are those associated with head injuries; and with the increase in traffic accidents they are becoming more frequent. When an individual is knocked out by a blow on the head, as consciousness recovers there may be a period of confusion before apparent normal response and behaviour are established. On subsequent investigation, however, it may be found that there is a post-traumatic amnesia (P.T.A.), not only for the period of unconsciousness and confusion, but also for a time when behaviour was regarded by onlookers as entirely normal. With any severe injury, there is also usually a short period before the injury for which memory is lost – the so-called retrograde amnesia (R.A.). These amnesias are interesting, both because of their variable form and content and also because their time of onset can usually be accurately gauged and their duration measured. R.A.'s in particular present interesting problems for any theory of the cerebral mechanism of memory, because they may include periods for which memory was known to be functioning normally – registration, retention and often recall of experiences all having actually occurred – during a period subsequently covered by a complete amnesia.

ASSESSMENT OF LENGTH OF AMNESIAS

In assessing traumatic amnesia, it is usual to measure the P.T.A. as a period between the injury and the subsequent resumption of normal continuous memory. This will, of course, include any period of unconsciousness and possibly of confusion. The circumstances of a head injury will often allow this to be measured accurately. However, it can only be assessed adequately after any confusion or disorientation has fully cleared. Indeed, it is always best to reassess amnesia a little time after apparent full recovery, as the patient's responses, even to questions involving short-term memory, may at the time appear quite normal, during a period subsequently found to be included in the amnesia. This is a not uncommon source of error in underestimating P.T.A. The patient is asked shortly after injury whether he remembers some occurrence in hospital, such as a visit to the x-ray department or the dressing of a wound, and may seem to recall this at the time. Normal memory is therefore regarded as re-established at this point. Subsequently, it may be found that the patient is quite unable to recall the whole period, including the questions and the answers he correctly gave. Periods of normal sleep and of impaired consciousness due to drugs, may, on the other hand, lead to a false overestimate. Fortunately, the routine of hospital life usually allows an accurate final check on the resumption of normal continuous memory.

This assessment is important because there is much evidence to suggest that the true length of the P.T.A. bears a direct relationship to the severity of brain injury inflicted. Thus, length of P.T.A. correlates with severity and persistence of neurological signs and symptoms, and with subsequent working capacity. This was well illustrated in a series of cases of closed head injuries in military personnel during World War II, reported by Russell and Nathan (1946). Brooks (1976) has also studied this point in a series of 82 patients all of whom had a P.T.A. of at least two and many of over 28 days, thus constituting a group of severe head injuries. All showed persisting defects of memory compared with a control group. He used as his measure the Wechsler memory scale (which probably includes more than just memory changes) and found that defects were linked to length of P.T.A. and increasing age, but noted no correlation with persisting focal neurological signs, including dysphasia, or with the presence of skull fracture, sometimes regarded as a measure of severity of brain damage. Both length of time off duty and loss of efficiency on return to duty were clearly related to the length of P.T.A. Indeed, this measure can be accepted as the single most useful guide to the severity of the underlying brain injury.

There is however some evidence (Fodor, 1972) to suggest that when cognitive deficits, other than memory, are shown on formal testing in the acute phase of head injury, these correlated with severity of injury as judged by neurological signs and symptoms more closely than did memory function. A difficulty in interpreting this type of evidence is the inevitably rather restricted nature of the memory tests which may bear little relation to what is measured by P.T.A. Moreover while general intelligence tests such as Wechsler Adult Intelligence Scales (W.A.I.S.) given to patients during their period of P.T.A. show results significantly lower than in a matched group tested after recovery from P.T.A., retesting the same patients after their period of P.T.A. has ended shows improvement in scores to the level of control group (Mandleberg and Brooks, 1975). There is therefore no convincing evidence to invalidate length of P.T.A. as a main prognostic guide to severity of brain injury.

The R.A. is taken as the time between the injury and the last clear memory that the patient recalls before this. There are pitfalls in assessing this also. In the circumstances of some head injuries, preceding events may be so routine as hardly to require notice or remembering. Thus, the scenes of a familiar car journey undertaken daily may be difficult to recall as a particular occasion, even without the intervention of a head injury. This may lead to a false lengthening of R.A. when no special event precedes the accident, or possibly to a false shortening if details recalled are those of the often repeated journey in general, rather than the particular one in which the injury occurred. Careful questioning and checking with those who witnessed the injury will usually overcome this difficulty. An assessment shortly after the injury may be quite misleading. R.A. seems to be especially influenced by even mild degrees of confusion, and a shrinkage of R.A. during the days following injury is not uncommon, even during a period which is subsequently part of the final P.T.A. Final estimates should be made when P.T.A. is stabilized and when there is clinical evidence of maximal recovery of cerebral function. The importance of actual assessment of all forms of traumatic amnesia cannot be too much stressed. Not only do they provide a valuable indication of the seriousness of injury and possible prognosis for the individual patient, but they also supply facts for the interpretation of memory mechanisms and, unless these facts are accurate, the interpretation is valueless. Thus, as with P.T.A., the R.A. must be assessed only when the patient has recovered fully from any clouding of consciousness.

R.A.'s are, in general, much shorter than P.T.A.'s; indeed, the great majority of the former are only of a few seconds' duration. There is some relation between length of P.T.A. and R.A. R.A.'s of more than a few minutes are rare when the P.T.A. is less than 24 hours; and it is only when P.T.A. is running into days or weeks that R.A.'s of over half an hour are likely to occur. This relationship is also well shown in Russell and Nathan's figures. It too is presumably related to the severity of the underlying brain injury.

A further factor which has to be allowed for is a possible psychogenic prolongation of either of these amnesias. The circumstances of head injury often include medicolegal considerations of compensation. Loss of memory and loss of personal identity are to the layman commonly associated — often in a rather dramatic manner — with head injuries. Since a long amnesia may imply more severe disability, both hysterical mechanisms and frank malingering may prolong the patient's own assessment of his loss of memory. Careful questioning may reveal inconsistencies in the story which suggest a false amnesia. Sometimes also, an apparent amnesia may be reduced or abolished in the drowsy and uninhibited state produced by light barbiturate narcosis. The technique used is similar to that of 'narcoanalysis'. The patient is given a slow and carefully graded intravenous injection of some anaesthetic such as Pentothal. As a state of drowsy euphoria is induced, the period of apparent amnesia is re-examined. Events and experiences thus recalled may thereafter be permanently remembered. The value of this procedure in recovering an hysterical or malingered amnesia is not as great as was thought when it was first employed two or three decades ago, both because such amnesias are not necessarily recovered in this way, and because some genuinely organic block to memory may possibly be overcome in the twilight state. Thus, Russell and Nathan (1946) found a reduction of amnesia in the R.A. or P.T.A. in only 12 out of 40 cases investigated, and the reduction was trivial in amount and did not appear to include any items likely to have been hysterically repressed. Provided that a detailed examination is made, with the fullest possible information already available to the examiner of the events and experiences supposedly included in the amnesia, narco-analysis is unlikely to give more information than can be obtained in the normal waking state. Psychogenic prolongation, unrevealed by such a careful waking examination, must be regarded as a rare cause of error in assessing organic traumatic amnesias.

P.T.A.'s may vary from minutes to days or even weeks. In injuries which have not inflicted gross brain damage, P.T.A.'s of a few minutes or a few hours are usual. When they extend to more than 24 hours there are usually evidences, in prolonged periods of complete uncon-sciousness and in focal neurological signs, of more severe brain damage. Very rarely, they occupy periods of weeks and, in such cases, coma and stupor and gross neurological deficits with local evidence of brain damage are all prominent. In such cases, permanent neurological deficits, including intellectual loss and personality change, are the rule. Without such supporting evidence, very prolonged amnesias are unlikely to be genuine.

In any injury which causes complete loss of consciousness an R.A. of a few seconds almost always occurs. Longer R.A.'s are related to other evidences of severe brain injury, including long P.T.A.'s. R.A.'s of more than a few minutes are rare with P.T.A.'s of less than 24 hours; while R.A.'s of more than an hour are almost always associated with P.T.A.'s of several days. As has been said, the majority of R.A.'s are of seconds only.

Case 1. A man of 32 suffered a severe head injury and multiple limb and trunk injuries in a road accident. He was comatose and completely unresponsive for some two weeks, requiring intravenous nourishment and assisted respiration for part of this time. The final assessment of his P.T.A. made three months later, was some three weeks. When his R.A. was first assessed at this time, he could recall nothing for about six months before his injury. During the next few weeks, his R.A. contracted to about 48 hours. However, even this R.A. was patchy and there was a complete and dense R.A. of only about two hours.

When examined again 18 months after the injury, he had a slight left hemiparesis with sensory loss. He was euphoric and inconsequential in con-versation and could not maintain the thread of his talk for more than a few minutes. He was liable to sudden inappropriate outbursts of anger, laughter or tears. Intellectually he was mildly demented, and quite unable to continue his previous work as a theological student. His friends and relatives regarded him as an entirely changed person. He was considered to have both a traumatic intellectual impairment and personality change. His P.T.A. and R.A. at this time remained unchanged from the earlier assessment.

This case illustrates the result of a very severe brain injury. The following is a much milder and more usual example.

Case 2. A boy of 18 was involved in a motor cycle accident. A right frontal laceration required stitching, but there were no other physical injuries. He was completely unconscious for about 20 minutes and thereafter appeared aware of his environment and gave his personal details correctly. However, an assessment of amnesia some ten days later showed that he had an R.A. of about 30 seconds and a P.T.A. of one to two hours.

VARIETIES OF P.T.A.

P.T.A.'s usually follow immediately on the head injury and its more obvious neurological consequences. They commonly end quite sharply with the return of continuous memory, often after a period of natural sleep. Continuous memory may, however, be resumed with some relative highlight of experience – the visit of some near relative to hospital, some unusual ward happening or some unpleasant personal experience, such as the painful dressing of a wound. Sometimes these experiences are retained in isolation as islands of memory before continuous memory is resumed. Their isolation from the temporal sequence of events gives them a confused unreal quality, though they may be vividly recalled.

> *Case 3.* A man of 22 was injured in a motor cycle accident. He suffered a scalp laceration and fractured a right tibia and fibula. He was unconscious for half an hour. On coming round, he appeared aware of his surroundings and answered questions correctly. However, when assessment of his amnesia was made a week later, his R.A. was momentary but he could only recall one incident during the first two days after injury. He had a vivid impression of his mother's face looking down on him and asking him what had happened to his clothes. This was corroborated as a true but isolated memory, occurring in the first 24 posttraumatic hours. Normal continuous memory was resumed after some 48 hours.

Occasionally the P.T.A. is delayed, usually by only a few moments. Some brief experience after the injury is recalled, often in unreal isolation, and sometimes in an inaccurate and confused way; thereafter, a dense amnesia ensues until memory is resumed at the end of the P.T.A. This delayed P.T.A. is uncommon and tends to occur in the more severe injuries.

> *Case 4.* A boy of 18 skidded in a car and hit a telegraph pole. He suffered scalp and facial lacerations, a fractured skull and broken leg. He recalled clearly switching off the engine and forcing open a jammed car door, both of which were subsequently corroborated. Thereafter, he could recall nothing until he came round in hospital some 48 hours later.

Sometimes the content of this immediate post-traumatic retained memory is a highly emotionally tinged experience. Russell and Nathan (1946) record an incidence in which a motor cyclist's machine caught fire, and he recalled trying to put it out before he became amnesic. It is possible that in such cases, the environmental stimulus may be so great that memory and attention are momentarily reinforced, perhaps by the spread of afferent impulses to pathways not normally used. However, in such cases, and in others where vivid perceptions or other unusually strong afferent impulses cannot be invoked, the neurological mechanism of the P.T.A. must initially differ from that usually occurring in immediate association with a complete concussion.

A somewhat different form of delayed amnesia is that seen following trauma which causes epidural haemorrhage. Here, following a head injury which involves a rupture of the middle meningeal artery, the patient has a brief period of concussion from which full recovery seems to occur, and he may then appear entirely lucid for a period of minutes or even hours. Then consciousness is again rapidly lost, and unless operation is immediately undertaken to stop the haemorrhage and evacuate the epidural clot, death from cerebral compression ensues. When recovery occurs following successful operation, the experiences of the lucid interval may be accurately recalled, or they may be hazy and confused. Sometimes they appear to be involved in an amnesia which may be considered as either a delayed post-traumatic result of the initial injury, or a retrograde effect of the injury from secondary cerebral compression. The latter seems more likely. Here the neurological mechanism involved is clearly different from that of simple concussion, and there is evidence that a compression of the brain stem is the effective agent.

PARAMNESIA AND CONFABULATION

During a period of P.T.A. the circumstances surrounding the injury may lead to false reminiscence. Details of a previous injury may be accurately given with reference to the current injury. If the general setting of the earlier occurrence is similar to the current one, it may be difficult to detect the error, and the patient will erroneously be thought to have recovered from his P.T.A. Discrepancies may, however, be found between the known circumstances and the patient's account, and if the interval between the two injuries is long, inaccuracies in dates and personal age may give clues. This type of paramnesia probably involves a substantial disorientation in time. However, the period during which it operates, and in which the patient is giving apparently accurate and coherent replies to questions involving memory, may subsequently become part of a dense and persistent P.T.A. It must, therefore, involve something more than simple temporal disorientation.

Case 5. A despatch rider of 22 was concussed in a motor cycle accident. Following a period of complete unconsciousness, he was confused and drowsy for two to three days, and after treatment at a local hospital was transferred ten days later to a special head injury unit. When seen at that time he gave details of his accident, including its locale and the incidents leading up to it, and an account of his journey from the first hospital. He gave his name and army number correctly, but persistently have his age wrongly. At clinical examination he appeared to be rational and fully orientated. It finally transpired, however, that he was giving details of an accident he had had before joining the army some two years previously, and that the description of his journey to the second hospital was also a false reminiscence. It is interesting that he gave his age correctly for the earlier accident, yet also gave his unit and army number, which he did not possess at the time. His final P.T.A. was assessed as 12 days. It involved the period of time of false reminiscence and the first two days of his stay in the second hospital.

Such discrepancies as this are common in this type of paramnesia. When taxed with them the patient may sometimes flatly deny them, or may give some superficial and implausible explanation. Such cases may be regarded as showing limited confabulation, in the sense that loss of the normal environment of a given incident of memory may cause it to be presented as a confabulatory experience or pseudo-reminiscence. Sometimes, however, a florid confabulatory syndrome may occur during the course of a P.T.A. In some instances there is little in the way of general abnormality of behaviour, and their social reactions in the limited environment of a hospital ward may be largely normal. There is often an unresolved conflict between their general behaviour, which is appropriate to a patient in hospital, and their response to questions, responses which suggest that they are not in hospital and that any physical disability of which there is evidence is not due to the injury or accident which is known to have occurred. In this setting, the explanatory confabulation may often be profuse, versatile and amusing. Such traumatic Korsakoff syndromes are more likely to occur in the setting of a severe brain injury, with consequent prolonged P.T.A. and R.A. and other neurological signs of brain injury. However, if a careful search is made, some aspects of this pseudo-reminiscence may be found for a brief period following lesser head injuries, and it may be simply the result of some degree of temporal disorientation, for this constitutes the most accurate parameter of minor degrees of confusion in amnesia. The content of confabulation will obviously reflect personal and emotional factors in the biography of the individual, but it is probable that the readiness with which confabulation occurs at all also represents previous personality traits and individual idiosyncrasies in the use of memory, rather than in factors purely dependent on the site and extent of brain injury.

A florid confabulatory syndrome, as opposed to the brief and isolated paramnesias, is rare in traumatic amnesia. Of 1 931 cases of closed head injury observed at a special centre during World War II, only 38 cases were recorded. Of these, only six showed confabulation persisting for more than two or three days. However, all did offer some pseudo-reminiscence either spontaneously or in reply to questions, for a period for which they were, on objective evidence, quite amnesic; and this occurred at a time when there was no evidence from their general behaviour of any drowsiness or confusion. A common, almost constant finding was a rather facile euphoria, which tended to disappear as recovery proceeded. In all cases where it was possible to check on this, the content of confabulation was found to consist of actual experiences, though somewhat altered in minor details. Their content was factual but their context completely inaccurate. All such cases had evidence of severe brain injury as shown by abnormal neurological signs, blood in the cerebrospinal fluid, fractured skulls or ventricular dilatation on air-encephalograms and long final P.T.A.'s. The latter are given in Table 1 for 37 cases; one patient died 27 days after injury and is not included.

TABLE 7

	Length of P.T.A. in days			
	<7	7–14	15–20	>21
No. of cases	4	6	5	22

The following example illustrates the features of a severe case. The discrepancy between normal behaviour in everyday ward activities and extreme confabulation is well shown. This is an important distinction from cases where confabulation occurs simply as part of a general traumatic confusion, which is seen during recovery from the majority of severe head injuries.

Case 6. An army sergeant of 24 was injured in a car accident in England. He responded to questions within 24 hours, but was confused and drowsy for some days longer. Eighteen days after injury he was transferred by ambulance to a special head-injury centre. He was then alert and co-operative and answered questions readily. He knew all his personal details accurately but gave the date incorrectly, and when asked where he was replied, 'I couldn't tell you the name of the hospital, but I have been here twice before for treatment'. In fact he had never been there before. He knew that he had been injured in a car accident, but said that he had just been flown over from France in a servicing plane and gave details of the journey. He was well enough to be up and about in the ward and his behaviour was helpful, friendly but rather euphoric. He would engage in long confabulatory talks with other patients, but rapidly learned the hospital routine and knew his way to the canteen, recreation room etc. Five weeks after injury, he knew the name of the hospital but said that he had been in a large number of hospitals before this one. Spontaneous confabulation had now ceased but, asked about what he had been doing that morning, he replied that he had been out getting a car, though in fact he had not left the hospital. The contrast between his confabulation and general behaviour was well shown by an occasion on which he had been playing cards in the ward and had actually won the game, but immediately after, when interviewed by a medical officer, gave an elaborate confabulatory account of his morning's activities. During the earlier days of his confabulation he had a short-term memory defect as well, and could not recall items of news read a few hours before, or details of a film seen on the previous day. His performance in memory tests involving the delayed recall of a simple story was also defective, though digit retention was average. His final P.T.A. assessed three months after injury was about six weeks. He returned to full duties with his unit six months after injury, and was reported as performing them efficiently

His incorrect statement that he had been in several hospitals since his injury, and the equally unfounded claim to have been in his present hospital on two previous occasions both probably represent what has been termed *reduplicative paramnesia* (Pick, 1915; Paterson and Zangwill, 1944). Current memories are related to some place other than the present location. There is a failure of identification or recognition with some disorientation of time sequence, a type of disability seen in more florid form in Korsakoff states.

Linked with such confabulatory states, and illustrating the point that they do contain real experiences, are the occasional instances in which the circumstances of the injury are recalled but in a confused manner, and are then woven into a delusional system to account for the injury which the patient is aware that he has suffered. Such systematized paramnesias may take on a persecutory and paranoid tinge. An example is quoted by Russell (1935) in which a patient involved in a motor cycle accident with a dog, subsequently ascribed his injuries to an attack by the dog and further elaborated this by suggesting the dog's owner had also attacked him. These delusions were short-lived in this case and cleared as his post-traumatic confusion receded. However, they may occasionally persist and give rise to false accusations and legal difficulties.

Very rarely, isolated circumstances related to the injury, while not recalled as normal memories or even isolated islands, may suddenly appear unheralded in consciousness, usually as a clear visual impression, less often accompanied by auditory impressions. When this occurs, its abrupt and hallucinatory quality and stereotyped pattern make it probable that it is an epileptic phenomenon rather than a variation of traumatic amnesia (Hooper, McGregor and Nathan, 1945).

TRAUMATIC AUTOMATISM

In the examples so far discussed, P.T.A. has followed on a period of concussion or loss of consciousness. However, this is not always so. A blow on the head may interrupt memory, partially or completely, but no complete cessation of activity may occur. This is usually associated with injury during the course of some simple routine or repetitive activity, when its continuance in a state of automatism is possible. Injuries on the field of sport are the common setting.

> *Case 7.* A man of 21, captain of his university boxing team, during a four-round contest received several blows on the head. However, he was not knocked out nor did he appear dazed or abnormal to his seconds. They only remarked that he was fighting badly during the last round. He himself had no recollection of the last half of the third round nor of the last round. He came round in the dressing room looking at a bruised eye in the mirror and had a considerable throbbing headache for the rest of that evening. He could not judge the onset of his amnesia accurately but its end was sharply defined. It lasted between 15 and 20 minutes and during it he had shaken hands with his opponent, spoken to some of his friends and prepared himself for a shower.

Similar incidents are seen on the football field. The causative injury may produce a momentary knock-out or a short period of obviously dazed behaviour, and thereafter the individual may continue the game for periods of up to an hour or so, with no memory of it afterwards. In such instances, play may be erratic and obviously confused and it is here that examples of players scoring against their own side are recorded. Here, as in other head injuries, there may be short periods of R.A. as well as P.T.A.

RETROGRADE AMNESIAS

Unlike P.T.A.'s, R.A.'s are much more stereotyped. The vast majority of them extend for a period of a few seconds to a minute before the injury. One widely accepted explanation for this is that a short time is required for the physiological processes of embedding or consolidation of the original perception—the laying down of the engram as it were—to occur, and that the injury interferes with this process.

There is little factual information as to the nature of the process. In animals however, a biochemical change has been shown to occur for a short period following electroshock of above seizure intensity (Cotman *et al.*, 1971). A short-lasting inhibition of normal synthesis of brain protein, with an increase in its precursor l-leucine was observed. The significance of this for the clinical situation is doubtful, though induced seizures in animals are known to produce R.A.

Occasionally there may be no R.A., even with an injury which causes a substantial P.T.A. of 24 hours or more. It is probable that a number of cases where no R.A. is recorded are due to inaccurate observation, because brief R.A.'s may be readily missed, unless very detailed knowledge of the circumstances of the injury are known to the examiner. However, it must be accepted that some instances of no R.A. following a fairly severe head injury have been recorded. The fact that they are very rare in blunt or closed head injuries does not obviate the need to explain them.

Although a brief R.A. is considered almost the rule in head injuries, the assessment of this is usually made some time after the event. Lynch and Yarnell (1973) examined six 'concussed' football players within less than three minutes of their injury. All recalled immediate retrograde events, including the concussive impact, even though confused or disorientated at the time—one case had suffered 30 seconds loss of consciousness. When re-interrogated three to 20 minutes later, all had an R.A. which was permanent for the injury and parts of the preceding game. The authors suggest from their observation that the decay-time for immediate memory must be 3 to 20 minutes. The opportunity to study immediate recall in concussion is rare and the confirmation that this follows the pattern seen in T.G.A. is of considerable interest.

An earlier observation of Fisher (1966) mimics even more closely the T.G.A. syndrome. A woman of 41 fell and suffered an apparently trivial occipital injury. There was no loss of consciousness and she got up immediately. However she showed a memory impairment for her whereabouts and reasons for being there, with loss of memorizing and a memory span reduced to about one minute. There was a variable but prolonged R.A. A full examination three hours later showed no neurological abnormality and a blood pressure 150/100. Twenty-four hours later memory function was normal but a permanent post-traumatic amnesia of ten hours with a retrograde of one to two seconds remained.

Very occasionally, there may be a long R.A. of days, weeks or months. In these cases the brain injury has usually been severe, and the P.T.A. also correspondingly long. Long R.A.'s always tend to be viewed with suspicion as psychogenic, and especially so when there is no evidence of severe brain injury. The difficulty is sometimes increased, because despite an inability to recall events for a period before injury, the patient may still be able to use skills and experience which were learnt during the period supposedly covered by the R.A. Despite these objections, however, there are a few well attested cases of such prolonged R.A.'s. One case recorded by Symonds (1962) had a persistent R.A. of one year. Although in such cases the R.A. is more complete for events shortly preceding the injury, the amnesia may include some events which appear objectively memorable throughout the whole period. It is always difficult to be certain that *all* the events of a long period in the past are forgotten, but substantial memory loss has been established. It is not easy to postulate a physiological explanation for such amnesias. In those where the loss is more patchy and perhaps only certain incidents are forgotten, a dynamic forgetting based on emotional considerations — some process of inhibition — may be invoked, but this does not appear to apply to the type we are considering here.

As with P.T.A., R.A., though much less commonly, may also show islands of memory within the general loss. However, the preserved memories seem to have no specially memorable qualities, and other and more important events are not retained. It is of course possible that the remembered experiences may have had some special importance in the personal biography of the individual. Another explanation may be that such islands are really factitious, in the sense that they only occur when the R.A. is estimated before all the elements of general post-traumatic confusion have fully cleared. They may simply represent a persisting temporal disorientation, which is in fact the most delicate and readily disturbed part of normal full orientation, and in general the last to recover following head injury. Measuring R.A. while some degree of temporal disorientation is present may result in misplacement of events which are remembered but incorrectly located in the personal time sequence.

It has also been remarked that R.A. — unlike P.T.A. — tends to show spontaneous shrinkage. Where R.A.'s are longer than the common minute or less (which they almost always are in the early stages), they show a marked tendency to shrink in the hours, days or weeks following recovery of consciousness. During the period of manifest confusion the R.A. may at first be relatively long (sometimes months or even years), but progressively shortens as confusion clears. This has been studied by Williams and Zangwill (Zangwill, 1964), who noted that the first step is commonly the emergence of an isolated recollection, often of an event which occurred 15–30 minutes before the accident, and which the patient accepts as his 'last memory' before finding himself in hospital. These 'last memories', which are often of quite trivial events, act as a kind of anchor in the reconstitution of continuous memory. They are often said to possess a curiously remote, sometimes almost depersonalized, character and are occasionally at first mislocalized in time. As recovery proceeds, further recollections emerge and gradually become related both to one another and to the general context of pre-traumatic memory.

Unlike what is often supposed, memories rarely return in strict chronological sequence, from the more remote to the more recent. 'Islands of memory' emerge in a haphazard manner and are gradually related in time to the 'last memory', such that a more or less continuous record of recent past experiences is eventually reformed. This appears to depend partly on the spontaneous rearousal of associative links and partly on the patient's own effort at recall. Although information provided by others may play some part in this, it by no means always serves to recall to the patient the content of the amnesic period, suggesting that the pattern of shrinkage is in large part endogenous. Psychogenic factors (for example, the emotional significance of particular events) appear to play little part in governing either the scope of the amnesia or the time-order of recovery. Assessment of the emotional factor is not easy, since it may be subtle and personal and not dependent on the objective and seemingly memorable quality of an experience: nevertheless, any substantial recovery of R.A. under barbiturate hypnosis, which would be expected to reduce such factors of an inhibitory kind, is rare.

Any analysis of these amnesias in terms of registration, retention and recall is perforce rather speculative. However, R.A.'s of longer than a few minutes must involve a defect of either recall or retention since registration is known to have occurred. If recall is at fault, then it cannot be a defect of any general mechanism of recall, because recall of other experiences both before and after the R.A. period is intact. If retention is the fault, it must be one which affects continuing and not initial retention since, again, retention is often known to have occurred for a while in the pre-traumatic period. Moreover, it must at times affect retention in a very selective and patchy manner. The suggestion that only more recent and therefore less securely retained memories are affected is not always true. Considerations such as these, make any explanation – either anatomical or psychological – of R.A. a crucial point in any coherent theory of memory.

In a detailed study of 24 cases of R.A., Wasterlain (1971) suggested a population with bimodal distribution: 20 R.A.'s of one minute or less segregating in a number of clinical features from four with R.A. of over ten minutes. Such a distribution is implicit in the widely held view to which this author subscribes that brief R.A.'s involve a defect of consolidation. However his invocation of a defect of retrieval for the more prolonged group leaves unexplained the qualitative and quantitative vagaries of prolonged R.A.

So far as P.T.A. is concerned, it seems likely that registration and retention are chiefly at fault. Registration may not be absent but simply defective, and this may be primarily at perceptual level. The factor of attention in a quantitative sense, in relation both to registration and retention, may here be important. That registration and retention for a limited time can occur during a period of P.T.A. has been shown, not only by simple clinical observations, but also by short-term memory tests. What appears to be defective is more prolonged retention. However, in this context the formal segregation of memory into these traditional components may be irrelevant.

RESIDUAL MEMORY DEFECT

Apart from R.A. and P.T.A., as defined above, careful enquiry often discloses some residual weakness of memory, in spite of otherwise full recovery from the psychological after-effects of head injury. This is of two kinds: first, there is some degree of impairment in memory for current events and in the general efficiency of memory function. And secondly, there may be defects in recall of events antedating the injury, and well outside the scope of the R.A. as conventionally defined. Although the degree of impairment is often minimal, and is easily missed on clinical examination, it may constitute a genuine minor disability for some time after the patient is restored to normal, active life.

As regards the first type of residual memory defect, it is evident for the most part subjectively, though it can often be demonstrated objectively by the use of appropriate tests of learning capacity (Zangwill, 1943, 1946a). Indeed, the degree of impairment shown on such tests often contrasts strikingly with the otherwise excellent restitution of higher psychological function. Patients who exhibit such a disability complain that they have difficulty in remembering the names of people they have recently met, that they are prone to forget to carry out instructions or even their own intentions, and in general that they display an excessive degree of absent-mindedness in the small matters of daily life. These difficulties form part and parcel of the post-concussional syndrome (Symonds, 1940, 1962), and should not be dismissed as due merely to anxiety or self-distrust. Although they may of course be exacerbated by anxiety, and even provide a nucleus for the development of post-traumatic neurosis, their origin should be ascribed to a persisting minor degree of cerebral dysfunction.

Some degree of persisting defect in recall of events which occurred well before the head injury, sometimes weeks or even months previously, is not infrequently observed, especially after injury of any appreciable severity. In a study by Williams and Zangwill (1952), defects of this character were ascertained in no fewer than 16 out of 24 unselected cases of head injury of varying severity. Their incidence appeared to bear a definite relation to the severity of the injury (as assessed in terms of duration of R.A. and P.T.A.), but the numbers were unfortunately too small to permit of statistical analysis. With the milder head injuries, the defect took the form of a vagueness of recollection for events which had taken place during the week or so preceding the accident, and on occasion, outright memory gaps of which the patient was clearly aware. These memory failures appeared too outspoken and too constant to attribute to ordinary processes of forgetting. In the more severe cases, memory for events which had occurred up to about a year before the accident was found to remain appreciably defective, what one might call 'islands of amnesia' in an otherwise coherent memory record. For example, one patient on returning home was quite unable to recall that her house had been redecorated about six months before her accident and expressed much surprise at its spick-and-span appearance. Another patient failed to recall many of his activities at work in the month or so before the accident, though he had described them fully to his parents at the time and the latter remembered them well. In general, recollection of the weeks or months preceding a severe head injury was often found to be vague and somewhat sketchy. Although these patchy residual amnesias may clear up, to some extent at least, the possibility of some degree of permanent residual memory weakness for more recent pre-traumatic events, as is found after recovery from tuberculous meningitis (Williams and Smith, 1954), cannot be wholly discounted.

AMNESIAS AFTER PENETRATING BRAIN WOUNDS

We have so far discussed entirely the traumatic amnesias arising from blunt or closed head injuries. This is understandable because with penetrating brain wounds, amnesia is, in general, rare and short lived. This general observation must have important implications for the cerebral mechanisms involved in amnesia. A blunt head injury causes a generalized shift of intracranial contents, with a number of oscillatory pressure waves passing through them. The process involves a banging of certain areas of brain against the containing skull. The areas involved will differ with the site and direction of the blow. With the common injury to the front of the head, the frontal and temporal poles and the brainstem in the region of the tentorial hiatus will be especially involved. In addition, tearing of meninges, and of small superficial and deep blood vessels may occur. Tearing of subcortical white fibre tracts in the hemispheres has also been demonstrated in such cases (Strich, 1956). All these rather widespread injuries, which may vary greatly in intensity from case to case, may be invoked as a pathological background to amnesias associated with concussion.

When amnesias do occur in penetrating brain wounds, they are usually a part of a general dementia dependent on severe and widespread damage, particularly to the dominant hemisphere. Rare cases are, however, reported in which severe and permanent defects of memorizing occur. In such cases, the R.A. is often very long and the P.T.A. also extensive, but the assessment of both may be difficult because memorizing from the time of wounding onwards may be defective.

> *Case 8.* A good example was a soldier who suffered a left temporal penetrating brain wound, the missile probably crossing the mid-line. As a result, he had an unusual type of deafness which suggested a lesion of both primary auditory areas, a type of cortical deafness. He was also dysphasic for a time. Later, however, the most striking disability was a severe and persistent difficulty in remembering current events. He attempted to overcome this in everyday life and work by keeping a small notebook as an *aide-memoire*. However, this too he was continuously mislaying. His final P.T.A. was of some weeks' duration and his R.A. difficult to assess, but involving at least some experiences and learnt material from months before his injury.

Here and in other similar cases, the site of injury was probably the temporal lobes, possibly mainly of the dominant hemisphere (Russell, 1948). There is tentative evidence also to suggest that similar defects of memorizing may follow injury involving the fornix system bilaterally. In such cases, the defect is not so much of a circumscribed amnesic period, whether post-traumatic or retrograde, but rather of some continuing defect in the process of remembering. The anatomical siting of injury has to be derived from indirect evidence until full autopsy studies are available, but it seems to conform to that derived from similarly localized disease processes in the brain.

A study by Jahro (1973) provides more definite evidence. He found 11 cases of a total of 1 556 penetrating brain wounds from the Second World War which showed a persisting memory defect of Korsakoff type. Only seven of the 11 were accepted as clearcut examples, the others being contaminated by more general intellectual changes or dysphasia. They were followed for periods of three to ten years. All seven showed marked persistent defects of memorizing with an effective memory span reduced to less than ten minutes. R.A. was long. Though early R.A. showed shrinkage, the final defect was from four years to one month in six cases. In one case however the florid condition only developed 18 years after wounding during a febrile illness with intracranial infection. All cases showed a notable disorientation in time and this remained in two cases where some improvement in memorizing allowed recall of isolated events. One case showed substantial recovery over a two-year period and this included a shrinkage of retrograde amnesia from an initial one year to seconds only.

These cases once more illustrate the association of a memorizing defect with prolonged R.A., and the important part played by temporal disorientation in the defect.

Such cases are rare in brain wound survivors and the site of causative lesion may explain this. It was derived from stereotactic measurements on x-rays, by the site of wound and missile track, and in two cases these localizations were confirmed at autopsy. In six of the seven, bilateral diencephalic lesions were indicated and proximity to the mammillary bodies was important. Wounds in this area are likely to be fatal. Fornix-cingulate lesions seemed ineffective, but in one case bilateral rostral hippocampal lesions appeared to be responsible.

This careful and detailed study in subjects where diffuse brain pathology was absent, is a valuable confirmation of the anatomical siting now increasingly accepted as the basis for persisting loss of memorizing.

Although the current view of amnesia in penetrating brain wounds is that it occurs only with wounds in special situations, this may need reconsidering. In a number of patients with localized penetrating brain wounds in a variety of situations and with no evidence of a general concussive effect, an assessment of P.T.A. some years after injury may reveal an amnesia of days, or even weeks, which was not recognized a few weeks after the injury. Such amnesias are not simply part of a general forgetting of the past, since experiences both before injury and after the amnesic period may be accurately recalled. Evidence of this sort is hard to come by, as it requires that the assessor of a P.T.A. long after injury should have some personal knowledge of the circumstances of the earlier post-traumatic period. This condition was sometimes fulfilled in World War II when medical officers in charge of early battle casualties subsequently reviewed their own cases for pensions purposes years later. This, at present, is the only rather unsatisfactory source of evidence on this point. If these observations are accepted, they would imply that even local brain wounds may have some widespread effect on psychological function in the early post-traumatic period.

6 Temporal Lobe Amnesia

Susan D. Iversen

INTRODUCTION

In the first edition of Whitty and Zangwill's *Amnesia,* Brenda Milner contributed a chapter entitled 'Amnesia following operation on the temporal lobes'. The year was 1966 and at that time Milner consolidated her observations of the previous 10 years on amnesias of temporal lobe origin.

As early as 1957 she had published with Scoville the initial observations on the unique patient, H.M., who shortly before had sustained, for the relief of severe epilepsy, a radical bilateral removal of the medial temporal cortex including the underlying limbic structures (amygdala, hippocampi and their associated fibre connections). It was apparent that there was a degree of retrograde amnesia in this patient. The death of a favourite uncle some three years previously was not recalled and information in use immediately before the operation, such as the layout of the hospital wards and the faces of the medical staff, was forgotten. By contrast, some vivid memories of the distant past appeared to be present. However it was in memories of events occurring after the operation (i.e. anterograde effects) that the amnesia showed its severity and specificity. Cursory observation of H.M. quickly revealed a clear pattern of memory dysfunction. H.M. could retain new information as long as his attention was not diverted from it; in other words he had intact short-term memory. However, if he was distracted then no permanent or long-term memory of the event was ever made. This was clearly true of verbal and non-verbal information in all sensory modalities. As, under normal everyday conditions, attention has to be shifted from one event to another, it was not surprising to find that

H.M. was apparently making no record of ongoing events. Half an hour after eating lunch, he could not remember a single item he had eaten or indeed remember that he had had lunch. These anecdotal reports of H.M.'s memory illustrate most dramatically the paradox of intact short-term memory together with a total inability to make any permanent record of that information. Consider, for example, H.M.'s response to the direction to remember the numbers '584'. In the absence of distraction he was able to retain this for about 15 minutes, apparently by working out elaborate mnemonic schemes. Milner (1970) reports that when asked how he had been able to retain the number for so long, he replied:

'It's easy. You just remember 8. You see 5, 8 and 4 add to 17. You remember 8, subtract it from 17 and it leaves 9. Divide 9 in half and you get 5 and 4 and there you are: 584. Easy.'

A minute or so later, H.M. was unable to recall either the number 584 or any of the associated complex train of thought; in fact he did not know that he had been given a number to remember because, in the meantime, the examiner had introduced a new topic.

Theoretical exponents of two-process models of memory have also found it useful to refer to the clear neuropsychological evidence of a dissociation of short- and long-term memory in H.M. For example, in presenting their two-process model of memory Atkinson and Shiffrin (1968) write:

We ask the reader to accept our Model (two-process) provisionally until its power to deal with data becomes clear. Still some justification of our decision would seem indicated at this point. For this reason, we turn to what is perhaps the single most convincing demonstration of a dichotomy in the memory system: the effect of hippocampus lesions reported by Milner.

LATER EXPERIMENTAL STUDIES OF H.M. ILLUSTRATING THE LONG-TERM MEMORY IMPAIRMENT

Subsequently a variety of experimenters have probed the mnemonic capacities of H.M. Except in some details the original picture of a global amnesia has remained intact. An extensive follow-up study on H.M. was published by Milner, Corkin and Teuber in 1968.

The earlier results implied that H.M. was unable to store information presented in either the visual or the auditory mode under normal conditions of interference. The supra-modal nature of his impairment was further strengthened by Corkin's (1965) studies with a tactile maze-learning task. Milner (1965) had reported that with a 28-choice-point visual stepping-stone stylus maze, H.M. failed to reduce his error score in 215 trials. The large number of choice points presumably created a high level of interference which prevented rehearsal of any mnemonic strategy which might have facilitated the learning of the correct route. Corkin introduced a tactile analogue of the visual maze. An aluminium stylus maze was used, which was placed inside a wooden frame. The frame was open on the experimenter's side, but was covered on the subject's side by a black cloth curtain which concealed the maze from view. The subject was first allowed to feel the perimeter of the apparatus with both hands. Then, his preferred hand (holding the stylus) was guided by the experimenter to the starting area, to the finish, and back to the start, thus providing a general orientation in the maze. The instructions were to find the correct path from start to finish. Each time the subject entered a blind alley, a bell was rung which signalled him to move back. He was prevented mechanically from retracing the correct path and was warned against making repetitive errors within a single trial, that is, retracing the incorrect path. Training took place on two consecutive days, proceeding in blocks of 10 trials to a criterion of 3 consecutive errorless runs or until 50 trials had been completed.

H.M.'s learning curve together with those of two other patients (P.B. and F.C.) with left medial temporal resections plus right temporal dysfunction from the Penfield and Milner series (1958) (*see* page 143) are illustrated in *Figure 11(a)*. No reduction in errors was observed over 80 trials in H.M. although his mean time to complete the maze decreased (*Figure 11(b)*). This probably indicates growing familiarity with the motor requirements of this task. The impairment on the maze tasks cannot be attributed to perseveration of errors at particular choice points. Frontal lesions which produce perseverative tendencies impair acquisition of the multichoice mazes (Milner, 1965; Corkin, 1965) but they also impair performance on the Wisconsin Card Sorting Test (Milner, 1963). In the latter task cards are sorted by colour, shape or number. A particular sorting strategy has to be maintained for a number of trials and then relinquished for a different strategy. Frontal lesions result in perseveration of sorting strategies and the patient is rarely able to shift from the initial strategy and sorts the whole pack of cards in the same way. As we shall see later, H.M. behaves normally on this task.

Virtually identical groups of right and left cortically-damaged patients have been tested on the visual (Milner, 1965) and tactile (Corkin, 1965) mazes and there is a high correlation between performance on the two tasks. That successful performance on these tasks depends on memory rather than perception, is borne out by the obser-

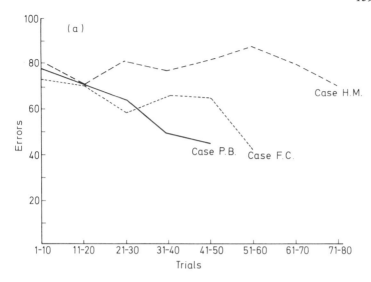

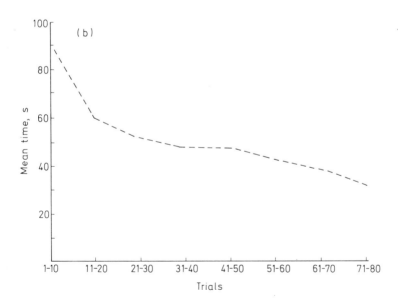

Figure 11(a) Learning curves for patients with bilateral hippocampal damage: total errors for consecutive blocks of 10 trials; (b) Case H.M.: mean time scores for consecutive blocks of 10 trials. (Reproduced by permission from Corkin, 1965)

vation that right temporal lobe lesions only impair performance if the underlying hippocampus is included in the removal. This is true both for the visual and tactile mazes.

Another paradigm which has proved useful for distinguishing perceptual and mnemonic disturbances is the Recurring Figure Test. The test was originally devised by Kimura (1963) for comparing the visual disorders associated with right and left temporal lobe lesions. In this task, the subject is shown a series of 160 cards (presented one at a time for 3 seconds), on each of which an unfamiliar figure is drawn; this may be either an irregular nonsense pattern or a regular geometric design. Eight of these figures are repeated in every block of 20 cards, interspersed at random with figures which occur only once. The first 20 cards constitute an inspection series, to which the subject is not required to respond verbally; thereafter, for each of the 140 test cards, he has to say 'Yes' if he thinks that the pattern has appeared before, and 'No' if he thinks that it has not. Mnemonic difficulties would be expected to result in impairment on this task and the high interference engendered by the new stimuli at the recognition stage should make it a very sensitive test of anterograde amnesia. With such an impairment the errors should be made to both the familiar and unfamiliar stimuli whereas perceptual disorders would tend to accentuate errors only to the unfamiliar stimuli (i.e. false positive errors). It has been reported that H.M. is severely impaired with both verbal and non-verbal items on the visual recurring figure test. The test has since been used in the auditory (Milner and Teuber, 1968) and tactile modalities (Corkin, cited in Milner and Teuber, 1968). Snatches of bird song were used for the auditory task and wire configurations modelled on the Kimura nonsense line-drawings for the tactile task. H.M. is impaired on both of these forms of the recurring figure test strengthening further the supra-modal nature of his amnesic impairment.

Konorski (1959) devised a rather different paradigm for assessing memory performance, the delayed paired-comparison task, which Prisko (1963) adapted for studying patients with temporal lobe damage. Five different kinds of stimuli were used, clicks and flashes of different presentation rate, tones, nonsense patterns and shades of red. On the task two stimuli of a given class are presented in succession, the interstimulus interval varying from 0 − 60 seconds. The subject is asked to say if the second stimulus is the same or different from the first. H.M. was tested on these tasks and was severely impaired as soon as the delay condition was introduced. Virtually no retention was seen at 60-second inter-stimulus delays. This test was originally conceived of as a measure of short-term memory but it is clear that successful performance depends on something more than the ability to retain an impression of a stimulus for 60 seconds. Even without direct interference in the intra-trial delay period the repetition of a limited number of similar stimuli would be expected to create considerable interference. Such factors must override the ability of H.M. to bridge delays with STM rehearsal strategies. This is brought out by his performance on a *delayed* matching task which was used by Sidman, Stoddard and Mohr, (1968). The subject faces a matrix of 9 panels in a 3 X 3 array. A circle and eight ellipses, varying in their axes ratios from 0.74 to 0.91 were the stimuli. On a given trial, a sample appeared on the centre panel and simultaneously, or after a varying delay, the surrounding panels lit up presenting the sample together with the seven remaining stimuli from the range. The subject was required to press the surround panel bearing the matching stimulus to the sample. Under simultaneous conditions (the sample and choice stimulus are on together) H.M. showed normal stimulus control as measured by a sharp generalization gradient. However, as soon as the sample was removed prior to the appearance of the surrounding stimuli, his performance deteriorated and at 32-second delays, the generalization gradient was flat. These results could be construed to indicate that H.M. shows a short-term memory impairment. However, the interpretation is countered by strong evidence to the contrary (*see* pages 150–159). Furthermore, when trigrams (combinations of three consonants) were used as the stimuli, H.M. achieved matching delays of 40 seconds. As was inferred in the case of the Prisko test, the results with non-verbal visual stimuli suggest that performance on this task also cannot be dependent solely on STM for the sample stimulus. Milner has suggested that the tendency to verbalize might be the important additional variable which distorts the intent of these tasks in the non-verbal mode.

However, this appears unlikely as far as the Prisko delayed comparison task is concerned. A tactile analogue of this was devised by Milner and Taylor (1972) involving wire shapes similar to those used by Corkin in the Recurring Tactile Figure Test. The difficulty shown by amnesic patients like H.M. on delayed comparison tasks was verified by the observation that although he was again able to match at zero delay, his performance delayed rapidly as soon as a delay was introduced. Patients with cerebral commissure section have been studied to find out which hemisphere performs best on the tactile matching task. Surprisingly, the right hemisphere was found to be markedly superior to the left (Milner and Taylor, 1972). As no access to verbal mediating centres was possible in these commissurectomized patients, it must be assumed that delayed matching is performed successfully without verbal coding and thus the supposed necessity for such coding can hardly be invoked to account for H.M.'s impairment.

Another possibility, considered below (pages 155–159), is that non-verbal stimuli do not have access to STM in the way that verbal stimuli do. Rather, they are handled entirely by long-term memory. If this were so then amnesics would be expected to fail on the Prisko test, and on the Sidman test with geometric drawings virtually irrespective of delay.

The selective anterograde amnesia in H.M. is not associated with any general intellectual impairment. Indeed, H.M.'s Intelligence Quotient is marginally improved (Preoperative on the Wechsler-Bellevue Intelligence Scale, 104; two years postoperative, 112; and in 1962 a value of 118 was recorded) since the operation, presumably because he is suffering markedly fewer epileptic seizures and less intensive drug therapy is required. This fact has made H.M. a particularly valuable patient to those interested in the normal organization of memory processes because the amnesias seen most frequently in the clinic tend to be associated with more widespread cognitive losses.

The body of results obtained with H.M. has probably been the single most important impetus to the growing interest amongst theorists in the use of dysfunctions of memory as a way of understanding the normal processes. The particular pattern of results obtained with H.M. (and it must be stressed that they are a peculiar and unique set of results) have helped other experimenters, studying what are invariably less homogeneous forms of amnesia, to define their questions and design their experiments as we shall see later in this chapter.

FURTHER CASES OF GLOBAL AMNESIA ASSOCIATED WITH TEMPORAL LOBE PATHOLOGY

This review has begun with a detailed description of H.M. because the neuroanatomical damage in this patient was specified at surgery and the global amnesia is so severe. He is a unique case. However, Milner (1966) cited other isolated classical cases from the literature in which severe medial temporal damage (of varying aetiology), had been associated with global amnesia. In addition there are the cases of the Scoville series (Scoville and Milner, 1957) who, except for H.M., were diagnosed as severely psychotic at the time temporal lobe surgery was undertaken. Indeed, the surgery was invoked in an effort to improve their psychiatric condition. One of these cases has been included in some of the Montreal tests and showed anterograde amnesia after the operation albeit not as severe as in the case of the one epileptic, H.M. This may be because their psychiatric illness made formal psychological testing less satisfactory.

Secondly, Milner has been concerned with the description of two further temporal lobe amnesics, who were given, for the treatment of epilepsy, *unilateral* left temporal lesions which encroached upon medial limbic structures. These patients (F.C. and P.B.) were found to have profound anterograde amnesia, which led Penfield and Milner (1958) to suggest that the remaining medial temporal structures of the right hemisphere were also damaged in these patients, both of whom had a long-standing epileptic condition. Abnormal EEG activity in the right temporal region indicated this might be so. In fact this has proved to be the case in one of these patients who subsequently died and was neuroanatomically assessed. Both of these patients have been tested by Milner and her associates on a variety of the long-term memory tasks which H.M. fails. Dimsdale, Logue and Piercy (1964) described a similar case of amnesia after unilateral temporal lobectomy including limbic structures. In this case surgery was performed on the *right* hemisphere and EEG abnormality observed in the left. This lady (N.T.) is the most important case in Warrington's series and has been tested extensively. Finally, Teuber, Milner and Vaughan (1968) have studied a patient with a bilateral stab wound in the base of the brain. The amnesia was assessed on many of the tests used with H.M. and appeared remarkably similar although not so severe.

In addition to these surgical cases, five postencephalitic patients have been studied in some detail and found to exhibit the now familiar amnesic pattern seen in surgical cases. Starr and Phillips (1970) formally tested a case almost six years after an acute attack of encephalitis and found a severe anterograde amnesia. A very similar picture emerges from Cermak's (1976) study of a postencephalitic patient (S.S.) two years after his illness. Drachman and Arbit (1966) tested three post-encephalitic cases and H.M. on their Expanded Digit Span Experiments. The pattern of memory loss was qualitatively similar in the two classes of patient. The detailed testing of all of these patients provides an increasingly complete picture of what can and cannot be remembered by the temporal lobe amnesic. Other vascular and neoplasist cases are mentioned in the neuropathology section but in most cases the amnesia has not been assessed in a range of formal situations.

RESIDUAL LEARNING CAPACITY IN AMNESIA

From anecdotal observations it was correctly perceived that H.M. had no perceptual or STM disorder. However, the initial impression that, despite intact perceptual coding and STM, H.M. had a *total* inability to form new memories, was already questioned by Milner (1966). She noted that he was able to learn to trace accurately a star shape when his drawing and the star stimulus were seen only reflected in a mirror. This learning curve was normal over a 3-day period, each new session being started at the same level attained in the pprevious session. Over the last ten years there has been added support for the notion that H.M. and other related temporal lobe amnesics have at least four reasonably intact cognitive abilities:

(1) Perceptual analysis and encoding
(2) STM
(3) *Motor* learning and memory
(4) Concept formation and instruction-following.

Furthermore, the fact that these abilities are intact in the absence of long-term memory says something about the neural substrates mediating these abilities and about the functional structure of normal cognitive abilities. Some of the latter reasoning has been useful to theorists of human learning and memory and supports the contention that studies of amnesia may, as we shall see later, provide useful information on normal cognition.

(1) Intact perceptual analysis and encoding in amnesias

Except for an inexplicable reduction in pain sensitivity (which may have predated the operation) there has never been any indication that H.M. suffers from basic sensory disorders. Information is apparently received and coded normally.

A variety of tests have been used to assess perceptual ability in amnesics. H.M., unlike patients with right parietotemporal lesions (*see* page 176), was reported by Milner, Corkin and Teuber (1968) to detect quickly anomalous features in cartoon drawings (Milner, 1958); on tests of tachistoscopic letter recognition (Dorff, Mirsky and Mishkin, 1965) and on letter masking (tested by Schiller) his performance is considered to be equivalent to that of normal subjects with the same acuity.

Schiller (reported in Milner, Corkin and Teuber, 1968) has studied metacontrast in H.M. Two stimuli (a disc and a ring) were briefly (10 s) exposed one after another, the disc always preceding the ring. At inter-stimulus intervals greater than 10 ms, H.M. was able always to see the disc and this is in accord with the performance of normal subjects.

Cermak (1976) has used a rather similar test from Oscar-Berman, Goodglass and Cherlow (1973) to assess rate of visual processing in amnesics. Identification of a target stimulus was modified by presentation of a second masking stimulus shortly afterwards. The minimum inter-stimulus interval which allowed correct recognition in S.S. fell within the normal range. A test of Glosser (Butters *et al.*, 1975) was used to assess the rate of audioverbal processing. The subject was required to report when a particular number was presented through the headphones and when a particular combination of numbers appeared dichotically with a brief (1.2 s) interpair interval. S.S. was excellent on both tasks indicating normal rates of auditory processing from the sensory register. Visuospatial skills are also intact as evidenced by excellent performance on timed-tasks such as the Block-Design subtest of the Wechsler scale and a modification of Hebb's triangular block task. The Mooney 'closure' task is a particularly sensitive test of visual perceptual ability. In this task, the subject has to organize a face out of a chaotic black and white pattern with incomplete contours. Forty-four faces are included in the test and the subject is asked to give the sex and approximate age of the person whose face he sees. H.M. responded quickly and accurately to this difficult perceptual task making only four errors and completing the series in less than seven minutes. This performance level was superior to that observed in age-matched control subjects (Milner, Corkin and Teuber, 1968).

However, the dividing line between a test which is purely perceptual and one in which memory comes to play a role is narrow, as indicated by H.M.'s failure on a modified form of the Gottschaldt Hidden-Figure Task (Milner, Corkin and Teuber, 1968). In the task particular geometric patterns have to be discovered and traced within a network of embedding and overlapping lines. This is clearly a complex task taxing several cognitive functions as it proves difficult for subjects with cortical damage in widely different areas. It is possible that the need to keep one particular geometric figure in mind, whilst analysing another more complex figure, might overtax H.M.'s short-term memory with a consequent slowing of performance and increase in error score.

All of the examples of normal perceptual functions cited so far involve visual cues. Milner (1966) has reported that H.M. and the two amnesics from the Penfield and Milner (1958) study can also register auditory signals. On the Seashore Tonal Memory Test, a short melody of three to five notes is played twice in rapid succession and the subject is required to say which note changes at the second playing. On this task H.M.'s performance was normal.

More recently it has been found that amnesics show a degree of perceptual/motor learning if the material to be remembered is of a particular kind or presented in a manner which capitalizes on the residual mnemonic capacity of the subject. For example, Milner (1965) originally found that whereas H.M. showed abysmal performance on a 28-choice-point visual maze, he did show, after a great deal of testing, some learning when the maze was reduced to 3 choice-points (Milner, Corkin and Teuber, 1968). He reached three consecutive errorless runs after 155 trials given in blocks of 4×25 trials per day. He was retested on days 3, 5, 8 and 14 and showed some retention. Presumably a modicum of success is seen on this task because the amount of information to be stored comes well within the limit of the STM span. However, when it is pointed out that normal subjects learn the 28-choice-point maze in 17 trials and retain it perfectly after 24 hours, the paucity of H.M.'s residual learning capacity is emphasized. Similar results (Milner, Corkin and Teuber, 1968) were obtained with H.M. on a shortened form of an equivalent tactual maze (Corkin, 1965), although the degree of learning was less impressive than on the visual analogue. Starr and Phillips' case was an accomplished pianist. He was taught to play a new melody by ear. Next day he could not remember having learned the piece nor its name but when the first few notes were hummed, he quickly played the piece correctly. This is another example of successful perceptual/motor learning. Cermak, (1976) has tested his postencephalitic case on a finger maze similar to that described by Corkin. This patient learned with some difficulty an 8-point maze but was able to retain it quite well over a 2-month period.

Another perceptual learning task on which H.M. shows some success is the Gollin Incomplete-Pictures' Task (Milner, Corkin and Teuber, 1968) in which the subject is presented with increasingly complete line drawings of a common object and is asked to say when it is recognized. H.M. was presented with 5 sets of 20 drawings, Set 1, containing the most fragmented and Set 5 the completed drawings. Set 1 was presented, followed by 2 and so on and the subject asked to say on every trial what he thought the line drawings represented. The sets of cards were presented until all 20 objects were named correctly. H.M. made 21 errors to criterion and matched normal subjects made a mean of 25.5 errors, a result which again illustrates the intactness of H.M.'s perceptual abilities. After a one-hour delay occupied with neurological testing and questions on recent events, H.M. successfully re-did the test now making only 11 errors. Clearly some retention had been shown, albeit less than in the controls who now made only 3.6 errors. Warrington and Weiskrantz (1968a) had originally used the Gollin test on amnesics and found the rapid perceptual identification and, at that time, unexpected evidence of some long-term memory in such patients. It has been a matter of some dispute as to whether this test facilitates residual learning capacities in amnesics because the *perceptual* nature of the material enhances perceptual analysis and hence storage or because the fragmented drawings act as recognition probes making it easier for amnesics to retrieve what little information they are able to get into long-term storage. Normal subjects remember better under recognition conditions and Warrington and Weiskrantz have devised a series of elegant tests in which recognition is aided by presentation of partial information in both normals and amnesics.

As we shall see, motor learning is normal in amnesics (pages 159–161), which suggests the possibility that the shortened mazes or Gollin material are handled partly by coding of motor responses. However, if this were so, it is difficult to understand why learning is still relatively poor on these maze tests while direct motor learning is so excellent.

Encoding processes

It is not appropriate to dwell on this topic or attempt to review the results as it is a time of active experimentation and as is usual at such times, conflicting results are appearing. It is clear that temporal lobe amnesics are able to organize incoming information using some of the encoding strategies which are known to be used beneficially in normal memory processing. It appears that severe Korsakoff patients suffer a generalized deficiency for using such encoding strategies. Butters and his collaborators (1975) have used a range of interesting new tests on such patients to support this view and reiterate that *their* Korsakoff patients do have such defects in addition to impairment in other aspects of memory. The Korsakoff pattern of deficits on virtually all aspects of information processing is admirably illustrated in the recent Cermak study (1976). What is in dispute is whether or not temporal lobe amnesics have similar difficulties. On balance it would appear they do not.

Warrington and Weiskrantz (1971) attacked this question directly, when a variety of isolated observations on amnesics began to suggest that a basic encoding disorder could explain their striking difficulty in the permanent storage of information. The frequent occurrence of prior-test intrusion in verbal recall has been commented on in several studies. Warrington and Weiskrantz were finding that partial information techniques (such as the Gollin test) improved retention in amnesics perhaps, it was suggested, by eliminating incorrect responses. These incorrect responses would be made under free recall conditions because amnesics fail to categorize separately 'new' and 'old' items or because of their tendency to overgeneralize among the alternative items in store. By contrast, other comments in the literature could be interpreted to indicate that amnesics are able to organize information. The subsequent experiments of Warrington and Weiskrantz (1971) were not an unqualified success because on two of the categorization tests, the normal results were unexpected and this made it difficult to evaluate amnesic performance. However, they repeated Talland's (1965) perceptual classification test in which a standard geometrical shape was presented and the subject asked to inspect 40 similar shapes and say if they were 'like' or 'not like' the standard. This was repeated with other designs when the standard was not present. Secondly, the task was extended to a condition when the subject was required to say which of the stimuli were *identical* with the standard which again was displayed or had to be memorized. Amnesics showed normal categorization. In the next test the ability to remember an unusual event better than frequently occurring events was also found to be true of amnesics. In addition they showed better retention of verbal material under 'cued' than under free recall conditions (as Cermak (1976) subsequently also found) indicating that amnesics are able to gain some advantage from semantic categorization and therefore must be capable of such encoding. Other experiments support Warrington and Weiskrantz' view. Weingartner (1968) reported that patients with large left temporal lobe removals which encroached upon the amygdala and hippocampus showed better verbal recall on lists of related words than on equivalent lists of random words, and Starr and Phillips (1970) found that the best verbal recall in their patient was recorded when he was given a list of ten words and told to arrange them in any order that made sense to him. The arrangements he used are shown in Table 8 together with the order in which they were retained. After 4 trials retention of these words was still perfect.

Baddeley and Warrington (1973) adopted the method of category clustering (Bousfield, 1953) to assess phonemic, semantic and visual imagery encoding in amnesic patients. Although the overall levels of performance were significantly higher in the control subjects, the amnesic subjects (like controls) benefited both from phonemic and taxonomic clustering and the degree of advantage afforded by this phonemic clustering was not significantly different in the two groups. By contrast, amnesics were not aided by visual imagery although the controls were.

It has been convincingly shown in normal subjects (Paivio, 1969) that the use of visual imagery can facilitate the recall of words. Jones (1974) has used this 'trick' significantly to influence the 'verbal' memory of patients with left temporal lobe removals. H.M. and a patient with

TABLE 8

Arrangements of words used by S.S. on 4 trials under the free study technique. To the right of the Table the immediate reproduction performance is presented indicating excellent retention (reproduced by permission from Starr and Phillips, 1970)

Free study technique

Trials	Arrangement of words by patient		Reproductions			

1. *Pleasant*   *Unpleasant*   *Immediate*

heart	hung	cheap	type	heat	
school	cheap	sky	clear	hung	Corr. = 7
clear	heat	post	(boat)	(roll)	Errors = 2
sky	fail				
type					
post					

When shown all 10 cards again he recognized those he left out and classified them:

Fail = Unpleasant
School = Pleasant
Heart = Pleasant

2. *clear sky* –get *cheap heat.* clear   school   post
In school a certain *type* of sky   type
student will *fail* if he gets cheap   fail   Corr. = 8
hung up on a certain heat   Errors = 0
kind of problem.
(made up above para-
graph leaving out 2 of
10 words).

3. Same as number 2   clear   post   school
sky   hung   type   Corr. = 10
cheap   ·   fail   Errors = 0
heat   heart

4. When we have a *clear*   clear   school   hung
sky, we have *cheap*   sky   type   post   Corr. = 10
heat. In *school* a *type*   cheap   fail   Errors = 0
of student that a *fail*   heat   heart
grade would break
his *heart.*
So they went on a picnic
and *hung* their lunch pail
on a *post.*

---

a bilateral medial temporal lesion associated with a tumour (spreading bilaterally) and its surgical treatment were also tested. Both of these patients with global amnesia were clearly able to use visual imagery but forgot the visual images as quickly as the word pairs which generated the images. Lackner (1974) has looked at linguistic processing in H.M.

using a click distraction test devised by Fodor and Bever (1965). H.M. was required to listen to 10-word sentences which were interrupted by the occurrence of a click and he was asked to repeat the sentences and say where the click occurred. Like normal subjects, H.M. showed a tendency to hear clicks presented during a sentence displaced into or toward the nearest syntactic break regardless of whether the click precedes or follows the clause break. On 7 occasions H.M. was unable to repeat an entire sentence and give the click location. On 6 of these sentences an interesting pattern is evident. H.M. repeated them to the major *syntactic* break and then stopped. The places at which H.M. stopped in the sentences were not random; instead they were a function of the syntactic structure of the sentences. These breaks in ongoing processing reveal the structural units of H.M.'s linguistic processing which appear to be in terms of constituent structure clauses, as in normal subjects. H.M. is also able to hold and process the overall structure of a sentence in order to detect ambiguity.

However, when this problem is investigated more thoroughly there may be certain encoding conditions where amnesics do show impairment. For example, Cermak's (1976) patient S.S. showed an equivalent impairment to that of the Korsakoff patients on a task developed by Underwood (1965) to measure the type of encoding subjects *spontaneously* perform on particular words during the presentation of a list of words. The subject is required to detect repetitions within a list of 60 words. While 6 words are actually repeated within the list, there are also 6 homonyms, 6 associates, 6 synonyms and 6 randomly chosen neutral words. The nature of the *false* recognition errors (subject says it is a repeat which it isn't) indicates the preferred encoding strategy. On this task S.S. showed homonym and associate errors indicating that acoustic and association coding strategies were spontaneously more likely than semantic coding. However, S.S. like Korsakoff patients can benefit from semantic coding if *directed* by the experimenter to do so. Should such results be construed to indicate a deficiency in encoding? Probably not, as a great deal of information is presented rapidly during the task and amnesic patients could fail to show the normal pattern of responses, not because encoding did not occur but simply because of the inadequacy of long-term memory. In short, it is difficult to assess encoding without a task structure which in its own right is so difficult that it is putting pressure on the basic amnesic disability in the patients.

(2) Intact short-term memory

As Drachman and Arbit (1966) have pointed out, the term short *versus* long can be rather misleading when considering memory function.

Short-term memory is characterized not so much by its duration as by its limited capacity. A small amount of information in the absence of interference could, theoretically, be held for long periods by a short-term verbal rehearsal system. As soon as the amount of information or the level of interference increases, the short-term store reveals its limitations and, if information cannot be passed to another form of storage, that information is lost. Thus in H.M. amounts of information within the span of STM can be held for long periods when there is no interference. In the everyday conditions of high interference, an intact STM could mediate little effective memory as evidenced by H.M.'s 'everyday' mnemonic performance.

H.M. has subsequently been tested on more formal tasks considered to assess short-term memory. He was included in a group of five amnesics tested by Drachman and Arbit (1966). The remaining patients were also, on clinical grounds, thought to have sustained bilateral medial temporal damage related to epileptic, encephalitic or haemorrhagic disease. In addition to the Wechsler memory scale, extended digit and paired light-span tests were devised. The tests consisted of two portions, a subspan and a supraspan phase. In the subspan phase of the digit test, random non-ordered series of digits beginning with five-digit lengths were presented by tape recorder at the rate of one digit per second. Three different series of each length were presented to each subject; if one or more of the three were repeated correctly, the next longer series was attempted. When a subject failed to repeat correctly any of the three series of a given length, the number of digits in the next lower series was considered to be his 'digit holding span' (DHS). In the supraspan phase the subject was then presented with a different series of the same length as the one he had previously failed to repeat. Repetitions of the series (training trials) alternated with attempts by the subject to reproduce the series (testing trials) until a criterion of one perfect recall was achieved. No subject was allowed more than 25 trials to reach criterion, and the test was discontinued if this number of trials was reached without success. When a subject reached criterion, he was given successively longer series in the same fashion until he had correctly repeated each series up to 20 digits or failed. A subject's digit storage capacity was recorded as the longest series that he could repeat within 25 trials or where he had reached the maximum, as '20+'. The extended paired-lights span paralleled the extended digit span test but utilized visual-spatial memoranda rather than auditory-verbal ones. A display and response panel placed before the subject contained two horizontal rows of ten lights each, one above the other. The lower lights also functioned as pushbuttons which the subject could press to indicate his responses.

Each presentation consisted of a training trial and a testing trial. In the training trial one upper and one lower light were simultaneously illuminated for one second, followed by a second paired-light display, etc, until all pairs in a given series had been presented. In the testing trial only the upper (cue) light was illuminated, and the subject had to respond by pressing the previously associated lower (response) light. Following each response, another cue light was illuminated until all pairs in the memorandum had been tested. The sub- and supraspan testing followed the same general pattern as that used in the extended digit span test.

The amnesic patients achieved a digit-holding span of 7.00 items compared with a score of 8.30 in the control subjects. This difference was not significant. By contrast, under the repeated-trial extended digit span test they recorded a digit storage capacity of 12 compared with 20 or greater for all the control subjects. If the number of learning trials to achieve criterion on a given span are considered, the amnesics require significantly longer even on span lengths which they are eventually able to learn. A similar pattern of results was obtained on an extended paired-light span test. The light pair holding span was not different for the two groups but on extended spans, the amnesics achieved a maximum of 5.5 pairs whereas the controls achieved 10 or more pairs. Again the amnesics required at least twice the control number of training trials on the spans they could learn and on the more extended spans showed virtually no improvement over the 25 trials of testing on a given span. The view that medial temporal pathology was the crucial common neurological feature in these patients was illustrated by the performance of an additional case with a lower IQ than that of the amnesics, who had bilateral neocortical damage to the lateral surface of the temporal lobe. This lady achieved an extended digit span of more than 20 items and a light pair span capacity of 10+, both scores equivalent to those achieved by non-brain-damaged patients.

The experimental psychology literature has provided other powerful tests with which to dissociate sub- and supraspan information handling processes. For example the sparing of short-term memory in H.M. was also investigated by Wickelgren (1968) using the 'probe-digit' technique. The items in the different experiments are single-digit numbers, three-digit numbers, or pure tones and the retention intervals varied from 0.25–8 seconds. On each trial a ready signal preceded by 1 second the presentation of the information to be remembered. With the single-digit test, a list of 8 digits was presented at 3 digits/per second followed by a *single test digit*. H.M. was required to say if that digit had occurred in the initial list. In the second experiment, lists (5 or 7 items) of 3-digit numbers were tested in the same way. Finally with the tone test, a standard tone was presented and followed by an interference tone. The test tone was played and H.M. was asked to say if it was the same or different in pitch from the first tone. Wickelgren and Norman (1966) had previously studied normal subjects on these tests and found that the curves of memory decay against time for single and 3-digit items could be accounted for by a single trace decay theory of STM. An additional component (assumed to be due to involvement of LTM) was required to explain the nature of the relationship between time and memory for pure tone. If H.M. had only short-term memory, then the results obtained with all stimuli should fit the theoretical single exponential decaying STM trace. This proved to be the case (*Figure 12*)

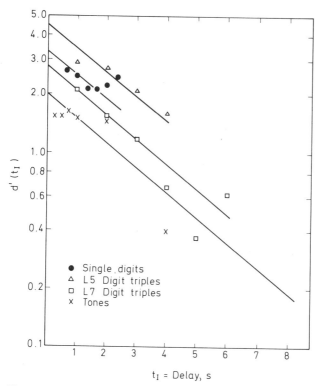

Figure 12. Rate of decay of four kinds of information in H.M. *According to strength theory (which predicts that information is handled and lost by a single process log* (d'(t_I)) *is a linear function of* t_I. *For the four kinds of information the results of H.M. fit a single exponentially decaying trace. (Reproduced by permission from Wickelgren, 1968)*

for all stimuli retention decreased over time and the *rate* of decay was approximately the same in the four stimulus conditions studied.

Baddeley and Warrington (1970) tested a group of amnesics on a wide range of tests validated as ways of quantifying short- as opposed to long-term memory in normal subjects. One patient (N.T.) had sustained a unilateral temporal lobectomy but exhibited symptoms closely analagous to H.M. and is inferred to have bilateral medial temporal involvement and four were carefully selected Korsakoff patients showing no dementia.

The tasks used were:
  (a) Free recall (Glanzer and Cunitz, 1966)
  (b) The Peterson and Peterson test (1959)
  (c) Proactive interference on the Peterson and Peterson test
  (d) Minimal paired-associate learning (Peterson, 1966)
  (e) Digit span
  (f) Hebb recurring digit test (Hebb, 1961)

(a) In the free-recall technique, the subjects are presented with a list of words which may be recalled in any order. Normal subjects recall, with a high probability, the last few items presented, a phenomenon termed the 'recency effect'. The later items are, presumably, still accessible from short-term stores when recall is demanded, whereas the other items are already dependent on the successful transfer to long-term memory for their recall. This involvement of both short- and long-term process is borne out by the observation that if recall is delayed by 20–30 seconds the 'recency effect' disappears and then all retention is dependent on long-term storage.

On delayed recall and on the initial items of the immediate recall list, amnesics showed poor retention. But in line with the hypothesis that they have intact STM, performance on the last items under immediate recall conditions was normal, i.e. they show the 'recency effect'.

(b) The Peterson and Peterson test (1959) assesses the rate of decay in short-term memory by requiring the subject to recall a list of three-letter words immediately or after a variable delay (5–60 s) occupied with counting aloud. Amnesics and normal subjects show virtually identical rates of decay indicating again the intact STM properties of amnesics.

(c) Keppel and Underwood (1962) found that after the first trial on the Peterson test more forgetting was seen on account, they hypothesized, of proactive interference from the previous words used in the earlier trials. This effect disappears if 2–3 minutes elapse between the trials indicating that the information loss from short-term memory is responsible (Loess and Waugh, 1967). As predicted amnesics and normals showed the same pattern of information loss, again indicating normal STM processes in amnesics.

(e) Digit span performance was normal in amnesics as expected.

(d) and (f) The results on these tests did not support the theory that amnesics have intact STM and deficient LTM. However, there are grounds for questioning what test (d) was actually measuring and no adequate explanation exists for the normal performance of the amnesics on this task. Finally, the normals showed poor learning on the Hebb test making a comparison with the amnesics tenuous.

Therefore, on balance, the study of Baddeley and Warrington (1970) stands as further clear support for intact STM in amnesics. Until recently the evidence of intact STM had been collected on tasks exclusively involving *verbal* information. Can amnesics hold non-verbal information equally well in short-term memory? Prisko (1963) found that H.M. could not retain the auditory and visual stimuli in her matching task as soon as a delay was introduced, and with delays of 60 seconds performance was reduced to chance level. Similarly Sidman, Stoddard and Mohr, (1968) found that in 8-choice matching-to-sample of circle/ellipse stimuli performance in H.M. deteriorated very rapidly as soon as the delay condition was introduced. Some explanations of these unexpected results have already been considered (page 141). However, Warrington and Baddeley (1974) point out that in these experiments controls showed no forgetting at any delays tested suggesting either that the task is dependent on LTM rather than STM or that performance is so good that forgetting is masked by a ceiling effect. Furthermore, even without delay the amnesics did not perform as well as controls, which may mean that the basic impairment on these particular tasks can be attributed to an encoding deficit. In fact in both experiments, the stimuli to be coded were somewhat abstruse shades of red, *rates* of click and light, for example. To gain further information on this point, they tested amnesics on memory for a position of a dot on a line, after various delays occupied with mental arithmetic. Controls and amnesics showed similar forgetting over the 5–60-second delay range. Furthermore, the amnesics would learn to reproduce a pattern of five random located dots just as easily as controls but unlike controls quickly forgot their positions after a short delay. These results are in agreement with Wickelgren's demonstration that amnesics show normal STM and forgetting for the pitch of pure tones.

The claim that STM is intact in temporal lobe amnesics does not, therefore, rest solely on the performance of H.M. In addition to the

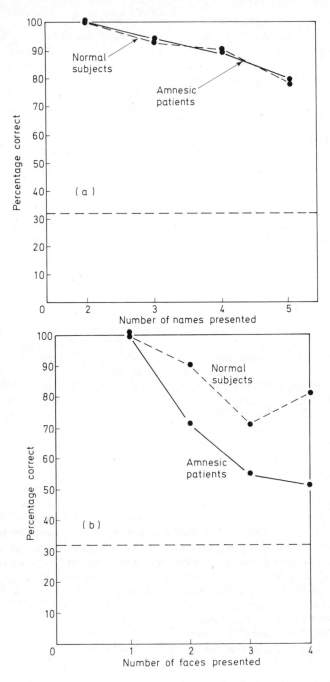

patients tested by Warrington and her collaborators, some of the individual amnesic cases in the literature (*see* page 164) have been tested formally in STM situations and provide supporting evidence. The encephalic case described by Starr and Phillips (1970) was tested with the Peterson technique and showed normal ST forgetting. Very recently Cermak (1976) has done extensive testing on a similar patient. He reports normal performance on a range of tests for assessing the properties of short-term memory including : (i) Peterson test; (ii) Massed *vs* distributed and high *vs* low interference conditions on the Peterson test (Cermak and Butters, 1972); (iii) Release from proactive interference in STM for words (Wickens, 1970) by distractor of different taxonomic category (Cermak, Butters and Moreines (1974).

However, in several independent studies, amnesics have been found to be impaired on certain tests of STM. The studies of Prisko and Sidman, Stoddard and Mohr on H.M. have already been mentioned and some explanations of these puzzling results have been considered. The amnesic described by Cermak (1976) was more severely impaired on the recall of irregular geometrical shapes (*non-verbal*) tested on a Peterson-type paradigm, than on the same test with verbal information. Could it be significant that these experiments have all used non-verbal stimuli? Recent experiments by Warrington and Taylor (1973) bear on this point. They tested five amnesics on the immediate recognition of unfamiliar faces and surnames. Strings of 1, 2, 3 and 4 faces or 2, 3, 4 and 5 surnames were presented singly at a 3-second rate. *Immediate* recognition was tested by presenting the test stimuli together with two 'new' stimuli for each 'old' one. For each string length (1, 2, 3, 4 and 5) 2, 4, 6, 8, 10 'new' stimuli, respectively, were presented in order that the probability of guessing correctly was constant for each string length.

On each trial immediately after seeing the test stimuli, the subject was required to point out the 'old' stimuli from a random array of 'old' and 'new' stimuli. With immediate recall name recognition was excellent in both groups (*Figure 13(a)*) but on face recognition the amnesics showed a severe impairment on string lengths of 2 and greater (*Figure 13(b)*). Under delay conditions normal subjects showed no decrement in the recognition of 3 face strings at 30 seconds delay (*Figure 14*), although the typical forgetting is seen with names over this period. This normal result leads Warrington and Taylor to suggest

Figure 13(a) Immediate recognition memory span for surnames (reproduced by permission from Warrington and Taylor, 1973); (b) immediate recognition memory span for faces (reproduced by permission from Warrington and Taylor, 1973)

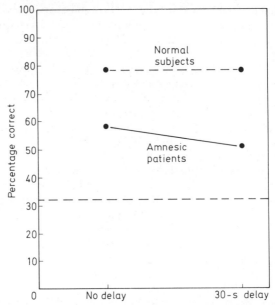

Figure 14. Memory for three faces with immediate and delayed recognition. (Reproduced by permission from Warrington and Taylor, 1973)

that whereas verbal information is handled by a two-process memory system (STM/LTM) *certain* non-verbal information is not handled at all by STM but is retained solely by LTM. If this is so it is easy to explain why normals do not give evidence of short-term forgetting with faces and why, paradoxically, amnesic patients are impaired whether there is a delay or not.

For the purpose of argument one can suggest that if an amnesic can't do it, it must involve LTM and *vice versa*. The results can then be used to formulate the following flow model for memory processing.

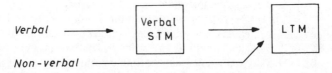

Such a model illustrates how performance of amnesics can give a vital clue to the normal process. This is clearly a very attractive general dictum but we do need to look at many more non-verbal tasks before coming to any definite conclusion that non-verbal memory does not involve a primary or ST memory process. This point has important implications for animal studies. In non-verbal organisms, STM would not be expected to exist according to Warrington and Taylor's (1973) argument. Animals would have only a long-term memory and all information would be processed directly by this unitary mechanism. The principal challenge to successful storage and retrieval would then be interference and a medial temporal lesion should make it difficult for animals to perform well in interference-rich situations.

However, situation tasks modelled on the sub/supraspan idea would not be relevant to animals, both kinds of tasks being handled similarly, nor would tasks with long intertrial intervals filled with distraction be of any particular relevance (Orbach, Milner and Rasmussen, 1960). Such tasks were modelled on the observation in H.M. that as soon as his attention was shifted information was lost (presumably from the short-term verbal handling mechanism). Also explicable would be the observation in hippocampal lesion monkeys (Correll and Scoville, 1970) that time in memory appears a relative unimportant variable.' As we have seen in normal people, time is also unimportant for the memory of stimuli which are not processed by STM (Sidman, Stoddard and Mohr, 1968; Warrington and Taylor, 1973).

The final implication of this model relates to the controversy concerning the *nature* of temporal lobe amnesia (discussed further on page 169). If non-verbal information is processed independently of STM and if amnesics show poor memory of such information, then a basic difficulty in transferring information from STM to LTM can hardly be invoked as a total explanation of amnesia. Rather, such information must be adequately handled in long-term memory which stores and retrieves that information. The common occurrence of intrusion errors in amnesics is seen as good evidence that information *is* stored but is erratically retrieved.

However, more studies of non-verbal STM memory in normal and amnesic patients is required to add weight to these tentative speculations. Even on the existing literature, it is not possible to state that STM is *never* invoked for the holding of non-verbal information. For the pitch of pure tones and the position of a dot on a line, normal short-term forgetting curves have been reported (Wickelgren, 1968; Warrington and Baddeley, 1974).

(3) Intact motor learning in amnesics

Milner's 1968 prediction that motor learning was intact in H.M. has been borne out by formal studies. Corkin (1968) tested H.M. on some specific motor tasks: rotary pursuit, bimanual tracking and tapping. In rotary pursuit a stylus was held in either hand and directed to a target. Contact had to be maintained as the target rotated. On the tracking task, a stylus was held in each hand and an asymmetric tract had to be followed as it appeared in a $^3/_8$ inch high horizontal slot. The tapping task required sequential tapping of four marked sectors of a circle with either hand separately or bimanually. On all these tasks, H.M.'s performance improved significantly over the daily testing sessions. Furthermore, when retention was tested on the rotary pursuit task several days after the end of training, H.M. showed perfect retention.

Experiments on other amnesic cases bear out these results. Starr and Phillips' (1970) case could learn Porteus mazes and remember them for two weeks. Performance was not normal but substantially better than on verbal memory tasks. Brooks and Baddeley (1976) have subsequently tested a group of patients including three postencephalitic amnesics and confirm the results of the Starr and Phillips patient. Whereas verbal paired-associate learning showed a severe deficit, pursuit rotor performance and perceptual motor learning on Porteus maze tests and jigsaw puzzle assembly was much less severely impaired, particularly when test criterion was in terms of time rather than errors. In the Starr and Phillips study the mazes were copied on to plywood and the paths indicated by strings, thus kinaesthetic and proprioceptive information was available to the blindfolded subject. The number of choice-points were considerable in the more difficult mazes, therefore it is surprising that the amnesic performed so well, whereas H.M. is reported by Corkin (1965a) to be unable to learn the full stylus-stepping maze she uses and does not perform terribly well even when number of choice-points is reduced to 5 points. It cannot be as Brooks and Baddeley (1976) suggest that visual mazes are failed by amnesics because they cannot use visual imagery as a mediating response. There are clearly some tactile mazes where they also fail and where imagery has not been invoked to explain normal performance. Presumably the physical design of the apparatus and the nature of the interference determines whether a particular task is handled by motor or sensory associative learning strategies. In the visual and tactile mazes used by the Montreal group both learning processes are presumably involved. However, if a maze can be handled as a motor learning task, then one would predict virtually perfect performance in amnesics as on pure motor learning tasks they are normal.

Finally, it may be noted in H.M. and the other cases of severe global amnesia, that testers have commented upon the fact that the patients can clearly follow instructions accurately and remember 'what to do' in testing situations, even in cases where they do not show any improvement on the task itself. Corkin notes that H.M. holds out his hands for the testing of sensory threshold with the von Frey hairs and that on the motor tasks he clearly remembers the apparatus from day to day (although he cannot remember how well he did with it). He can say what he is supposed to do on the rotary pursuit and bimanual-tracking test. Starr and Phillips' (1970) case could always remember what to do when he sat down at the Porteus maze task. 'He would close his eyes, raise his finger in the air and say "Those puzzles".'

The demonstration of intact motor learning in the absence of any other form of long-term memory, is neurological evidence in favour of the theory that motor memory is dissociable from other mnemonic processes (Adams, 1967). This view was put forward on the basis of experimental work with normal subjects. Motor memory is not inter-ference-sensitive in the same way that verbal associative memory is. This could account for the surprisingly good motor memory of amnesics. In other words, motor memory does depend on medial temporal structures but because interference is not a threat to storage, the rudiment of function remaining in amnesics is sufficient for storage. It has been stressed that interference is the variable which is so devastating to the amnesic. However, a more likely explanation is that motor learning is not dependent on neural substrates in the medial temporal region but on other brain areas which are intact in amnesics. This alternative site has not been identified. There are no reports to my knowledge of patients with selective brain damage associated specifically with motor learning disability. Neurological theorists have considered, not unnaturally, that the motor substrates of the brain are likely to be involved. Marr (1969) for example, produced a mathematical theory of cerebellar function which could account for motor learning and memory. Bloomfield and Marr (1970) and Gilbert (1975), more recently, proposed that the noradrenergic innervation of the cerebellum from the locus coeruleus is a crucial feature of a motor memory mechanism. These speculations await further investigation, although Mason and Iversen (1976) have found that, contrary to Gilbert's suggestion, locus coeruleus lesions in the rat do not impair the ability to learn a complex new movement.

(4) Concept formation

Several experimenters have commented on the fact that H.M. appears to be able to form concepts. One of the clearest examples is provided by Milner's (1969) observation that H.M. performs well on the Wisconsin Card Sorting Task, in which successful performance depends on shifting between sorting categories based on shape, colour and number. He was tested shortly after his operation in 1955 and again in 1962. On both occasions he achieved the criterion of 10 consecutive correct responses for each of the three categories twice in the 84 cards of the test. The notable feature of his performance was the lack of perseverative errors to an incorrect sorting strategy. Presumably he quickly forgot a strategy if it was said not to be appropriate or in other words his sensitivity to interference helped him to lose irrelevant information. The two unilateral

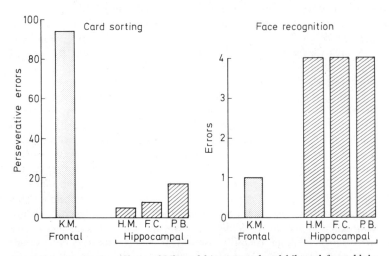

Figure 15. Contrasting effects of bilateral hippocampal and bilateral frontal lobe lesions on the performance of two tasks: the Wisconsin Card Sorting Test and a delayed face recognition task (Milner, 1968b). K.M. has sustained bilateral removal of the anterior portion of both frontal lobes, for post-traumatic epilepsy. P.B. and F.C. each had left temporal lobectomies, with persisting EEG abnormalities in the right temporal lobe (Penfield and Milner, 1958); H.M. is the case of bilateral mesial temporal lobe excision. K.M.'s lesion impairs sorting behaviour but not memory for faces; the bilateral mesial temporal lobe lesions have the converse effects.

temporal lobe cases from the Penfield and Milner (1958) study show similar success on this task (*Figure 15, left*). By contrast a bilateral frontal patient was severely impaired. However, when delayed (90-s) retention of face pictures was studied a completely opposite pattern of results was obtained (*Figure 15, right*). The amnesics now showed a characteristically high number of errors whereas the frontal patient could remember the pictures accurately.

Oscar-Berman (1973) has used an interesting concept formation task for studying Korsakoff patients. The subject was presented with a series

Set 1 Set 2

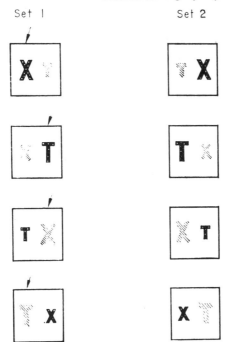

Figure 16. Examples of stimuli used in the Levinian (Hypothesis) analysis. Stimuli in Set 1 are outcome stimuli, and stimuli in Set 2 are blank-trials stimuli. Arrows over correct outcome stimuli were used in the Memory-Aid condition. 'Large' would be the correct hypothesis as indicated by the arrows in Set 1, and therefore, the correct responses to Set 2 stimuli would be RLLR. Examples of incorrect hypotheses are RRLL (the letter X), LLLL (the position left) RLRL (the dark colour), etc. Absence of an hypothesis appears as any combination of three responses to one side of the cards and one response to the other side (e.g. LLLR, RLRR, etc) (Reproduced by permission from Oscar-Berman, 1973)

of 16-trial two-choice visual discrimination problems. The two stimuli differed along the dimensions of colour, size, form and position; on any problem, there were two cues representing each dimension (e.g. red and blue, large and small, T and X, left and right). Thus, there were eight different combinations of stimulus pairs (two internally orthogonal sets of four stimulus arrays, each set differing only in the left-right position of the cues). An example of two such orthogonal sets of stimuli can be seen in *Figure 16*. On each of the 16 trials, the subject was asked to select one of the two stimuli as that which the experimenter had preselected as correct, and he was told that the 'correct aspect' of the stimulus would be the same throughout that problem. It was his task to discover which of the eight cues was the relevant one. On four orthogonal trials (trials 1, 6, 11 and 16, called outcome trials) the subject was given verbal feedback about the correctness of his choice; on the remaining 12 trials (the other set of four internally-orthogonal stimuli, presented three times in random orders), no such feedback was given (called blank trials). Half of the outcome trials were pre-designated by the experimenter as correct, and half were predesignated incorrect. That is, the experimenter said 'correct' or 'wrong' in a prearranged order and regardless of the subject's response. Each of the eight correct-wrong orders which can occur on the first three outcome trials was assigned to each of the first eight problems and then again to each of the last eight problems. On trial 16 of each problem, the subject was told 'correct' on half the problems, and nothing was said on the other half. From patterns of the subject's responses on sets of blank trials, she determined which hypotheses, if any, he was using for problem solution.

On this problem Cermak's patient S.S. solved 69 per cent of the problems compared with a mean of 47 per cent in control subjects, This improved to 100 per cent under the 'memory aid' condition when the subject could refer back to previous outcomes (i.e. Trials 1, 6, or 11 as the task progressed). S.S. appeared to be able to actively retain prior outcomes and was able to switch hypotheses effectively when learning that previous ones were inappropriate.

TEMPORAL LOBE PATHOLOGY ASSOCIATED WITH AMNESIA

It is now generally accepted that *bilateral* hippocampal damage is responsible for H.M.'s global amnesia. The surgeon's notes recorded that the suction lesion made in H.M. involved bilaterally the amygdala, the hippocampus throughout most of its extent and encroachment into deep temporal-lobe white matter. Quite early it was established that selective bilateral amygdalectomy did not result in global amnesia. Scoville used bilateral amygdalectomy for the treatment of abnormal behaviour and did not report any associated amnesia. This has been verified more recently by Narabayashi *et al.* (1963) who have carried out bilateral stereotoxic amygdalectomy in 21 patients without evidence of memory disturbance.

At the time H.M.'s condition was discovered and studied, surgeons at the Montreal Neurological Institute had been performing temporal lobectomies for the relief of epilepsy. Surgery to the left temporal lobe tended to be less radical in the late 1940s and early 1950s as the extent of the language area in the temporal lobe, particularly in the medial surface, was not fully understood. The accumulating evidence on these unilateral lesions was that generalized memory disorders were not seen after unilateral temporal lobe lesions, even when they did encroach upon the hippocampus. These observations seemed to emphasize further the significance of the bilateral damage in H.M. However, in 1958 Penfield and Milner presented a report on two cases with unilateral temporal lobe removal which did show generalized amnesia similar to that observed in H.M.

For a number of years it was inferred that bilateral damage would be seen in these patients at autopsy. One, an engineer, suffered from repeated epileptic fits associated with automatism and confusion. Electroencephalographic examination revealed a focus of abnormality in the left temporal lobe, A removal was made in the anterior temporal lobe which spared the uncus and hippocampal lobe. Epileptic seizures recurred after some years and, evidence was found of remaining abnormal tissues in the left temporal lobe region. A second operation was, therefore, performed which extended the left temporal lobe removal to include the uncus and the anterior half of the hippocampus and its overlying tissue. After this second operation profound amnesia was observed despite no deterioration of intelligence or language disorders. The surgeons were forced to conclude that damage to the right hippocampal zone must have existed prior to the surgery on the left hemisphere. A second patient was recorded in the Montreal series, who showed severe amnesia after a left radical temporal-lobe removal including most of the hippocampus.

Milner referred to these cases in the 1966 review and commented that patient 1, the engineer, had died in 1964 from a pulmonary embolism and, at autopsy, preliminary inspection of the brain indeed revealed severe damage to the medial temporal structures of the right hemisphere, confirming Penfield's prediction. More detailed neuro-pathological information on this patient has since become available (Penfield and Mathieson, 1974). In the right temporal lobe, the amygdala, the cortex of the superior, middle and inferior temporal lobe, the occipitotemporal and parahippocampal gyri were normal. By contrast, the hippocampus was shrunken, the normal laminar structure of the pyramidal cell groups indistinct. On microscopic examination a marked loss of neurones was observed. The thalamus, hypothalamus, diencephalon, basal ganglia, cerebellum and brainstem appeared normal.

This kind of histological pattern in the hippocampus has been termed 'Ammon horn sclerosis' by Spielmeyer (1930), and Sano and Malamud (1953) found that 29 out of 50 institutionalized epileptics showed such damage at autopsy. Hippocampal damage of this kind is frequently produced by birth trauma and may be intensified by lack of oxygen associated with the apnoea in certain forms of epilepsy.

Bilateral hippocampal damage has also been noted as a dominant feature of the neuropathology at autopsy in a group of related cases with vascular lesions of the temporal lobe, all of whom showed antero-grade amnesia (although this was not extensively or formally tested). Penfield and Mathieson (1974) list three such cases (Glees and Griffith (1952); Victor *et al.* (1961) and De Jong, Tabashi and Olson (1969).

Despite the apparent parsimony of the picture a few riders should be added. In fact we understand very little about the neural basis of long-term memory. A few questions and comments may serve as useful comments on this problem.

(a)   Why is it that ancient memories are said to be relatively intact?

Presumably because they are coded in substrates outside the hippocampus.

Penfield and Mathieson (1974) have commented that the extent of retrograde amnesia varied in the Penfield and Milner (1958) unilateral temporal-lobe series although the severity of the antero-grade amnesia was equal. He notes that the antero—postero extent of the hippocampal lesion varied in these patients and the second case who sustained a one-stage left-medial temporal lesion almost certainly had a larger lesion extending considerably more posteriorly in the hippocampus. It is suggested that the hippocampus has access to a widespread diencephalic substrate for memory storage and that during the span of life experience the hippocampal-diencephalic substrate is programmed and fixed in an orderly fashion involving initially the posterior hippocampus. As time passes more anterior hippocampal tissue is involved in the actual holding of previous experiences. Thus it would be predicted that anterograde with only minimal retrograde amnesia would be seen after a discrete anterior hippocampal lesion and that the retrograde amnesia would become more severe as the damage extended posteriorly. This indeed is the pattern in the two unilateral cases (P.N. and F.C.) of the Penfield and Milner (1958) study.

(b)   Is it significant that deep temporal lobe fibres were damaged in H.M. and the Montreal patients?

Bickford *et al.* (1958) found in patients that electrical stimulation of deep temporal lobe fibres prevented memories being formed.

The duration of the anterograde amnesia varied with the strength and duration of the current.

(c) In discussing cases like H.M. attention has always been directed to the body of the hippocampus itself. However, the hippocampus functions through its afferent and efferent pathways and amnesia may not be essentially a processing disorder but a disconnection syndrome. This comment generates two points. Firstly, that Van Buren and Borke (1972), when they examined sections of brain from three patients who showed global amnesia before death, felt bound to point out that in addition to hippocampal damage, widespread involvement of white matter and diencephalic structures was observed. Surprisingly these were not Korsakoff patients; the lesions were due to vascular damage.

Secondly, interesting cases cush as the one described by Teuber, Milner and Vaughan (1968) illustrate the point that the hippocampus should be considered as part of a wide neural circuitry in regard to its mnemonic role. They describe a patient who sustained a stab wound in the medial aspect of the base of the brain and showed a global amnesia qualitatively very similar to that described in H.M. and the unilateral temporal lobe patients of the Penfield and Milner (1958) series. By comparison with other published cases, it is concluded, that in this case the damage is likely to be focused on central gyri rather than the penduncle. However, the fact that this was a very discrete lesion and that the hippocampi and overlying cortex were certainly not involved led Teuber, Milner and Vaughan (1968) to comment 'amnesic syndromes can be produced by interfering with diverse parts of the complex anatomical system'.

As neuropathological evidence is not available on most of patients whose mnemonic performance forms the basis of this review, one cannot be categorical about the exact spectrum of neural damage which produces the condition we have described in this article as temporal lobe amnesia. This is a global amnesia for new information but it is clearly not associated with generalized cognitive loss, many functions being largely intact as discussed on pages 143–164. In addition to these formal performance measures the patients are motivated, are quick to follow instructions, have insight into their condition and adopt what strategies they can to overcome it.

Korsakoff psychosis is not to be included in this category of patient. As Cermak's comparative study shows, Korsakoff patients, although they have a global amnesia are also impaired on certain measures of encoding and STM (Cermak and colleagues, 1971, 1973 and 1974). Also they do not show the motivation and awareness of the temporal lobe cases. Clearly many (if not all) Korsakoff patients have bilateral damage to medial temporal structures but in addition there is usually more widespread diencephalic damage to midline structures and the fibre pathways interconnecting them. It would clearly be wrong to use temporal lobe cases and *unselected* Korsakoff patients as a homogenous amnesic group and hope to define the exact nature of the amnesic syndrome. However, it would appear that carefully selected Korsakoff patients, who do not show dementia, exhibit an amnesic condition virtually identical with temporal lobe amnesia as illustrated by Warrington's case material. The encephalitic cases which have been described in detail also show this highly selective amnesia. These patients almost certainly have virus-induced damage in a range of mid-line structures, including the hippocampus. However, in terms of their psychological deficits such patients have been grouped with the classic case, H.M. (*see* Drachman and Arbit, 1966). One must suppose that there is, in these patients, crucial and restricted hippocampal damage. However, there are other encephalitic cases with a different spectrum of damage which show a more general cognitive disorder. Such patients might resemble the Korsakoff case more closely than the temporal lobe case. A variety of CNS (central nervous system) diseases could, at least, theoretically produce what one might call the 'hippocampal amnesia'. As Cermak (1976) has commented 'It is most likely the case that the area of the brain affected . . . is far more important in determining the behavioural deficits exhibited than is the nature of the patient's disease.'

It is also possible that we shall need to reverse the dictum that *bilateral* medial temporal damage is a prerequisite for global amnesia. Mnemonic processing is especially related to language and, in particular, STM may have a unique role to play in verbal memory. Thus massive dominant hemisphere lesions might be expected to produce a particularly devastating amnesia. Geschwind (personal communication) believes that *acute* lesions of this kind (e.g. vascular infarcts) to the left hemisphere rather than surgical lesions are able to produce profound amnesia. He described such a case (Geschwind and Fusillo, 1966) who subsequently was included in the neuropathological study of Van Buren and Borke (1972) referred to earlier. Patients of this kind are likely to be more common in routine neurological services than cases with bilateral damage of the kind we have been discussing, and may provide interesting material for study. Geschwind maintains that *acute lesions* to the normal brain result in more severe cognitive disorders than surgical lesions to brains which, invariably, have been dysfunctional for very many years before surgery. This would be the case in epileptics and probably in many neoplasm cases.

Our knowledge of amnesia and normal memory can only benefit from detailed *comparative* studies of these various neurological cases.

WHAT IS THE FUNDAMENTAL DEFICIT IN TEMPORAL LOBE AMNESIA?

This question is included to complete the coverage of the review. However, it will not be dealt with in detail, as it has been considered by Piercy in an excellent and scholarly review in this volume. It is also an area fraught with controversy at present and it is clearly not the appropriate time for an 'outsider' to comment. It is an issue which will take time and effort to resolve. There are, firstly, methodological problems and traps. Secondly, as indicated in the previous section, pure temporal lobe amnesics are rare. Other neurological material must be used in the study of amnesia. However, the spectra of deficits clearly do vary in the different amnesic conditions. It is not clear at present how to accommodate all of this different information into a definitive statement on the nature of amnesia.

Some mention of this work should be made since one of the aims of the review is to record developments in the study of temporal lobe amnesia which have occurred since the first edition of this book was published. In that volume Weiskrantz (1966) contributed a thoughtful and provocative article on experimental approaches to the study of amnesia, in which he proposed a model of the neural basis of memory. He pointed out that failure to recall could be caused either by loss of information due to faulty storage or to inaccessibility of the stored information at the time of retrieval. He proposed that treatments such as electroconvulsive shock (ECS) could raise background noise in the CNS, making items of stored information indistinguishable from background noise. He was, at that time, impressed by observation in the rat that a learned habit was apparently forgotten 24 hours after ECS, but if retention was not tested until several days after such treatment, the learned habit reappeared. The ECS had, in some way, made the learned response temporarily unavailable.

In 1968, Warrington and Weiskrantz presented, for the first time, some experiments on amnesic subjects which suggested that new information was reaching the memory store but was unavailable at the time of recall. They noted that amnesics often reproduce items from earlier lists when they are performing in verbal recall situations. Testing memory by recognition or with partial information techniques, in which a 'clue' is given at the time of recall, greatly improves the memory performance of amnesics. A number of interesting experiments followed which have been reviewed by Warrington and Weiskrantz (1973). The suggestion is that amnesics do, indeed, store information but that the new items are easily interfered with by other information thus preventing accurate recall. Testing techniques which cut down on the levels of interference or enhance the discriminability of the required item by 'cueing' techniques are beneficial to the amnesic. Starr and Phillips (1970) 'in their encephalitic case' also raised the possibility of a retrieval deficit, pointing out that changing the manner of retrieval from recall to recognition resulted in improvement in memory performance for some items. They also note that 'The patients in the course of recalling one set of items, report items from other lists presented at an earlier date even though they would be unable to recall the earlier lists if directly questioned. We take this evidence to indicate that these patients are indeed capable of transferring verbal items into long-term storage.' By contrast, techniques which purposely increase the likelihood of

TABLE 9

Examples of semantically and phonetically related paired-word associate stimuli used in the experiment by Winocur and Weiskrantz (1976).

A. Semantic		B. Phonetic	
Stimulus	*Response*	*Stimulus*	*Response*
chair	bench	hair	fair
bowl	plate	class	mass
break	destroy	treat	heat
cook	bake	blame	shame
wool	cotton	gain	rain
earth	soil	dear	fear
ask	inquire	corn	horn
wealth	fortune	steam	dream
army	soldier	pray	clay
doctor	nurse	gold	told
laugh	happy	wall	call
metal	steel	sail	mail

confusion between different items impede amnesics further. It has been pointed out by several authors (*see* Iversen, 1976, for review) that it is exactly under such testing conditions that hippocampal lesioned animals show deficits — discrimination reversals, spatial reversal, discrimination with many negative cues, concurrent learning of discrimination tasks. Winocur and Weiskrantz (1976) model a recent task for amnesics on these animal observations. Verbal paired-associate learning is very difficult for amnesics but they found that lists of semantically related words were learned with equal ease by amnesics and controls (Table 9). On recall of list 1, after 1, 2 and 4 exposures respectively, amnesics made 3.8, 3.5 and 2.2 errors compared with 3.5, 2.2 and 1.5 errors in controls. Rhyming pair-associated word lists were also learned by amnesics. However, if after learning a list of semantically related words amnesics were asked to learn a second list which included the words from the first list with different non-semantically related words (e.g. silent—quiet becomes silent—yellow), amnesics were quite unable to learn the second list and showed many intrusion errors from the first list. Thus the use of related word-pairs cuts down on interference and facilitates learning in amnesics.

Unfortunately the effect of retrieval aids has not been systematically looked at in the surgical temporal-lobe amnesic cases. Milner commented in 1968 that 'Against this attractive hypothesis (retrieval) one can adduce two points: first, these same patients do show normal recall for many remote events antedating the onset of their amnesia . . .' Clearly it is difficult to explain why this would be so if a basic retrieval impairment existed. Retrieval of old and new information should be difficult. Although it is widely claimed that amnesics can remember old events, Sanders and Warrington (1971) have suggested this claim should be scrutinized with more rigorous long-term memory evaluation than has been used to date. The temporal lobe surgical case of Dimsdale, Logue and Piercy (1964) is reported to have a 10-year retrograde amnesia and the postencephalitic patients of the Rose and Symonds (1960) series, retrograde amnesia of 2—30 years extent. The impression that old memories are intact may arise from the fact that families often provide this information and refer to particular highlights in the family experience which have been repeated and discussed frequently. Furthermore, there is no independent way of evaluating exactly how detailed the memory of the amnesic is for these remote events. Using a technique devised by Warrington and Silberstein (1970) and expanded by Sanders and Warrington (1971) to assess memory for events and photographs over a 38-year period, Sanders and Warrington (1971) find that the five amnesics they studied, including the Dimsdale case, showed as severe deficits in recalling remote as recent events — an observation which supports the retrieval hypothesis.

Although not all may agree with Warrington and Weiskrantz (1974) that 'it seems difficult to sustain the credibility of the hypothesis that the amnesic deficit is one of consolidation', the importance of interference at the retrieval stage cannot be denied and is worthy of further investigation.

MATERIAL SPECIFIC MEMORY LOSS ASSOCIATED WITH UNILATERAL TEMPORAL LOBE DYSFUNCTION

Global amnesia appears to be associated with a profile of bilateral medial-temporal damage. It was generally considered that unilateral damage did not result in severe amnesia largely because the intact medial-temporal structures compensated and 'took over' to a large extent the functions of the damaged side. As Penfield commented (in Penfield and Mathieson, 1974) 'I've concluded, then, that under normal conditions removal of one hippocampal area would not produce the memory loss, that one hippocampus can duplicate the work of the other, and that, normally, either can carry on when its fellow is removed'.

Early unilateral temporal lobe lesion studies

In her 1966 review Milner noted that left temporal-lobe lesions impair the learning and retention of verbal material irrespective both of the method of measuring retention adopted and the modality of presentation

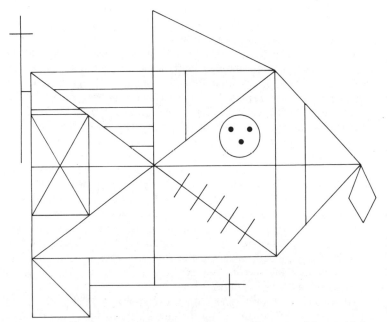

Figure 17. Illustration of the Rey—Osterieth figure (Reproduced by permission of Harper and Row Publishers Inc., Copyright L. Weiskrantz, from Milner and Teuber, 1968)

(visual and auditory). The patients report difficulty in remembering names, conversations, what has been read in the newspaper or books. One of the important advances in the last ten years has been the demonstration that unilateral temporal-lobe lesions produce highly specific memory disorders, depending on whether the dominant or non-dominant temporal lobe is damaged. It was originally recognized that dominant hemisphere lesions impaired both the perception and memory of verbal information. By contrast, right temporal-lobe damage impedes the memory for non-verbal material such as unfamiliar faces (Milner, 1968; Warrington and James, 1967a: de Renzi and Spinnler, 1966) and tunes (Shankweiler, 1966). On the recurring-figure memory test devised by Kimura (1963) squiggly line drawings are forgotten

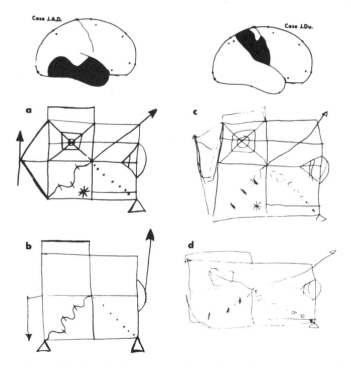

Figure 18. Reproductions of the Taylor figure by two patients with different posterior cortical excisions for epilepsy. Case J.A.D., right temporal lobectomy. Case J. Du., right parietal lobectomy. Above: lateral extent of removal. Below: a and c, copy from model; b and d, delayed recall. (Reproduced by permission of Harper and Row Publishers Inc., Copyright L. Weiskrantz, from Milner and Teuber, 1968)

whereas words or line drawings of common objects are not. The supramodel nature of the unilateral temporal-lobe deficit has been emphasized by the demonstration of equivalent impairment on auditory and tactile forms of the recurring figure test. Further compelling evidence of impaired memory for patterned visual stimuli after right temporal lobectomy comes from studies using the Rey—Osterieth pattern (*Figure 17*) (Work of Taylor cited in Milner, 1969). The patient is asked to copy the design as accurately as he can. Forty minutes later, without previous warning, he is then asked to draw the figure again but this time from memory. Right temporal lobe patients are hardly impaired on initial reproduction but they show a disproportionate loss of accurate reproduction when compared with the left temporal group.

TABLE 10

Specific defects as related to side and site of cortical epileptogenic lesion (Reproduced by permission from Milner, 1969)

Epileptogenic lesion	Card sorting categories	Delayed verbal recall		Picture anomalies	
	Mean	*Mean*	*Range*	*Mean*	*Range*
Left frontal	2.2	14.9	11–19	26.0	17–30
Right frontal	2.1	14.2	11–22.5	25.8	19–32
Left temporal	4.6	10.5	2–17.5	27.8	21–32
Right temporal	3.5	13.6	6.5–19	20.7	10–29
Left parietocentral	4.5	18.3	16–22.5	29.0	22–34

Right temporal lobe patients are also impaired on both the visual (Milner, 1965) and tactile (Corkin, 1965a) forms of the maze described earlier and the severity of the impairment correlates with the degree of involvement of the hippocampus.

Head injury cases who develop a localized epileptic focus have also been studied (Milner, 1969). Similar, albeit less severe, verbal and nonverbal memory loss can be seen in patients with active epileptic foci in the left or right hemisphere (Table 10) which have not been treated surgically. Furthermore, a *transient* specific temporal-lobe amnesia is seen after injection of sodium amytal into one or other carotid artery. Patients with vascular or neoplastic damage confined to one of the hemispheres have frequently been used (e.g. Warrington and James, 1967b; de Renzi, Faglioni and Spinnler, 1968) as the subjects in the studies which demonstrate a verbal/non-verbal memory dissociation between the hemispheres. Patients with such selective memory loss do not have difficulty in remembering daily events, because, although one form of memory may be deficient, other forms of coding are intact and form the basis of adequate day-to-day memory.

The study of facial memory referred to earlier has generated a degree of controversy. Both de Renzi and his colleagues (1966, 1968) and Milner (1968b) have studied the memory for faces and obtained an impairment after right temporal-lobe lesions. However, de Renzi argued that the deficit was one of higher order perception rather than memory, as severe deficits were seen under conditions of immediate recall as well as delayed recall. By contrast, Milner did not find a deficit in the right anterior temporal group under immediate recall conditions. De Renzi argues for a perceptual interpretation pointing out that a poor perceptual trace will result in inadequate memory. Milner argues, however, for a major mnemonic involvement in facial recognition task, because of the finding that the deficit increases in severity when a lesion encroaches upon the hippocampus.

Experiments by Dee and Fotenot (1973) support the view that the superiority of the right hemisphere in handling non-verbal visual information is associated with a superiority in the memory for such stimuli, rather than in the perception *per se*. In agreement with Kimura (1966) they find that tachistoscopically-presented complex visual forms are more accurately recognized when projected to the left, than to the right, visual field. Recognition was tested not by requiring the subject to choose amongst a large number of alternative stimuli but by presenting a single stimulus in central vision and asking whether or not it was the same as the target form. The delay between target presentation and choice varied from 0—20 seconds. At 0 seconds delay successful performance depends on perception and no field difference was found. As the delay increased, left-field superiority became apparent. Such results are consistent with Milner's finding that right temporal lobe lesions affect the memory for faces but not their perception.

Interestingly in the same issue of *Neuropsychologia* that Dee and Fotenot's article appeared, Hines, Satz and Clementino (1973) reported that similarly, the right visual field advantage for verbal information (also demonstrated by Kimura and Dee and Fotenot) is apparently concerned with a memory advantage rather than a perceptual advantage. They found that increasing the number of pairs of letters to be remembered or the interstimulus interval influenced performance, whereas varying the stimulus presentation time did not. However, the importance of right hemisphere perceptual functions can be demonstrated under certain testing conditions. In independent studies both de Renzi and

Milner have reported visual perceptual disorders after right temporal or parietotemporal lesions. Milner (1968b) finds severe deficits on the McGill Picture Anomaly Series, on the Hebb Block Design Test, on the recognition of tachistoscopically presented line drawings and de Renzi and colleagues (1968, 1971) on the perception of visual-spatial relationships. The discrepancy of facial recognition may arise from the fact that the test depends on both perception and memory and thus lesions involving both posterior parietotemporal and anterior temporal lobe tissue would be expected to show a deficit on both immediate and delayed recognition. Lesions confined to more anterior temporal-lobe regions would affect only the memory of the visual material. As Milner (1968b) comments 'removals limited to the right anterior temporal-lobe region tend to produce defects in recall that exceed those in perception, even though this may not be the case for more posterior lesions of the right hemisphere'. This is borne out by the observations of de Renzi, Faglioni and Spinnler (1968) that their right lesion group with visual field deficits (indicating deep posterior damage) are most severely impaired on the facial recognition task and by the study of Warrington and Rabin (1970a) on a large number of right vascular and neoplasm cases which concluded that on measures of visual perceptual-matching, the right parietal sub-group was the most severely impaired.

In the monkey the dissociation of perception and memory in the temporal lobe was resolved experimentally by the finding that bilateral lesions to the posterior ventral temporal lobe produced severe perceptual disorders, whereas anterior ventral temporal lobe lesions left perception relatively unaffected but severely impaired behaviour on visual memory tasks. Warrington and Rabin (1970b) have described results which suggest that it may be impossible to show a similar dissociation in patients with right parietotemporal lesions. Matched groups of patients with left and right lesions were tested on:

(a) a set of perceptual tests (Warrington and Rabin, 1970a) in which subjects were required to judge whether two visual stimuli (slope of line, position of dot, size of gap in a contour) were the same or different.

(b) Kimura Recurring Memory Test using four types of test stimuli: arrangement of dots, with and without a boundary, meaningless shape silhouettes and silhouette drawings of flowers, chosen to minimize verbal labelling. In the analysis of the results, the left and right lesions were divided into two groups, those with parietal and those with temporal lobe foci. Both groups were impaired on the recurring memory task but the temporal group made false negative errors, whereas the parietal group made false positive errors.

When correlations of perceptual and memory performance were calculated, a positive correlation was found only for the parietal group suggesting that their impairment on the memory task unlike that of the temporal group may have a perceptual basis. This is in agreement with their earlier findings that parietal but not temporal lesions impaired performance on measures of visual perceptual ability (Warrington and James, 1967b; Warrington and Rabin, 1970a). Newcombe and Russell (1969) tested 81 men with Second World War missile wounds of 20-year standing of either the right or left hemisphere. The right lesion group was impaired on both the Mooney Face-Closure Task and a visual stylus maze. In this study there was again indication of a dissociation between perception and memory in that there was no overlap between patients most severely impaired in 'closure' and those most severely impaired in maze-learning.

This dissociation of perception and long-term memory with right parietotemporal lesions can probably explain the apparent discrepancy between Milner's and de Renzi's results on facial recognition discussed earlier.

An interesting aside is afforded by the additional result that in the Warrington and Rabin study, rather surprisingly, lesions of the left hemisphere and in particular the parietal region also impair performance on immediate visual memory and on the recurring figure test. Warrington and Rabin speculate that this unexpected mnemonic deficit from the left parietal group is due to a deficit in *short-term* memory, which in independent studies has been demonstrated on more classic short-term memory tests such as the digit span (Warrington and Shallice, 1969). The recurring figure test involves STM and LTM and thus lesions to both the *left parietal* region and the *right anterior* temporal lobe produce deficits. It is not clear if the left parietal STM syndrome is restricted to *verbal*, particularly audioverbal, information, but even if it is one could quite reasonably say that the figures used by Warrington and Rabin have some potential for verbal coding.

More recent studies of unilateral temporal-lobe amnesia

Within the last five years attempts have been made to investigate more directly the inferences made on the basis of the earlier studies notably of (a) a verbal/non verbal distinction between the hemispheres, and (b) a correlation of severity of impairment with degree of hippocampal involvement; inferences, based on different groups of patients tested on a large assortment of tasks. Large numbers of well matched patients from the Montreal population with left or right lesions of varying extent have now been tested on pairs of complementary tasks specifically designed to test mnemonic capacity under identical conditions in both verbal and non-verbal modes. Corsi (1972) is responsible for the execution of these elegant studies which Milner has referred to in several recent reviews (1970, 1971, 1973).

Tests were chosen on which normal performance must depend on the ability to transfer information from the working memory to a more permanent store. The first pair of tests derived from a recurring digit test devised by Hebb (1961). In this, subjects attempted to memorize lists of numbers which exceeded the span by one digit. Lists were devised so that, unknown to the subject, one list recurred regularly. Although subjects did not apparently notice this, memory for the repeating list was better than for the remaining lists, presumably because it had been rehearsed through long-term memory several times. A non-verbal analogue was devised in which the memory span for spatial positions was determined. The subject watched the experimenter tap a series of blocks arranged on a board and was then required to re-tap the sequence. Lists of positions one greater than the span were then presented, again with one sequence repeating. Memory for the sequence was again enhanced in normal subjects. Corsi found that left temporal lobe lesions impaired memory for the digit sequence test and not for the spatial position test and *vice versa* in the case of the right temporal lobe lesions. However, the number of patients was large in each group and was therefore divided into three groups depending on the extent of the temporal lobe damage and the involvement of the underlying hippocampus (and presumably deep temporal lobe white fibres). In both left and right lesion groups the severity of the memory impairment correlated with the anterior extent of the lesion and the degree of hippocampal involvement.

The second pair of tasks was derived from the Peterson and Peterson test, a now classic method for studying the transfer of information from short- to long-term memory. The subject is presented with a list of digits or trigrams and is required to repeat them after a delay occupied with verbal interference (usually counting aloud; for example, backwards in threes from a given number). Interference impedes the transfer of information from STM to LTM. Patients with left temporal lobe damage show lower recall scores than right temporal lobe cases on this task. The non-verbal analogue was derived from a test of Posner (1966) in which the subject is required to remember a marked position on a line after a delay occupied with a number game. Right temporal lobe damage impairs this form of the test and again the severity of the deficit correlates with the extent of hippocampal involvement in the lesion.

Electroconvulsive therapy and memory disorders

Electroconvulsive shock proved a useful technique for studying the temporal and dynamic characteristics of information storage in the rat. It was of course clear that psychiatric patients receiving electroconvulsive therapy (ECT) also suffered amnesia after the shock. Inglis (1970) wrote that 'some of the transient side-effects of electroconvulsive therapy on humans resemble, in kind if not in degree, those more severe and chronic learning defects that are known to appear as an accidental result of temporal lobectomy in man'. This theory was backed by the observations that:

(i) ECT electrodes are typically placed over the temporal lobe.

(ii) ECT produces local electrical charges as well as a generalized widespread activity. The severity of the amnesia does not correlate with the clinical efficacy of the treatment suggesting that the two electrical effects may be dissociated.

(iii) After temporal lobe stimulation (particularly in the region of the amygdala) in conscious patients 'he seems to be deprived of the ability of making a memory record . . . but only when stimulation was followed by epileptic after-discharge' (Penfield, 1958, p. 215).

(iv) the hippocampus has a *very low* threshold for electrically induced convulsion.

In earlier times bilateral ECT was the common clinical practice. In recent years it has been clinically verified that the unilateral treatment is far more desirable from the point of view of the patient. A series of studies have now been published in which such a regime has been used and the results indicate that material specific memory loss is associated with the dominant and non-dominant hemispheric ECT. This material adds weight to the theory of a verbal/non-verbal dissociation between the hemispheres and thus ECT patients provide a large and valuable group of subjects for studying the amnesic syndrome.

A useful and extensive review of this work has recently been published by d'Elia (1970). The volume includes the clinical validation for the use of unilateral, as opposed to bilateral ECT, but this matter is not of concern here. Once unilateral treatment became acceptable, comparisons were made of the relative virtues of dominant (D) *versus* non-dominant (N-D) ECT. The general consensus of evidence demonstrates that dominant ECT produces severe confusional and verbal memory deficits (d'Elia, 1970; Sutherland, Oliver and Knight, 1969; Annett, Hudson and Turner, 1973; Fleminger, Thorpe and Nott, 1970; Costello *et al.*, 1970) albeit not as severe as after bilateral ECT. Non-dominant ECT does not produce equivalent impairment. In view of the

evidence on unilateral temporal lobe lesions it should not be surprising
to find that N-D ECT has no effect on verbal memory. As a great deal
of human memory performance depends on verbal processing, D ECT
is clearly going to be the more devastating treatment. Clinically therefore N-D ECT is favoured. However, if appropriate and sensitive non-
verbal tests are used, it can be demonstrated that N-D ECT does indeed
produce anterograde amnesia as would be predicted from the surgical
cases discussed earlier. As non-verbal memory is not of such importance
to Man, N-D treatment is considered the more acceptable of the two.

The dissociation of verbal and non-verbal memory disorders after
D and N-D ECT has now been found in several studies. Cohen *et al.*
(1968) tested the effect of D, N-D and bilateral ECT on a word
association test and on the Forms Test and produced the first clear
hemispheric dissociation effect. On the word test the subject had to
learn to complete each of seven word-pairs when given the first member
of the pair: for example, to respond 'whistle' when given the stimulus

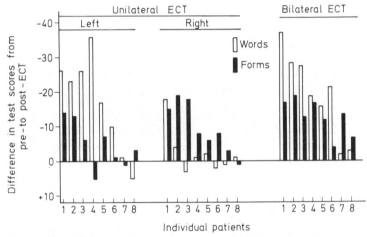

*Figure 19. Individual post-ECT decrements in word association and Forms Test
scores for all patients (Reproduced by permission from Cohen et al., 1968.
Copyright 1968 by the American Association for the Advancement of Science)*

word 'carpet'. The lack of a familiar associative connection between
the words was deliberate. On the non-verbal Forms Test the patients
were required to learn to complete, by drawing from memory, each of
seven designs when given a portion of the complete design. Seven trials
were given on each test. Eight patients were assigned to each ECT
group. On the day before the first treatment, they performed on the
tests and again on the day after the fifth treatment (spaced 2–3 days

apart). Every treatment resulted in a *grand-mal* seizure. The results of individual patients are illustrated in *Figure 19*. After bilateral ECT patients showed negative savings on both tests. After D(left)ECT the word test was more affected than the drawing task, whereas after N-D(right)ECT the reverse was true. Cohen and his colleagues (Berent, Cohen and Silverman, (1975) have presented data on additional D and N-D ECT cases which clearly substantiate the earlier findings. Halliday *et al.* (1968) tested more than 50 patients assigned to N-D, D and bilateral ECT groups. Learning and memory were assessed before and after the four ECT treatments and three months later. In one of the verbal tasks, the patients had to learn the meaning of five unfamiliar words and were scored in terms of the number of failures to give the correct meanings over five trials. One of the non-verbal tasks was the Rey – Davis peg-board (Zangwill, 1946b) in which the patient had to learn the different positions of a single fixed peg on each of a series of boards, each also bearing a number of movable pegs. The result with N-D and D ECT were as expected. D'Elia *et al.* (1976) have published equivalent results using a more extensive battery of tests. The four tests were: (1) 30-word-pair test; (2) 30-figure test; (3) 30-face test; (4) 30-geometrical figure test. The tests were conducted as follows.

(1) Word pairs were read out ten at a time and the subject was then asked to complete the pair after being presented with the first words of the pairs in a new order.

(2) This was derived from Cronholm and Molander (1960) and the subject was shown a picture of 30 common objects, which were pointed out and named. Immediately after presentation, the subject was asked to point out the objects which he recognized in a new picture, where the 30 objects are mixed with 30 others. After 3 hours the procedure is repeated with the first 30 objects distributed in a *different order* in a new picture mixed with the other 30 objects.

(3) Photographs of undergraduates (male and female) were the stimuli and the task structure was identical to that of (2).

(4) The geometrical figures were probably not completely 'non-verbal' but verbal labels could not easily be given to them. Again testing was as in (2).

The experiment was designed as an intra-individual crossover double-blind comparison in connection with the second and third treatments in the ECT series. Half the patients started with N-D and the other half with D ECT. The D ECT produced significantly poorer *delayed memory* on the word-test, whereas N-D ECT produced a significant effect on the delayed face test. The figure test did not differentiate the groups either in immediate or delayed memory testing, probably because the stimuli involved both verbal and non-verbal processing. Interestingly, the geometrical and face tests produced a significant deficit in the immediate memory for these stimuli after N-D ECT. This observation using ECT material supports the contention of de Renzi, (discussed on page 175) based on neurological cases, that the right temporal deficit is one primarily of higher perceptual processing rather than memory. This would explain why geometrical figures and faces are not very well remembered immediately after presentation whereas loss of verbal material handled by the left hemisphere is seen only after the 3-hour delay.

CONCLUSION

The last ten years have seen major advances in our understanding of the role of the temporal lobe in perception and memory. These studies have confirmed and extended the work of the previous decade in firmly establishing that the hippocampus has a unique role to play in the memory of ongoing experience. The other achievement has been the demonstration that lesions of the dominant hemisphere produce verbal deficits whereas equivalent damage of the non-dominant hemisphere results in disorders of non-verbal memory. In the process we have come to realize that we do not understand the terms 'verbal' and 'non-verbal' as clearly as we thought we did. No doubt this in its own right will lead to further advances. Furthermore, by studying the deficiencies in temporal lobe amnesia, we have found a new window on the processes of normal memory.

Acknowledgement

I am grateful to Dr Gregory Belenky for discussing with me the effects of electroconvulsive shock on memory function.

7 Memory Disorders Associated with Electroconvulsive Therapy

Moyra Williams

Convulsive therapy was first introduced by von Meduna in 1933, following observations that schizophrenic patients often became accessible and tractable after induced seizures. The chemical agents used by von Meduna in the early days were replaced in 1937 by electric currents passed through two electrodes placed on the forehead, an innovation introduced by Cerletti and Bini.

The usual method of administering the treatment (ECT) until the early 1960's is described in most psychiatric text-books (Mayer-Gross, Slater and Roth, 1960; Sargant and Slater, 1963; Kalinowsky and Hoch, 1961). Briefly, alternating electric current of 70 to 120 V is applied through temporal electrodes for 0.3 to 0.6 seconds, the aim being to produce a clinical seizure with the minimum amount of electric current. Treatments are usually given two to three times per week for two to four weeks, depending on symptoms.

In order to relieve the patients of anxiety over the onset of the seizure, and to minimize the risk of fractures, an anaesthetic (usually Pentothal or Brietal Sodium), followed immediately by a muscle relaxant (usually Scoline), are administered intravenously just prior to the passing of the current. Atropine may be given intravenously at the same time, or intramuscularly half an hour earlier. Patients who are particularly apprehensive may be given sodium amytal half an hour before the treatment, and those who become worried by the post-convulsive state may be given intravenous barbiturate after the fit. A number of variations in this basic procedure have been described and studied: up to 1950 ECT was usually applied without either anaesthetic or relaxants. Since the early 1960's variations in the placement of the electrodes have been given much attention, in some cases both electrodes being placed over one hemisphere only (Unilateral ECT), and in others the two electrodes being placed over the two frontal lobes (Bifrontal ECT). The effects of electrically induced convulsions have also been compared with those induced by chemical means, most frequently flurothyl or Indoklon (ICT — *see* Laurell, 1970). The differences observed will be discussed more fully later on.

Ever since ECT was first used, it has been noted that an adverse effect on memory is an almost invariable sequel. This has been of great concern to clinicians and has received considerable attention. The extent, duration and severity of the memory disorders following ECT depend on a number of variables, a description of which is the object of the present paper.

ASSESSMENT OF MEMORY

The degree and type of any memory disorder noted will depend largely on the functions measured and the means used to assess them. Some degree of memory is involved in most mental activity, and in clinical practice it is necessary to recognize at least four separate functions, since they may break down independently of one another. These are: (1) ability to take in and repeat material after a single exposure to it (short-term memory or memory span); (2) ability to retain it after long time intervals (long-term memory or retention); (3) ability to acquire skills or habits after repeated practice (learning); (4) ability to reproduce acquired skills as and when appropriate (for example, speech, manual dexterity, etc.). In addition to these functions, memory in the human subject has two aspects, the subjective and the objective.

Subjective sensations of memory impairment following ECT are often related to the symptoms of depression and may clear up with relief of the latter. They more often reflect ability to learn and to retain material for a short time than the ability to reproduce it after a longer interval (retention). Thus, Cronholm and Ottosson (1963a) tested 35 patients on three learning tasks which involved the immediate reproduction of visual and auditory stimuli. Their ability to reproduce the same material three hours later was compared with the immediate performance, the difference being regarded as a measure of 'forgetting'. These patients were tested before, and one week after the termination of a course of ECT, and at the second interview they were also asked to rate themselves according to whether they felt their memory was worse, the same, or better following the treatment. It was found that experience of improvement was reported by those patients whose depressive symptoms had been relieved, but not by the others, and furthermore, that the sensation of improvement was related to improvement in the immediate reproduction scores rather than to the longer-term retention.

A sense of impaired memory has often been reported by patients on account of inability to remember occasional remote experiences, even when such disorders are not apparent to any outside observer, and when learning and retention in test situations appear to be intact (Brody, 1944; Janis, 1950). This lack of the sense of familiarity appears to be similar to the phenomenon so commonly seen in other organic amnesic states, and described by Claparède (*see* MacCurdy, 1928) and discussed at some length by Baddeley (1975).

Objective evidence of memory disturbance following ECT has been measured by a variety of techniques. It is usually found that any form of prompting or reconstruction of the original situation (as in a recognition test), produces less evidence of impairment than tests of recall (Mayer-Gross, 1944). However, this is a feature of all aspects of memory function (*see* Piercy, Chapter 1 of this volume) and is not specific to the organic memory disorders.

On all tests, allowance has also to be made for the fact that different aspects of memory may be retained or impaired in isolation. An event which arouses a series of behavioural reactions may itself be forgotten, even though the reactions it aroused are retained in a person's repertoire. Again, the emotions aroused by a stimulus may persist and become associated with other stimuli, while the original stimulus is forgotten. Thus, Williams (1952) reports the case of a patient who was shown a series of pictures while in the confusional state after ECT, the first of which appeared to re-awaken a 'forgotten' traumatic incident from her youth. This picture was followed shortly afterwards by one of an innocuous chip basket. The following day the patient had no recollection of the traumatically-laden picture and, indeed, failed even to recognize it. She was, however, deeply disturbed that day, attributing her depression to 'wondering why you had shown me the picture of the basket'. Finally, isolated impressions may be retained, but without their spatial and temporal contexts, so that they are reported by the subjects as having been experienced at a different time (Williams and Zangwill, 1950). A similar phenomenon has been demonstrated in the performance of alcoholic Korsakoff patients by Huppert and Piercy (1976).

ASPECTS OF MEMORY AFFECTED BY BILATERAL ECT

ECT has an adverse effect on memory, both for events preceding the shock and for those experienced after it.

Memory for events preceding treatment

After every shock, patients experience a period of amnesia for the few seconds preceding it, similar to the retrograde amnesia following concussional head injuries. The events forgotten are usually independent of psychological importance, but are closely related to the onset of the seizure, those last experienced being most readily forgotten. The residual R.A. is seldom longer than a few seconds, but investigation has shown that the cut-off point is neither sharp nor sudden. Although most patients usually deny any recollection of visual stimuli presented to them within a few seconds before the onset of the seizure, it has been noted that such stimuli can frequently be picked out on a choice recognition test (Mayer-Gross, 1944) or can be recalled with prompting (Williams, 1950). Even so, most patients still fail to remember where and when they had seen the material, and the sequential nature of picture-sets or numbers tends to be missed.

Material learned by repetition is affected in the same way as isolated stimuli. Zubin and Barrera (1941), using paired associates composed of common household commodities with different brand names, found that if two sets of word-pairs were learned by subjects at 12-hour intervals and memory was tested some two hours after the second session, subjects remembered more of the second than of the first list. In a group of subjects given ECT immediately after the second learning task, no such differences were noted.

The degree to which an event or stimulus tends to be forgotten depends not only on the time of its occurrence, but also on (1) its nature, and (2) the efforts made to assimilate or 'encode' it (Dornbush and Williams, 1974). Familiar, easily-retained word-pairs are recalled more easily than unfamiliar ones (Williams, 1975), while pictures which a patient is expressly asked to remember are recalled more readily than those he is just asked to look at casually (Stones, 1970).

The effect of ECT on behavioural responses set up before it seems to be somewhat equivocal, but in general verbal responses elicited by visual stimuli immediately before ECT are elicited again more easily afterwards, in spite of the fact that the original stimuli have been forgotten.

As well as amnesia for test stimuli, many patients complain of forgetfulness for remote personal events. 'Gaps' of memory, particularly for a period of disturbed mental activity, may remain permanently (Ebtinger, 1958). Names of persons and places and habits of work are also vulnerable (Brody, 1944). These memory losses resemble closely those following concussional head injuries (Williams and Zangwill, 1952), and fall outside the scope of R.A. as conventionally assessed.

In the restitution of personal memories following ECT, as in those after head injuries, there is nearly always a considerable 'shrinkage' with the passage of time. On first regaining orientation, patients may be unable to remember a large part of their past lives, but the gaps gradually close as normal mental functions are restored. The pattern of shrinkage is not always strictly from past to present (Ebtinger, 1958), and consists rather of filling in between islands, as in the case after head injuries (Zangwill, 1964). Time may, however, be important in the recovery of the most recent pretreatment memories. Cronholm and Lagergren (1959) found that stimuli shown to subjects 60 seconds before treatment were recovered before those shown 15 seconds before it, and the latter, before those presented only 5 seconds prior to the shock. Kehlet and Lunn (1951), however, found no such shrinkage. Their subjects were shown three series of pictures 16 hours, half an hour and a few seconds before the shock. Examination half an hour and 2 hours after the shock showed no improvement in memory at the two retest sessions.

Retention and learning after treatment

Immediate effects of treatment

The early recovery of mental activity following each shock again shows many similarities to that after head injury. Patients pass through a stage similar to that seen in post-traumatic amnesia (P.T.A.), when they are disorientated, confused and unable to respond to questions in a coherent manner. Stimuli presented to them at this time are forgotten almost immediately, and after final recovery of orientation the patients claim total amnesia for events occurring at this time.

Studies by Dornbush, Abrams and Fink (1971) and by Stones (1973) show that the forgetting at this time is due to very rapid decline in availability of information after perfectly adequate perception. Thus, immediate reproduction of letters or digits is within normal limits, but the differences between basic and post-ECT performance increase as the retention interval is increased from 4 to 24 seconds.

The adverse effect of ECT on retention and learning passes off gradually (Zinkin and Birchnell, 1968; Miller, 1970) although some deterioration of performance compared with pretreatment level is usually seen for 4–6 hours. Zinkin and Birchnell failed to find any cumulative effect of successive treatments, but Brunschwig, Strain and Bidder (1971) found a steady decline in performance in some patients, though not in others. The degree of decline was found by them to be related to remission of depressive symptoms.

Although there are similarities in the patterns of retention and loss of information in the R.A. and P.T.A. caused by ECT (Williams, 1950; Zinkin and Birchnell, 1968), there are also some differences, especially with regard to material mediated by verbalization (Williams, 1973, 1977).

The restitution of memory for past events after each individual treatment is gradual and parallels that for learning. Patients almost invariably regain personal orientation (knowledge of name, occupation and home address) before that for place or time, the latter being the last to be restored in most instances (Lancaster, Steinart and Frost, 1958; d'Elia, 1974). It is usually considered that those habits most firmly established and most often practised are the first to be regained. This principle applies even to the restitution of vocabulary. Rochford and Williams (1962) asked 12 patients to name a series of simple common objects, the names of which were acquired at different ages by children, and were found to present different degrees of difficulty to patients with organic dysphasia. The names themselves represented different degrees of frequency of usage in the language as a whole. It was found that a very close parallel existed between 'difficulty' or rarity of word, and time elapsing between treatment and recall of it by the ECT patients. Whereas a comb (a frequently used word learned by children at the age of four years) could be named by 90 per cent of the patients within two minutes of them being able to give their own names, the teeth of the comb (rarely used and not learned by children until the age of 11 years) could not be named, on the average until 12 minutes later. Although this suggests a regression in terms of age, the authors suggest that age of acquisition and restitution of mental activity may both be related to, and dependent on, frequency and usage.

It is important to note that after unilateral non-dominant ECT, word-finding is not affected in this way (Pratt and Warrington, 1972), and the early post-ECT confusional state passes off much more quickly (Halliday, *et al.,* 1968; d'Elia, 1974). This will be discussed more fully later in this chapter.

Long-term effects of treatment

For some time after return of full consciousness and orientation, post-ECT patients often continue to experience gaps for pretreatment memories and defects of retention, although immediate memory span returns to its pretreatment level fairly quickly. Ability to learn new material is largely dependent on depressive symptoms (Cronholm,

Eriksson and Lindgren, 1961), but usually returns to its pretreatment level by two to three weeks after termination of the treatment (Zubin and Barrera, 1941). The main defects noted on psychological tests are similar to those seen in other organic amnesic states (*see* Piercy, Chapter 1 in this volume).

The length of time over which this defect persists is not easy to establish, and appears to depend largely on the individual subject. There is usually still some sign of retention defect one week after termination of a series of bi-weekly treatments (Hetherington, 1956; Cronholm and Blomquist, 1959), and some observers claim that recall of common words after interpolated learning of nonsense syllables does not return to normal until three weeks after termination of a course of ECT. Cronholm and Molander (1964), however, found complete restitution of all memory functions, including retention, in a group of 28 patients re-examined one month after the last electroshock treatment of a series. The mean number of treatments in this series was 5.3, and the period over which the treatment was given had a mean of 17.9 days.

VARIABLES AFFECTING MEMORY AFTER ECT

Intensity of electrical stimulation

Many variations have been tried in the manner of giving ECT. Mayer-Gross, Slater and Roth (1960) claim that there is little convincing evidence that modifications of wave-form, pulse-strength, duration and interval between pulses, and polarity, have different effects on post-convulsive confusion or on memory disturbances. Brengelman (1959) substantiates this view, but Cronholm and Ottosson (1963b) studied the effect of treatment with ultrabrief stimuli, as opposed to routine treatment, with pulses of longer duration, and compared both with the effect of routine treatment, accompanied by lidocaine to reduce and modify the seizure activity. They found that with the ultrabrief technique, R.A. as assessed by the patients' ability to recall material presented to them before treatment, was shorter than with the routine method. After lidocaine, more electrical energy had to be applied to induce a seizure than with the routine method, but the R.A. in patients so treated was no longer than after the routine method alone. Prolongation of the cerebral discharge by continuous insufflation of oxygen was found by Holmberg (1955) to increase both the therapeutic effects of treatment and the memory impairment, but Fink (1974) believes that hyperoxygenation before application of the current may reduce memory impairment.

It seems from these observations that the memory impairment itself may be related more closely to length and extent of cerebral discharge than to the energy used in producing it, but Ottosson (1960b) carried out another carefully controlled experiment to investigate this point, and found that impairment of memory was more closely related to intensity of stimulus than to length of cerebral discharge. This has been confirmed by more recent investigators in both animal and clinical studies (Fink, 1974; McGaugh, 1974).

Electrode placement

The effect of applying the electrodes to one side of the head only has attracted much attention. The effects of stimulating the non-dominant hemisphere only were first reported by Lancaster, Steinart and Frost (1958) who compared the return of orientation and memory for a sentence read to the patients immediately before treatment, in 28 patients receiving unilateral ECT, with that of 15 patients receiving bilateral ECT. It was noted that after unilateral ECT, orientation returned consistently earlier than after bilateral treatment, and that memory for the sentence was retained in significantly more cases. Cannicott (1962) studied 40 patients given unilateral non-dominant ECT, many of whom had previously had bilateral treatment. The nursing staff reported no post-ECT confusion in the unilateral group, and the patients themselves reported less memory impairment than after bilateral treatment. Typical descriptions by the patients were, 'The previous treatment affected recent events and current happenings . . . your system does not affect the memory so much' and, 'Last time I could not remember stupid little things like people's names . . . this time I just come home and carry on normally'.

It was not till 1968, however, that more carefully controlled studies began to be carried out comparing the effect of Unilateral Non-Dominant UND) with Unilateral Dominant (UD) and Bilateral (BiECT). Zinkin and Birchnell (1968) compared UND only with BiECT, and the only aspect of memory assessed by them was that for picture recognition. They found significant differences in favour of UND both in R.A. (recognition 2 hours after treatment of pictures seen 3 seconds before it) and in anterograde amnesia. In neither group of patients was the performance after two treatments any different from that after six (ruling out the possibility of cumulative effects), and in both groups performance fell off with increasing time-lapse between presentation of the stimulus and test — i.e. with retention interval. Both groups also showed improvement of performance with increasing time between shock and stimulus presentation; but whereas the UND group was back to its pretreatment level within two hours, the BiECT group still showed some deficits up to four hours later.

Halliday *et al.*, (1968) compared the performance of right-handed subjects receiving UND, UD and BiECT on three different tests; Picture Recall, Verbal Learning (word definitions), and Non-Verbal Learning (the Rey–Davis Board). Patients were tested before and after the termination of a full course of treatment and again some months later. It was found that patients receiving UND received slightly more treatment sessions than those receiving BiECT (several of those receiving UD found the experience so disturbing that they withdrew from the trial), but despite this their post-treatment learning deficit cleared up more quickly. As expected from the asymmetry of cerebral function (Inglis, 1969) they found that patients receiving left-sided ECT (UD) showed learning deficits predominantly in the verbal sphere (word definition) while those receiving right-sided UND showed them predominantly in the non-verbal sphere (Rey–Davis). The greatest difference between the three forms of treatment, however, lay in the speed with which personal orientation returned and general confusion cleared up after UND – a phenomenon greatly welcomed by the patients themselves.

D'Elia in 1970 described another well-controlled trial in which he found that although the average number of treatments needed for the relief of depressive symptoms was again slightly higher in the UND than in the BiECT group the ultimate therapeutic effect of both forms of treatment was the same. Both R.A. (assessed by the recall of personal data and word-pairs) and anterograde amnesia (measured by ability to recall personal experiences, world-news and word-pairs) were significantly less in the UND than in the BiECT group. In a subsequent study comparing UD with UND and BiECT, d'Elia (1974) found memory less disturbed in even UD than BiECT, although the difference did not reach significance in the verbal test (the learning of 30 Word-Pairs). A similar difference was reported by Dornbush, Abrams and Fink in 1971. In considering the possible reasons for these differences much attention has been paid to the part played by verbalization in retention and retrieval. Although the ability to name objects from pictures or verbal descriptions of them tends to return sooner after right-sided UND than after BiECT in right-handed subjects (Pratt and Warrington, 1972) there is a good deal of variation (Pratt, Warrington and Halliday, 1971). Clyma (1975) found that using this task to determine dominance, 12 per cent of a group of right-handed subjects referred for ECT showed a right hemisphere dominance. A point of interest was that this group consisted predominantly of personality disorders and did not show great relief from their depressive symptoms after the treatment, which raises speculations about the connections between mental illness and cerebral dominance as well as about the effect of ECT itself.

Why picture recognition should be more severely affected after bilateral than after unilateral right-sided treatment seems unclear, unless verbalization is commonly involved in the retrieval of pictures (Williams, 1973). Another possibility suggested by d'Elia is that in unilateral ECT there is less spread of current throughout the cerebrum, so that the unaffected hemisphere can 'take over' from the other.

A suggestion was put forward by Inglis (1969) that on theoretical grounds ECT given through electrodes applied to the frontal lobes should be as effective against depression as BiECT but cause less memory impairment. This was tried out by Abrams and Taylor (1973), but although they found less memory impairment after bifrontal ECT than after either UD or BiECT, the antidepressant effect of the treatment was not so good. They also found seizures difficult to elicit in three cases. Knowles (1973) overcame this latter difficulty by placing both electrodes in the midline fronto-central, 4–6 cm apart. Although he 'never failed to induce a convulsion with 65 volts for 6–8 seconds', he makes no mention of the therapeutic or amnesic effects of the treatment.

Number and interval of shocks

The treatment of some refractory conditions with ECT, applied two or three times per day for up to 34 treatments (Intensive ECT), was first described by Milligan (1946). By the end of such treatment, most patients showed 'complete regression', consisting of incontinence, dysarthria or muteness, rigidity and increased reflexes.

The number of treatments necessary to produce this state varied with individuals, and in one case took 65 single shocks. Emergence from the state usually took seven to ten days, but according to this author no lasting damage to cerebration occurred in 50 patients so treated. He mentions one patient, 'employed as a linguist in a government department who reports that she has no memory difficulties, but continues to express herself freely in five languages'. Russell and Jillett (1953) describe a different form of intensive ECT, in which an initial stimulus of 150 V for one second is immediately followed on the first day by seven further stimuli at intervals of 0.5 seconds, the number of extra stimuli being increased by one per day up to ten on the fourth day. The authors claim that the increased number of stimuli 'do not increase the severity of the fit, but render it smooth and short' and furthermore, that after intensive ECT, 'the degree of amnesia and confusion following treatment varies from case to case, but is no greater than that following a comparable number of ordinary ECT's. Stengel (1951), on the other hand, carried out a careful clinical study of ten patients receiving intensive ECT (two to four shocks on successive days for one to two weeks) and reported that in four of them, the residual R.A. for personal events extended far beyond that normally seen. One patient, who at first had forgotten all events and learning in her early childhood, gradually improved, but never recovered any memory for the three years preceding the beginning of the treatment. He notes that these patients did not show any other features of the organic amnesic syndrome (that is, confabulation or disorientation), and that all the patients who were left with massive and unremitting R.A. had shown marked hysterical tendencies before treatment was initiated.

On the basis that, as it usually takes 6–8 individual shocks to clear up a depressive illness, the quicker these could be given the better, Abrams and his colleagues (Abrams, 1974) tried administering these in a single day and under one anaesthetic instead of spaced out at three-to-four-day intervals. They found that the memory defect caused by this number was not significantly greater than after a single shock – a fact they felt might be explained by the absence of 'Turnover in cerebral amines'.

Alexander (1953) claimed that a non-convulsive stimulus applied immediately after a straight ECT (counter-shock) caused the subsequent memory defect to clear up more quickly than without it. This was also confirmed by Russell and Jillett (1953), but Cronholm and Ottosson (1961) found the immediate R.A. to be increased by such a procedure.

It is usually believed that, even if treatments are spaced at two-to-three-day intervals, return of memory functions will become progressively slowed up, and ultimate recovery retarded as the number of shocks increases. This belief is perhaps based on the finding that the convulsive threshold tends to rise after successive treatments (Kalinowsky and Hoch, 1961), so that the stimulus necessary to produce a seizure may have to be increased as a course of treatment progresses. Experimental work does not bear out the impression that memory impairment increases with the number of treatments given. Thorpe (1959) studied the ability of patients to learn ten three-letter nonsense syllables four hours after every treatment, for 20 successive treatments. The learning graphs showed some fluctuations for the first ten days, but thereafter showed a steady improvement up to the 20th day. Cronholm and Lagergren (1959) found that there was a trend towards more complete and more rapid recall of single numbers given to the patients just before the shock, from the first to the fourth treatments. Perlson (1945) has also described one patient who received a total of 248 individual shocks, without showing any residual impairment of cerebral function. It should be noted, however, that these observations all refer either to learning or to the retention of skills acquired before treatment was started. It is unfortunate that the aspect of memory most often disturbed by ECT, that of retention, has not been measured by these observers and no study has been published in which the retention defect after ECT has been related to number and frequency of treatments.

Concomitant medication

Brengelman (1959) concludes that no effect of the anaesthetic can be noted in the memory disorders following ECT; and as the memory disorders reported since the widespread use of anaesthetics and relaxants are very similar to those reported earlier, this conclusion seems justified. The only direct investigation of the effect of medication is that described by Cronholm and Molander (1957). Using the same battery of tests as had been used to measure the post-ECT memory disorders, they studied the effect of Evipan on retention, given one hour after initial presentation of the test material. No fall-off in memory was observed in these subjects, compared with that seen in a comparable group who received both Evipan and ECT.

In another study, Owen and Williams (1975) compared a group of women undergoing minor surgery necessitating anaesthesia with matched non-anaesthetized controls on the recall of pictures. No differences in either free or cued recall were observed.

Age and clinical diagnosis of patients

Although clinicians are usually reluctant to give ECT to elderly patients for fear of the treatment exacerbating the incipient effect of age, there is no evidence that the memory of older people is more adversely affected than that of younger subjects (Ottosson, 1970). This seems curious in view of the fact that stronger currents are required to induce seizures in older than younger subjects, and that, as already mentioned, the memory disturbance following ECT is directly related to current strength. The author suggests several explanations for the apparent anomaly: (1) the memory of older subjects being basically less good than that of younger ones has less to lose; (2) the extra energy may be taken up by extracerebral tissues and does not necessarily affect the brain; (3) the patients in the sample studied did not include any who showed signs of anteriosclerosis or senile dementia, and were therefore rather atypical. Ottosson further points out that the test was carried out after a single treatment only, and does not exclude the possibility of cumulative effects being greater in older subjects.

The retention defect caused by ECT appears to be largely independent of mental illness as such. The pretreatment performance of patients in the different diagnostic groups shows many characteristically different patterns, but pre- and post-shock memory functions were found by Cronholm and Lagergren (1959) to show the same quantitative and qualitative differences in all diagnostic groups. Where immediate memory span and learning are assessed, the situation is somewhat different. Improvement in performance commonly follows relief of depressive symptoms, but does not necessarily follow relief of other symptoms of mental disorder.

Stengel's observation (1951) that prolonged R.A.'s following intensive ECT in his group of patients all occurred in those with marked hysterical symptoms is noteworthy. He suggests that although none of these patients had shown hysterical amnesias prior to treatment, the physical disability suffered by them may have been used as an 'organic nucleus' for further symptom formation. The use of ECT in hysterical patients is now strongly condemned by most clinicians (Sargant and Slater, 1963), although Milligan (1946) found that the most satisfactory results of intensive ECT in his 50 subjects were in those patients who showed hysterical conversion symptoms.

COMPARISON BETWEEN MEMORY DISORDERS FOLLOWING ECT AND THOSE IN OTHER CONDITIONS

Some similarities between the memory changes following ECT and those following concussional head injuries have already been noted. Cronholm and Schalling (1963) compared the performance of a group of brain-injured (but not wholly incapacitated) subjects with that of patients receiving ECT, on a wide range of intellectual and memory tests. Both groups were found to show defects of retention in comparison with normal controls, but the brain-injured group also showed impairment on other tests of intelligence, whereas the patients receiving ECT did not.

Using the same material as had been used to test the memory of ECT patients, Williams (1953) found that patients after head injury showed much the same type of retention defect as did those after ECT.

Both groups showed similar responses to prompts and cues, having especial difficulty in spontaneous recall.

From a psychological point of view, the retention defect after ECT is very like that seen in Korsakoff states due to chronic alcoholism, or to brain disease involving particularly the area surrounding the floor and walls of the third ventricle (Whitty, 1962; *see* Chapter 8) or the hippocampal region (*see* Chapter 6). Here the picture is characterized by good preservation of intellect and personality, with marked impairment of recent memory, together with appreciable retrograde amnesia. In toxic-confusional states and in cases of cerebral atrophy, on the other hand, a generalized impairment of cerebral functions accompanies, and occasionally predominates over, that of memorizing and recall. In this connection, it is interesting to note that Cronholm, Eriksson and Lindgren (1961) compared the performance of workers exposed to high doses of carbon monoxide with a control group, on the same tests as had been used on the patients receiving ECT. There was no significant difference between the two groups on the tests of memory, but there was a suggestion that exposure to carbon monoxide had had an adverse effect on intellectual functions other than memory.

The question of whether the memory disorder following ECT is due to the seizure, or to the electrical disturbance causing it, has already been discussed briefly. Some light may be thrown on this by comparing the disorders following ECT with those following seizures due to other causes. In idiopathic epilepsy, some momentary loss of memory for events preceding the fit, together with some amnesia for the period after it (during which apparently purposeful activity may be carried out) is usually reported. Subsequent retention defects, of the sort seen after ECT, however, seem to be rare. After chemically induced seizures, the picture more closely resembles that after ECT. Sherman and Mergener (1942) reviewed the work published up to 1942, and themselves described a study carried out on ten patients who received a mixture of electrically and chemically induced shocks. They found no significant differences on any tests. Brody (1944), however, quotes the case of one patient who, throughout a course of Cardiazol treatment, had not complained of memory impairment during or after the treatment, but a subsequent course of ECT had to be terminated because her memory disturbance worried her so much. The effect of Metrazol on the reversal of habits was studied by Rodnick (1942). Subjects were taught two mutually exclusive habits (habit 1: moving the finger to the left at the sound of a signal; habit 2: moving it to the right). After Metrazol treatment, more patients reverted to the first habit than did a comparable group of patients receiving no treatment. It was concluded from this experiment that Metrazol had been responsible for wiping out the second habit and causing reversion to the first, but to what extent this could be related to other aspects of memory was not discussed. Indeed, the author himself talked more in terms of 'conflict resolution' than of memory impairment.

The finding that Speer's synthetized fluorinated ether, flurothyl (Indoklon) was epileptogenic but otherwise harmless started a wave of trials in which this substance replaced electricity in the treatment of depressive patients (Laurell, 1970; Small and Small, 1972; Small, 1974). Although its antidepressant effect was similar to that of bilateral ECT, it caused less impairment of memory, despite producing a much longer seizure. This is explained on the basis that chemically-induced seizures are probably primarily subcortical.

THE NATURE OF MEMORY AS SEEN THROUGH ITS BREAKDOWN AFTER ECT

The disorders of memory following ECT are regarded by clinicians as an unwanted side-effect of the treatment which all efforts should be made to reduce or eliminate. Perhaps it is for this reason that little use has been made of the experimental situation afforded by it to study the breakdown of memory in Man. Much work has been carried out on animals (McGaugh, 1974) but, as will be appreciated, many aspects of memory which can be studied in the human subject are closed to the animal psychologist. For example, the difference between repetition of a response and a sense of familiarity with or recognition of the stimuli originally arousing it are difficult to appreciate except by verbal report.

Some studies aimed at defining the different aspects of memory which may break down independently have already been described. Thus, it is frequently found that a raised threshold to recall precedes actual obliteration (Mayer-Gross, 1944), and that displacement of recalled material, together with fusions and distortions similar to those seen in normal subjects after time-lapse (Bartlett, 1932), are a feature of the paramnesias due to all forms of organic cerebral disturbance (Woods and Piercy, 1974; Huppert and Piercy, 1976).

It is also commonly observed that as in other organic amnesic states, behavioural patterns may be acquired even though the circumstances of their acquisition are forgotten. Some attention has also been paid to the sensory modality in which the stimulation is presented, and the relevance of this to hemispheric asymmetry as demonstrated by unilateral placement of the electrodes. However, little effort has been made by experimental or academic psychologists to investigate the human memory functions through studies involving the clinical application of ECT, though several have been made involving patients with organic amnesic states due to cerebral derangement from other causes (*see* Piercy, Chapter 1 in this volume). The situation presented to the psychologist by the clinical application of ECT would seem to present an ideal opportunity for testing out predictions based on various theoretical models as well as opportunities for obtaining more information about the factors actually concerned in memory itself; and it is hoped that before this 'unwanted side-effect' is entirely eliminated from the treatment of depression, psychologists will have learned something from it.

SUMMARY

(1) After an electrically induced convulsion, there is always some amnesia for (a) events preceding it (retrograde amnesia); and for (b) events experienced immediately after it (anterograde amnesia). The retrograde amnesia, which may at first be appreciable, rapidly shortens to its final brief duration (a few seconds). The defect of memory for current events clears rapidly after a single treatment, though some difficulty in retention (accelerated forgetting) may remain for some hours. Residual memory defect may, however persist for some weeks after termination of a course of treatment.

(2) The changes in memory functions caused by ECT are basically similar to those seen in other organic amnesic states.

(3) There is evidence that retention defect is related in some measure to the strength and duration of electrical stimulation and to the duration of the seizure. There is also evidence that confusion and memory defect are less marked following unilateral (non-dominant) than bilateral ECT, and that the type of item remembered is different.

(4) There is no good evidence that the acquisition of new habits or the execution of those acquired in the more remote past are significantly affected, even by a prolonged course of ECT.

(5) The opportunity for experimental studies of memory functions in Man afforded by ECT has been poorly utilized by experimental and theoretical scientists.

8 Neuropathology of Amnesic States

J.B. Brierley

The purpose of this selective review is to present and to discuss some of the considerable information that has been obtained from the neuropathological examination of the human brain in cases of amnesia. This evidence has led to the conclusion that the retention and perhaps, to some extent, the recall of sensory impressions and experience are dependent upon the structural integrity of certain small and relatively well-defined regions of the brain. This conclusion does not imply that the functions of retention and recall are carried out within these regions, any more than that the unconsciousness resulting from a small lesion in the upper brainstem justifies the conclusion that consciousness resides at this level.

The ability to receive a sensory impression, to retain it and to recall it at the appropriate moment, will be referred to as the process of memorizing. Some disturbance of this process is a salient feature of many of the disorders of memory that have an organic basis, and those that occur in hysteria and the functional psychoses will not be considered here. In clinical practice, four terms are commonly used to describe disorders of memorizing. The first is a defect of 'immediate memory' and is usually evinced by a reduced digit-retention span. The second term is a defect of 'recent' or 'short-term memory' or of 'memory for recent events'. Here the reduced retention span is one of hours or even days. A distinction between these two terms is not always made and Brown (1964), in a review of 'short-term memory', uses this latter term to describe retention for a period of seconds or minutes. It may be that the distinction between 'immediate' and 'recent memory' is more artificial than real, and due to the fact that the presentation of digits lends itself to easy quantitative assessment of retention. The retention times of everyday stimuli, however, may increase progressively from a period of a few seconds, without the sharp break implicit in the two terms.

A third term is a defect of 'remote' or 'long-term memory' or of memory for 'remote events'. The time span of this type extends from the events of a few months before the present time, back to those of childhood. There seems little reason to believe that 'short' and 'long-term' memories are subserved by different processes within the nervous system.

In the normal subject, it is evident that the greater part of the sensory impressions received in the course of a day will not be available to recall for more than a few minutes or even seconds. Progressively smaller fractions will be retained for progressively longer periods, and only a minority will remain to constitute remote events when recalled at some future date. The presence of damage within those portions of the brain that will be described later, can lead to an expansion of the territory of the 'normally forgotten', at the expense of that of the 'normally remembered'.

The characterization and the measurement of defects of memory are the task and the goal of the psychologist, but it must be noted that the psychological tests in current clinical use can define and measure a defect of memory for recent events when retention is reduced to a matter of minutes. If, however, the reduced retention span is a matter of weeks, the interval between the presentation of test material and the assessment of its recall will permit the intrusion of many uncontrollable external influences, which may affect recall itself. In such cases, the performance of the usual psychometric tests will be normal, and the evidence of a defect of memorizing is largely that of the patient himself (if insight is retained), his relatives and his immediate social contacts. A disability defined in this way, although less incapacitating, is no less real than one in which retention, reduced to a matter of minutes, can be given quantitative expression on the basis of psychological test scores.

A fourth term employed to define a particular disorder of memorizing is 'retrograde amnesia'. This term is relatively precise, in that it defines a period of time before an accident or an illness, for which the patient can recollect either none or only some fraction of the salient events.

There is now considerable evidence to show that some impairment of memory for recent events, and frequently some period of retrograde amnesia, are symptoms of damage within two topographically separate but interconnected regions of the brain. These are the mammillary bodies, together with certain thalamic nuclei in the diencephalon and the hippocampal formations within the temporal lobes. This conclusion is based upon the neuropathological study of cases in which the damage was more or less restricted to one or both of these regions. In the following discussion instances of restricted damage to these two regions will be considered first, and only brief reference will be made to the very large literature in which a pathological process, that is more or less diffuse, is accompanied by a disturbance of memorizing as only one of several mental symptoms.

THE MAMMILLARY BODIES AND THE THALAMI

Thiamine deficiency

Within the symptom complex of Korsakoff's psychosis, disorders of memory consist of a retrograde amnesia, which may cover a period of many years before the illness, and a defect of memory for recent events, which can be so severe that retention of new sensory material beyond a period of one or two minutes is not possible.

The psychosis was first described by Korsakoff in 1887 and the description was amplified in his two communications in 1889. The English translation of the last paper (1889a) was provided by Victor and Yakovlev (1955), from which it is apparent that Korsakoff had observed that a disorder of memory could exist as an isolated symptom in certain cases. He stated that, '. . . memory of recent events, those which have just happened is chiefly disturbed, whereas the remote past is remembered fairly well'.

It seems that Korsakoff attributed the total mental disturbance to a 'neuritis' of the subcortical fibres of association, but did not present neuropathological evidence to support this contention. Korsakoff was well aware that the psychosis was not confined to alcoholics, but could occur in a variety of conditions including uterine infections, puerperal septicaemia, typhus fever, tuberculosis, diabetes mellitus and intoxications by arsenic, lead, carbon monoxide and ergot.

It is interesting to note that Wernicke (1881) had described the neuropathological appearances in two chronic alcoholics and in one case of poisoning by sulphuric acid. The term 'superior, haemorrhagic polio-encephalitis' was applied to a neuropathological picture consisting of petechial haemorrhage in the walls of the third ventricle, in the grey matter around the cerebral aqueduct and in the floor of the fourth ventricle. Korsakoff appeared to be unaware of the observations of Wernicke, and it was Gudden (1896) who first appreciated the relationship between the neuropathology described by Wernicke and Korsakoff's psychosis. He reported the neuropathological alterations in the brains of five alcoholics and noted that the mammillary bodies were involved in each. Similar observations were made by Bonhoeffer (1899, 1901) from a study of the brains of alcoholics, and the important observation was made that the abnormalities were not typical of an inflammatory process.

Adequate proof of the correspondence between the neuropathological process underlying Korsakoff's psychosis and that described by Wernicke, was provided by Gamper (1928). In a detailed study of the brains of 16 alcoholics, lesions were shown to extend from the thalamus and hypothalamus to the lower brainstem. Although there was considerable variation in the number and severity of lesions from case to case, the mammillary bodies were involved in all, and there were no consistent changes in the cerebral cortex. In view of this careful study, it was surprising that the neuropathological investigation of five cases of Korsakoff's psychosis by Carmichael and Stern (1931) was restricted to the cerebral cortex. Some evidence of increased lipochrome and occasional chromatolysis was observed in cortical neurones, and no mention was made of the hypothalamus, thalamus or brainstem.

The detailed neuropathological study by Kant (1932) of the brains of 17 alcoholics, confirmed the involvement of structures between the anterior hypothalamus and the lower brainstem as described by Wernicke (1881). In two cases, only the mammillary bodies were affected.

The reports of Korsakoff's psychosis in association with gastric carcinoma (Neubürger, 1931), and with intractable vomiting (von Hosslin, 1905; Ely, 1922), were already pointers to an underlying metabolic link between such conditions and alcoholism. Prickett (1934) observed haemorrhagic lesions in the floor of the fourth ventricle of rats that had been fed a diet deficient in vitamin B_1 (thiamine), but the similarity between these lesions and those of Wernicke's encephalopathy was not recognized. Further instances of the occurrence of the Wernicke type of pathology in cases of malignant disease of the gastro-intestinal tract were published by Neubürger (1936, 1937) and by Környey (1938), but the presence of Korsakoff's psychosis was not reported in any of these cases. The fundamental biochemical disturbance responsible for the lesions in the brain, described by Wernicke (1881), was established by Alexander, Pijoan and Meyerson (1938). The typical lesions were observed in the brains of pigeons that had been fed a diet deficient in thiamine but containing an excess of vitamins A, B_2, C and D. It was suggested that thiamine possessed anti-angiodegenerative and anti-neuritic properties, as its absence could lead to the vascular changes within the regions of the brain delineated by Wernicke and to the peripheral neuropathy of beriberi. Alexander (1939, 1940) pointed out the essential similarity between the lesions in the brains of thiamine-deficient pigeons and those of Wernicke's encephalopathy occurring in man on the basis of alcoholism, and presented an excellent series of illustrations of both. Ferraro and Roizin (1941) reported similar changes in the brains of cats that had undergone a period of total starvation, and these changes were regarded as indirect evidence of the relationship between thiamine deficiency and the lesions in the brain.

An attempt to treat Korsakoff's psychosis by the administration of thiamine was made by Bowman, Goodhart and Jolliffe (1939). For an average period of 11 days, 51 cases were given a diet, the thiamine content of which was described as 'borderline'. Fifteen of these cases were considered to have recovered. Of the remaining 36 patients, 15 were given a diet rich in thiamine and 21 were given the same diet, supplemented by injections of the vitamin. On the diet alone, one patient recovered, while on the supplemented diet, ten recovered, but there was no record of memory function before and after treatment.

Additional evidence for the occurrence of Korsakoff's psychosis, on a basis other than alcoholism, was given by Campbell and Biggart (1939). Of a series of 12 cases, only one was an alcoholic; the remainder consisted of three cases of gastric carcinoma, one of chronic dyspepsia, two of hyperemesis gravidarum, two of macrocytic anaemia, one of bronchiectasis with cardiac failure, one of pyosalpinx with urinary infection and one of presumed pertussis. Each brain was submitted to detailed neuropathological examination and the distribution and severity of the lesions were tabulated. The mammillary bodies were involved in all 12 cases. In two, additional lesions were minor foci in some nuclei of the hypothalamus and brainstem. In five there was also involvement of the thalamus. It was concluded that the order of frequency of the lesions was: mammillary bodies (12), other hypothalamic nuclei (9), thalamus (7) and fornix (2). In this series, the clinical features, including disorders of memory, were not described in detail.

A further attempt to treat Korsakoff's psychosis by giving thiamine was described by Jolliffe, Wortis and Fein (1941). Of 27 cases, three were non-alcoholic and 25 exhibited a peripheral neuropathy. Fourteen died during the course of treatment and of the remainder 12 were left with a residual Korsakoff psychosis which was stated to have cleared in four cases, but unfortunately, no assessment of memory before and after treatment was recorded.

As a contribution to the definition of the neuropathological substrate of Korsakoff's psychosis, that of Rémy (1942) is outstanding. An alcoholic male patient, aged 60 years, became disorientated, ataxic and subject to visual hallucinations. He then improved somewhat and, for a period of ten years, remained in a state which was characterized by euphoria, confabulation and a gross defect of memory for recent events, which contrasted with the ability to recall remote events with fair accuracy. He died of carconoma of the larynx and his brain was examined in detail. Abnormalities were confined to the mammillary bodies, which were small and heavily gliosed. Their neuronal population was reduced and there was also some pallor of myelin staining in the origin of the mammillothalamic tracts.

The neuropathological findings in the brains of three cases of alcoholism associated with Korsakoff's psychosis were described by Benedek and Juba (1944). The mammillary bodies were involved in all three, there were small lesions in other hypothalamic nuclei in two cases but demyelination was the only alteration observed in the thalami. The nature and the severity of the amnesic component of the Korsakoff psychosis were not defined.

A series of 42 cases of 'Wernicke's disease' was investigated by Riggs and Boles (1944). Eighteen were alcoholics, prolonged vomiting had occurred in 11, the diet was inadequate in 7 and the remainder consisted of miscellaneous disorders. Twenty-nine brains were available for neuropathological study, but this was not complete in all. The mammillary bodies were affected in 21 out of 23, the dorsomedial nucleus of the thalamus in 23 out of 27 and the pulvinar of the thalamus in 10 out of 14. Lesions in the brainstem were observed in the majority. The psychiatric state, including disorders of memory, was not described in detail, and this was also true of the five cases (all alcoholics) studied by Bailey (1946), in which the typical Wernicke pathology was identified.

Delay and Brion (1954), after a full review of the literature, described the pathology in the brain of a single case of Korsakoff's psychosis. The patient, a woman of 59 and an alcoholic, exhibited a peripheral neuropathy. No particulars of the amnesia were given. The major neuropathological abnormalities lay in the mammillary bodies, in which there was a striking proliferation of blood vessels and of microglia, but a relatively slight loss of neurones. There were also a few foci of subependymal gliosis around the third ventricle, in the septal regions and around the posterior part of the aqueduct of Sylvius. This case was included in the series of eight alcoholics whose clinical (apart from details of the amnesia) and neuropathological features were described by Delay and his colleagues (1956). It was concluded that the mammillary bodies were never involved alone, but usually together with the dorsomedial nuclei of the thalamus, and/or more or less of the brainstem nuclei usually involved in Wernicke's encephalopathy. Attention was drawn to the fact that the eighth case, although presenting a typical Korsakoff psychosis, was the only one in which lesions were not present in the mammillary bodies. In a report which also lacks any reference to disorders of memory, Gruner (1956) described the neuropathological findings in a series of 17 cases of so-called alcoholic encephalopathy. There was a history of alcoholism in 13, four of which presented a typical Korsakoff psychosis, and in the brains of these four, alterations were restricted to the mammillary bodies.

'The relationship between the Wernicke and the Korsakoff syndrome' was the title of a paper by Malamud and Skillicorn (1956), in which a neuropathological analysis of the brains of 70 cases of Korsakoff's psychosis was presented. The 'periventricular and periaqueductal grey matter' was involved in all. In 57, the mammillary bodies were small and yellow on naked eye examination and histologically abnormal in 67. The dorsomedial nuclei of the thalami were involved in 37 cases and the pulvinar in three. Memory was impaired in every case, but this amnesia was not described in detail.

In a well illustrated publication, Delay, Brion and Elissalde (1958a) described the pathology in the brains of eight cases of Korsakoff's psychosis, all alcoholics. All suffered from a retrograde and an antero-grade amnesia, details of which were not presented. In each case the mammillary bodies were atrophic and yellow, but on microscopic examin-ation, loss of neurones was only slight. Damage elsewhere in the hypo-thalamus was present in one case and in the fornix of another. The thalamus, including its inner portions (but nuclei not specified) and its anterior nuclei, were normal in seven cases. In a second paper (Delay, Brion and Elissalde, 1958b), the relevant neuropathological literature was fully reviewed and the essential findings of previous investigators were presented in tabular form. The absence of consistent lesions in the cerebral cortex was stressed, as well as the almost invariable involve-ment of the mammillary bodies.

The only investigation in which the clinical features, the psychometric assessment of amnesia and the neuropathological data from a single series of cases have been brought together, is that of Adams, Collins and Victor (1962). In a series of 300 cases of Korsakoff's psychosis due to chronic alcoholism and malnutrition, the onset of the illness was usually rapid, so that within a few weeks or even days, the typical signs and symptoms of Wernicke's encephalopathy had appeared, often with the addition of polyneuritis. These symptoms responded rapidly to treatment with thiamine if this was begun with minimal delay. As the state of confusion disappeared, the Korsakoff psychosis became apparent. This could improve somewhat, but there was usually a grave defect of recent memory and there was little or no tendency to confabulate. Extensive psychological testing was carried out in 15 relatively acute, and in 24 chronic, cases and the results were compared with appropriate controls. The assessment of general intellectual functions was reported by Victor, Talland and Adams (1959), of concept formation by Talland (1959), and of the rate and mode of forgetting narrative material by Talland and Ekdall (1959). The defective memory for recent events involved all categories of material, but the degree of emotional colouring did not appear to be important. The period of retrograde amnesia could be greater than a year, and beyond this the recall of remote personal memories was also defective. No reliable details of memory for remote events could be obtained and the need for further study of this aspect of memory was emphasized.

Fifty-four brains from cases of this series were submitted to systematic neuropathological examination, and the lesions described by Wernicke were found to a greater or lesser extent in all. The neurological signs of oculomotor paralyses, nystagmus and ataxia could be explained on the basis of lesions in the brainstem and in the anterior lobe of the cerebellum. The psychiatric symptoms were correlated with lesions in the inner borders of the dorsomedial, anteroventral and pulvinar nuclei of the thalamus, the mammillary bodies and in the terminal few millimetres of the fornices. Minor and inconstant lesions were seen in other thalamic and hypothalamic nuclei. The cerebral cortex, corpus striatum, subthalamic and septal regions, cingulate gyrus, hippo-campi and the brainstem outside the 'Wernicke regions' were normal.

This brief survey of the literature relating to the neuropathological basis of Korsakoff's psychosis has shown that a particular pathological description can be correlated only exceptionally with an amnesia that has been defined with precision. The report of Adams, Collins and Victor (1962) is the only one that has gone some way towards providing this correlation, but even in this study the length of retrograde amnesia and the severity of the disorder of memory for recent events cannot be set beside the neuropathological findings in any one case. Until this has been done for a wide range of retrograde and anterograde amnesia, it will not be possible to define the minimal lesion responsible for either or both.

The conclusion which is justified at present is that, within the range of structures first enumerated by Wernicke, those of the brainstem and cerebellum are unrelated to amnesia, while at least some of those within the diencephalon can, if damaged, result in retrograde and anterograde amnesia. According to Adams, Collins and Victor (1962), the important loci of such lesions are the inner portions of the dorsomedial (that is, magnocellular division), anteroventral and pulvinar nuclei of the thalamus, the mammillary bodies and frequently the terminal portions of each fornix. The publications of Rémy (1942), Delay and Brion (1954) and of Gruner (1956) are, however, reminders that Korsakoff's psychosis can exist on the basis of damage that is confined almost entirely to the mammillary bodies.

It is apparent that neuropathological examination has been carried out almost entirely in those cases of Korsakoff's psychosis whose psychiatric disability necessitated admission to hospital. The possibility remains that a group of subjects may exist in which relatively minor diencephalic damage can be the basis of less florid amnesia, and one for which compensation is possible within society.

The neurological process itself is not one of inflammation and is restricted to one or more of the structures that have been considered above (which do not include the hippocampi). Its predilection for certain regions and its bilateral symmetry are features that remain unexplained. All neural elements (neurones, axis cylinders, blood vessels and glia) may be involved to a variable extent from case to case and from lesion to lesion. In some lesions, and particularly in the thalamus, a loss of nerve cells may be considerable, although the axis cylinders and the myelin sheaths may be well preserved. The mammillary bodies, although often shrunken. may show only a slight loss of neurones in their central portions, while demyelination may be conspicuous in the terminal portions of each fornix. Proliferation of the microglia is usually present but lipid phagocytes are infrequent. A proliferation of fibrous astrocytes is also common, so that, in a long-standing case, the shrunken mammillary bodies often contain a dense feltwork of glial fibres. The proliferation of blood vessels and the presence of haemorrhages, emphasized by earlier writers, are by no means invariable. A swelling and proliferation of the endothelial cells of capillaries renders them prominent, and is easily mistaken for an increase in capillary density. The haemorrhages which often enable the pathology to be recognized on naked eye examination are also neither invariable nor always agonal. The presence of haemosiderin around vessels and in macrophages is evidence that, in some cases, haemorrhage may have occurred at an earlier date.

Tumours

Cases in which a tumour of the third ventricle was associated with some disturbance of memory were reviewed by Weisenburg (1911) who came to the conclusion, however, that mental disorders including amnesia were attributable not to damage within the diencephalon, but to the effects of raised intracranial pressure upon the cerebral cortex. Since that date, there have been numerous reports of the occurrence of Korsakoff's psychosis or of some form of amnesia as a symptom of intrinsic tumours within the walls of the third ventricle (gliomas, ependymomas, medulloblastomas or secondary carcinomatous deposits) and of tumours compressing the floor or the walls of the third ventricle (pituitary adenomas, craniopharyngiomas and colloid cysts). The amnesia was not characterized with precision in the majority of these published cases. In earlier reports, such as those of Frazier (1936) and Love and Marshall (1950), the amnesia was regarded as evidence of invasion of the frontal lobe. The investigation of the case histories of 180 patients with verified intracranial lesions by Williams and Pennybacker (1954) is important, as the conclusion was reached that an impairment of memory was most common when the areas surrounding the floor and walls of the third ventricle were disturbed. Four patients of this series with obvious amnesia were submitted to psychological tests, which gave evidence of a defect of memory for recent and often for remote events. In two of these patients, an improvement in the defect of recent memory followed either removal of the tumour or the aspiration of fluid from it. Unfortunately, the details of this improvement were not recorded and there was no specific reference to the existence of retrograde amnesia. Two instances of Korsakoff's psychosis on the basis of secondary carcinomatous deposits confined almost entirely to the mammillary bodies, were described and illustrated by Örthner (1957).

The literature relating to psychological disturbances (including amnesia) associated with tumours of the diencephalon was well reviewed by Ajuriaguerra, Hécaen and Sadoun (1954) and by White and Cobb (1955).

The association between the Korsakoff syndrome and a retrochiasmal craniopharyngioma was described in 5 cases by Kahn and Crosby (1972). In four of the cases the amnesia cleared more or less completely after the tumour was removed, an effect attributed to restoration of function of the mammillary bodies.

In the opinion of the author, no cases have yet been reported in which pathologically verified lesions (neoplastic or otherwise), confined to the mammillothalamic tract or to the anterior nuclear group of the thalami, have been correlated with an accurately defined defect of memorizing. With regard to the dorsomedial thalamic nuclei, the bilateral stereotactic lesions (diameter 1 cm) placed in these structures by Spiegel and his colleagues (1955), produced only a transient impairment of memory for recent events. The precise extent of the lesions in each case is not known, but the inner magnocellular portion is unlikely to have escaped in every one. It is this portion of the dorsomedial nucleus that Adams, Collins and Victor (1962) consider to be concerned in the process of memorizing.

Trauma

Although some form of amnesia is a well-known consequence of head injury, it is only rarely that a particular type of amnesia can be correlated with a relatively circumscribed injury. Of the 1 000 cases of brain wounds surveyed by Russell (1971), 8 exhibited a Korsakoff-type of amnesia and in these it was believed that a metallic fragment had traversed the fornix and septum lucidum. Recently, Jarho (1973) reported an assessment of 1556 veterans who had sustained open brain injury during World War II in Finland. Eleven of these exhibited a 'Korsakoff amnesic syndrome' consisting of a non-specific disorder of recent memory (remote memory remaining intact), normal cognitive functions and disorientation in time. However, the amnesic syndrome '. . . ensued in immediate association with wounding' in only 6 cases and was regarded as 'borderline' in the others. The site of injury was determined by plotting the fragment's track from skull x-rays and its final position from a stereotactic brain atlas.

The injury was unilateral in three cases and the amnesia was border-line in each. In one, the fragment lay near the midline in the region of the optic chiasma.

Of the 8 instances of bilateral injury, 3 were borderline or of delayed onset. In each of the 5 with a typical amnesic syndrome the diencephalon was considered to have been involved, with interruption of the mammillo-thalamic tract or fornix bilaterally in 4 cases and involvement of both dorsomedial thalamic nuclei in 1.

Subarachnoid haemorrhage

One of the earliest reports of the occurrence of Korsakoff's psychosis in a case of subarachnoid haemorrhage is that of Flatau (1921). Since then, many further instances have been recorded and were well reviewed by Tarachow (1939). No pathological report has yet appeared to indicate whether the amnesia is due to damage within the diencephalon, the temporal lobes or both.

Symonds (1966) has drawn attention to the fact that the amnesia in tuberculosis meningitis, although severe at first, may clear up entirely. However, among such cases, it is possible to isolate those in which memory for recent events is normal while a substantial retrograde amnesia remains unchanged.

THE HIPPOCAMPAL FORMATION

Localized lesions

The only lesions in the temporal lobes having borders that are well defined (if not always known) are the results of surgical intervention. Many such lesions are relevant to the present theme as they are followed almost immediately by some recognizable amnesia which, if it persists for any length of time, may be described in clinical and psychological terms.

A grave defect of memory for recent events was reported by Scoville (1954), as the sequel of the bilateral removal of tissue along the inner borders of both temporal lobes. This operation was designed as a therapeutic procedure in certain cases of severe schizophrenia and was an extension of the technique of orbital undercutting. In 30 severely deteriorated cases, bilateral partial resection of the temporal lobes was carried out and combined, in some cases, with orbital undercutting. A purely temporal resection was also carried out in *one* epileptic whose seizures were resistant to medication. Improvement in the psychotic patients was slight. The seizures in the epileptic patient were reduced in frequency and Milner (1969) has reported that although intellectual functions are regarded as normal, the gross amnesia persists. There was no evidence of general intellectual impairment in those patients that were suitable for testing. A defect of memory for recent events was present in eight patients and was severe in three and moderate in five. The detailed analysis of this amnesia was reported by Scoville and Milner (1957). The first three patients were able to retain a three-figure number or a pair of unrelated words for only a few minutes. There was also evidence of a patchy retrograde amnesia for periods of up to three years. In these patients, the extent of tissue resection was from 5.5 to 8.0 cm posterior to the tips of the temporal lobes. In the second group of five patients there was a lesser impairment of memory for recent events. In these five patients the bilateral resection extended 5 to 6 cm posterior to the tips of the temporal lobes. It was concluded that the amnesia was related to the bilateral removal of the hippocampus and the hippocampal gyrus, and was more or less proportional to the amount of these structures removed, although it must be pointed out that the precise extent of these surgical ablations has not yet been verified by neuropathological examination. It was noted that bilateral resection of the uncus and amygdaloid nucleus alone did not result in amnesia.

A bilateral anterior temporal lobectomy was carried out by Petit-Dutaillis and his colleagues (1954), in an attempt to relieve severe psychomotor seizures in a male patient aged 24 years. The tip of the temporal lobe and the uncus of the right side were first removed, and five months later the tip of the left temporal lobe (excluding uncus and hippocampus) was resected. A retrograde amnesia for a period of several months shrank somewhat and then remained as a permanent feature, while a defect of memory for recent events was only transient.

The effects of the two-stage removal of the anterior 7 cm of the temporal lobes were described by Terzian and Ore (1955). A male patient, aged 19 years, had been subject to psychomotor and grand-mal seizures since childhood. The removal, on the left side, of the tip of the temporal lobe, the uncus, the amygdaloid nucleus and the anterior part of the hippocampus had no reported effect on memory and the seizures soon recommenced. The resection, 19 days later, of the corresponding regions of the right temporal lobe gave rise to what was regarded as the equivalent of the Klüver-Bucy syndrome. There was also an extensive patchy retrograde amnesia, a severe defect of memory for recent events and some disorientation in space, but the condition of the patient did not permit psychometric assessment.

Since 1955, the operation of temporal lobectomy has been confined, almost exclusively, to the treatment of temporal lobe epilepsy, and, in view of the warnings explicit and implicit in the above reports, has been confined to the temporal lobe of one side. The unilateral procedure, however, is not without effect upon memorizing. Milner and Penfield (1955) described a marked non-specific defect of memory for recent events in two instances of anterior temporal lobectomy on the dominant side. In one patient, this type of amnesia was the immediate effect of a resection, which included part of the hippocampus and the hippocampal gyrus. In the second case, memory was unaffected by the removal of the anterior 4 cm of the lobe, but when, five years later, the ipsilateral uncus, amygdaloid nucleus, hippocampus and hippocampal gyrus were resected, a retrograde amnesia for a period of three months before the operation and a defect of memory for recent events became apparent. In both these patients, memory for remote events seemed to be unimpaired. To account for these amnesias, it was assumed that damage must have been present in the hippocampal formation of the opposite side, so that the unilateral lobectomy had led to the manifestations of bilateral hippocampal damage. These were the only cases in a series of 90 in which unilateral temporal lobectomy had given rise to serious amnesia. It was noted, however, that the removal of the lobe on the dominant side frequently gave rise to a difficulty in the learning and retention of purely verbal material, while a defect of rapid visual identification could be a sequel of the removal of the non-dominant lobe.

Meyer and Yates (1955) and Meyer (1956) also presented evidence to show that anterior temporal lobectomy on the dominant side could result in a disorder of memorizing, which was described as a severely impaired ability to learn new verbal and auditory material. Attention was drawn to the fact that this defect, in minor degree, could often be recognized before the operation and was intensified by it. The original cases of Meyer and Yates (1955) have been reviewed by Blakemore and

Falconer (1966), and the auditory learning defect, present in all cases one year after the operation, had almost invariably disappeared within three years of the operation. The rate of its disappearance was influenced adversely by the continuation of seizures.

The statement by Walker (1957) that 10–15 per cent of unilateral temporal lobectomies of either side are followed by some disorder of memory, was not supported by detailed evidence. Of four cases submitted to unilateral temporal lobectomy, three exhibited a lasting defect of memory for recent events. The extent of tissue removed was not described in detail and the normality of the contralateral temporal lobe seemed reasonably certain in only one case.

Serafetinides and Falconer (1962) described a non-specific defect of recent memory in 6 out of 34 patients submitted to temporal lobectomy in the non-dominant hemisphere. In 4 out of these 6 patients, the results of psychometric testing were normal during a follow-up period of 2 to 9 years. The evidence of impaired memory came from each patient and from a near relative or friend, and showed that material of all categories was forgotten after a period ranging from hours to weeks. In no instance was this disability incapacitating and it was usually compensated for by *aides-memoires,* such as written lists and meticulous diaries. It was also stated that, in each of these patients, a spike discharge could be recorded from the sphenoidal electrode on the opposite side. This was interpreted as evidence of dysfunction of that lobe, but not necessarily a structural alteration.

This brief survey of the principal publications describing disorders of memorizing as a sequel of operations upon one or both temporal lobes, leads to the conclusion that the inner portions of these lobes and the hippocampal formation (that is, hippocampus and hippocampal gyrus) in particular are essential for normal memorizing. The apparent proportionality between the amount of the hippocampal formation that was removed and the severity of the ensuing defect of memory for recent events in the cases of Scoville (1954), remains the most convincing evidence that the hippocampal formation, rather than the tip of the lobe, the amygdaloid nucleus, the uncus and the superior, middle and inferior temporal gyri is the region participating in the retention and recall of recent events. The four cases of Bailey (1946), in which bilateral removal of the gyri of the outer aspects of the temporal lobes was without effect upon memorizing, are indirect evidence in support of this conclusion. As far as the fusiform gyri are concerned, Scoville's diagrams of the operative resection make it clear that at least the inner halves of these gyri were removed, as well as some portion of their central white matter.

Further verification of the extent of the relatively large volumes of tissue removed in the present-day operation of anterior temporal lobectomy, will undoubtedly appear in postmortem studies in the course of time. These will provide invaluable information in relation to the pathogenesis and symptomatology of temporal lobe epilepsy, but are unlikely to define the portions of the temporal lobes involved in the process of memorizing any more precisely than the few bilateral and largely hippocampal resections carried out by Scoville (1954).

Diffuse processes

Amnesia has been described as one, and occasionally the only, symptom of the destruction of tissue along the medial borders of the temporal lobes as a sequel of many different pathological processes. In most cases, the nature of the process is such that a clear line of demarcation between normal and abnormal tissue cannot be drawn. Further, the longer the interval between the inception of the process and death, the greater will be the secondary and often widespread changes, including gliosis, nerve fibre degeneration and the transsynaptic and retrograde degeneration of nerve cells, all of which make the task of delineating the limits of the original lesion difficult, if not impossible. These diffuse processes include vascular disease, neoplasia, systemic hypoxia, demyelinizing disease, meningitis and encephalitis. Brief reference will now be made to some of the more important examples of this group.

Vascular disease

The first recorded instance of amnesia as a symptom of medial temporal lobe damage was probably an example of vascular disease and was described by Bechterew (1900a). Bilateral softenings in the uncinate gyrus, hippocampus and subjacent white matter were seen in the brain of a patient who had exhibited apathy and a severe defect of memory during life.

Whether the case described by Glees and Griffith (1952) is an example of vascular disease is far from certain. A 73-year-old woman had exhibited a progressive defect of memory for recent events for a period of 15 years. She was confused, disorientated and agitated and died in a withdrawn and deteriorated state. In her brain, the tips of the temporal lobes were replaced by cyst-like cavities communicating with the lateral ventricles. The hippocampi, hippocampal gyri and portions of the lingual and fusiform gyri were absent on each side. Although the fibre content of each fornix was reduced to 22 per cent of normal, it was surprising that the mammillary bodies were considered to be normal.

A severe defect of memory for recent events (assessed by psychometric tests) and a retrograde amnesia were the results of proven vascular occlusion in the patient described in clinical and neuropathological detail by Victor and his colleagues (1961). A right-handed male patient, aged 59 years at death, suffered a stroke which left purely right-sided neurological residua. Two years later, a second stroke added further neurological signs and a marked amnesia. This consisted of an incomplete retrograde amnesia for a period of two and a half years before the second stroke, and a striking defect of immediate recall (reduced digit retention) and of the ability to learn new facts and skills. Memory for remote events seemed good and there was only a slight impairment of general intelligence. The patient died three and a half years after the second stroke and, at autopsy, marked atheroma of the vertebrobasilar arterial system was observed. There was also occlusion of both posterior cerebral arteries. In the left hemisphere there was extensive damage in the temporal and occipital lobes. In the former, the uncus, amygdaloid nucleus, anterior hippocampus and hippocampal gyrus were spared. More posteriorly, a softening in the white matter of the hippocampal gyrus expanded to involve the cortex in the floor of the collateral fissure and could be traced back to the occipital pole. There was considerable loss of nerve cells in the posterior part of the left hippocampus, marked narrowing of the fornix and a small gliosed mammillary body. On the right side, a smaller lesion involved the white matter of the hippocampal gyrus and could be traced back to the occipital pole. The right hippocampus was virtually intact, but there was a discrete lesion in the crus of the right fornix and softenings in the splenium of the corpus callosum and in the hippocampal commissure. There were recent infarcts in the posterior part of the diencephalon, the midbrain and the pons.

The defect of memorizing appearing after the second stroke was attributed to the superimposition of a lesion in the right fornix upon the pre-existing damage in the left hippocampal formation. However, the presence of neuronal loss in the mammillary bodies (and particularly the left) must imply that the amnesia in this case cannot be attributed to bilateral lesions of the hippocampal formation alone.

Systemic hypoxia

The diabetic patient described by Grünthal (1947) has often been quoted as an example of a defect of memory on the basis of bilateral hippocampal lesions due to hypoglycaemia. It seems, however, that no specific mention was made of memory function and the clinical state was one of severe dementia, following a period of insulin coma four months before death. The brain, weighing 1 024 g, showed a moderate cortical atrophy although, microscopically, the cortex was stated to show only a gliosis of the outer layers and some perivascular loss of nerve cells. There was a softening in each hippocampus, extending into the entorhinal region and narrowing and gliosis of the fornices. The mammillary bodies were described as normal.

Although amnesia has often been described as one symptom in patients surviving carbon monoxide poisoning, cardiac arrest and hypotension, there appears to be no report in which a well defined amnesia has been correlated with lesions restricted to the mamillary or hippocampal regions of the brain. This is not surprising, as the neuropathological alterations characteristic of hypoxia are almost always diffuse (Meyer, 1963; Brierley, 1965). The discrete cerebral and cerebellar lesions resulting from abrupt and severe hypotension are an exception to this rule, but such lesions almost invariably spare the Ammon's horns and the mammillary bodies (Brierley, 1965; Adams and his colleagues, 1966).

Encephalitis

Certain cases of encephalitis have attracted attention by virtue of their very striking amnesic sequelae and the relative concentration of the inflammatory process in the medial temporal and other portions of the limbic regions. In acute cases, the process is characterized by tissue necrosis and haemorrhage, affecting particularly the structures within the limbic lobes, that is, the uncus, amygdaloid nucleus, hippocampus, hippocampal and cingulate gyri and the posterior orbital regions. These alterations are typical of acute encephalitis due to the virus of herpes simplex, but this diagnosis is often only presumptive and, in the case of identification of the virus or of a positive serological test, rests upon the demonstration of typical Type 'A' intranuclear inclusion bodies in nerve cells and glia after death. About 70 per cent of these cases die within the first two weeks and among those that survive, disorders of memory may be conspicuous and include a retrograde amnesia and a defect of memory for recent events. Six adult cases were described by Drachman and Adams (1962), of which three survived. Two of these exhibited severe defects of memory, and in the three fatal cases, the medial temporal and orbital regions were involved asymmetrically in a necrotizing process and Type 'A' intranuclear inclusion bodies were identified in all three. In the non-fatal case of presumed inclusion-body encephalitis reported by Adams,

Collins and Victor (1962), a retrograde amnesia for a period of six years eventually shrank to one of a few weeks and was associated with a severe defect of memory for recent events.

Cases of acute encephalitis mainly affecting the temporal lobes, but without demonstrable inclusion bodies, have also been recorded (Fields and Blattner, 1958). In the majority of these, survival was from a few days to a few weeks, but was five months in one of seven apparently similar cases reported by Aszkanazy, Tom and Zeldowicz (1958). In this one case, mental deterioration was too great for any specific disorder of memory to be apparent.

The four non-fatal cases described by Rose and Symonds (1960) cannot be ascribed with certainty to either herpetic or non-herpetic acute encephalitis. The evidence for encephalitis included an increase in cells and protein in the cerebrospinal fluid of three cases, and the presence of a paretic Lange curve in two. After recovery from an initial febrile episode there was evidence of intellectual impairment in all cases, and a patchy retrograde amnesia of up to 30 years was described in three. In each case there was a defect of memory for recent events so severe that, in one case, the period of retention was reduced to 30 seconds.

Instances of subacute and presumably viral encephalitis were described by Brierley *et al.* (1960) in three male patients in the sixth decade of life. A marked impairment of memory was noted (but not described in detail) in two, but otherwise, the presenting psychiatric features showed little in common. In all, death took place in coma after a period of profound dementia. Neuropathological examination showed that the inflammatory process was concentrated in the limbic regions of the brain and in the mammillary bodies. No inclusion bodies were identified.

In a single case of subacute necrotizing encephalitis described by Beck and Corsellis (1963), a severe defect of memory for recent events appeared overnight in a male patient aged 59 years. There was no retrograde amnesia. Death took place 15 months later, and neuropathological examination showed that a subacute necrotizing process had destroyed the hippocampal formation of each side. The fornices were shrunken and gliotic and the mammillary bodies were yellow in colour and reduced to about half their normal size.

AGEING AND THE PRESENILE DEMENTIAS

A gradual failure of memory for recent events, often contrasting with a relative preservation of the ability to recall the events of childhood, is a well-known feature of a proportion of non-demented elderly subjects (Kral, 1958). There is as yet no satisfactory explanation for this amnesia in neuropathological terms. In such subjects, death is commonly due to causes outside the nervous system, and there is little likelihood of histological study of the brain. The only investigation of the brains of non-demented old people is that of Gellerstedt (1933), who observed senile plaques in 84 per cent of the brains of a series of 50 subjects. Attention was drawn to their frequency in the hippocampal formation. The psychiatric state of these subjects was not assessed in detail and there was no specific reference to amnesia.

In addition to senile plaques, the ageing brain may show alterations in the neurones and in the glia. Brody (1955) has reported a decrease in the number of neurones in the cerebral cortex with advancing age, and, in any one region, the loss is greater in the granular layers (II and IV). There is also a variable increase in the intracytoplasmic lipochrome, some loss of Nissl substance and an increased basophilia of the nucleus (McMenemy, 1963). The commonest change in the glia is an increase in fibrous astrocytes, particularly beneath the pial surface of the cortex and the ependymal lining of the ventricles. Neither the neuronal nor the glial alterations show any selective concentration in the hippocampal or mammillary regions.

Among the presenile dementias, Alzheimer's disease is most closely related to normal ageing, in that the amnesia which can be an isolated early symptom is an exaggeration of the senile defect of memory for recent events, and also because its neuropathological basis is an exaggeration of the process of normal ageing. Even so, it is only rarely that a striking amnesia of this type can be correlated with a high incidence of senile plaques and of neurofibril change in the hippocampal formations and in the mammillary bodies (Brierley, 1961). The amnesias encountered in arteriosclerotic dementia and in Pick's disease have an even less satisfactory explanation in neuropathological terms, and the very limited evidence for such correlations has been reviewed by Brierley (1961).

NEUROANATOMICAL ASPECTS

The hippocampal formation

This comprises the hippocampal (or parahippocampal) gyrus and the hippocampus (or Ammon's horn).

The hippocampal gyrus

This gyrus forms the medial edge of the temporal lobe and is continuous, laterally, with the fusiform gyrus in the floor of the collateral fissure.

At this point, it exhibits the six layers typical of neocortex, but passing medially, this lamination is lost and gives way, over the crest of the gyrus, to transitional or allocortex which is succeeded by the Islets of Calleja on the dorsal aspect. More laterally, these again give way to the entorhinal cortex, which consists of three layers continuous with those of the hippocampus itself.

The connections of the hippocampal gyrus are little known. It may receive fibres from the cingulate gyrus and, in the monkey, from the superior temporal gyrus and the insula (Adey and Meyer, 1952). The hippocampal gyrus is an important source of fibres to the hippocampus, and these fibres are derived from the entorhinal area on the dorsal aspect of the gyrus.

The hippocampus

This structure consists of a strip of three-layered allocortex, folded into the medial aspect of the temporal lobe so that the floor of the fold bulges into the medial wall of the inferior wall of the lateral ventricle. The lower limb of the fold is continuous with the entorhinal region of the hippocampal gyrus, and the upper limb turns downwards and laterally to expand into the endofolium, which lies within the curvature of the dentate gyrus (fascia dentata).

Afferent connections   There is no evidence, in Man, that direct fibres from the olfactory tracts enter the hippocampus. The major source of hippocampal afferents is the entorhinal cortex on the dorsal aspect of the hippocampal gyrus. This region gives rise to two main fibre tracts (Cajal, 1909; Lorente de No, 1934), the 'perforant' or 'direct temporo-ammonic pathway' and the 'alvear', 'crossed temporo-ammonic' or 'temporo-alvear pathway'. The perforant pathway, arising within the lateral portion of the entorhinal region, terminates among the apical dendrites of the pyramidal cell layer of the hippocampus and also among the neurones of the gyrus denatus. The 'alvear pathway', arising from the more medial part of the entorhinal region, is believed to cross to the opposite entorhinal cortex, and any contribution to the Ammon's horn itself is doubtful. Other afferent fibres arise in the septal region and pass backwards through the fornix to the hippocampus. Others may be derived from the medial forebrain bundle (Cragg, 1961), from the olfactory cortex or pyriform area (Cragg, 1961) and from the cingulate gyrus through the striae of Lancisi and the dorsal fornix. Commissural connections between the two hippocampi are considered to be less important in the primate than in lower forms.

Efferent connections The most important efferent pathway from the hippocampus is the fornix, through which the axons of the hippocampal pyramidal cells pass to the mamillary body and largely to its medial nucleus. Other efferent fibres pass via the postcommissural fornix to the tegmentum of the midbrain and pons, the amygdaloid nucleus and the anterior nuclear complex of the thalamus. Further details of the internal structure and the connections of the hippocampal formation have been reviewed by Powell (1959) and by Green (1964).

The mammillary bodies

In Man, the largest nuclear subdivision of the mammillary body is the medial mamillary nucleus, which forms the greater part of the structure. The largest group of afferent fibres to this nucleus is derived from the hippocampus via the postcommissural fornix. Further afferents ascend from the tegmentum of the midbrain in the mammillary penduncle, and others pass backwards from the anterior diencephalon in the medial mammillary nucleus and also receive afferent fibres from the orbital surface of the frontal lobe.

The principal efferent pathway from the mammillary body is the mammillothalamic tract which arises almost entirely from the medial mammillary nucleus and terminates in the anterior nuclear complex of the thalamus. Other efferent fibres constitute the mammillotegmental tract which terminates in the tegmentum of the upper brainstem.

The anterior nuclear complex of the thalamus

This complex consists of three nuclei, the anterodorsal, anteroventral and anteromedial nuclei.

Afferent connections pass to all three nuclei via the mammillothalamic tract and the anteromedial nucleus also receives a contribution of fibres from the postcommissural fornix.

Efferent fibres pass from this nuclear complex to the full extent of the cingulate gyrus on the medial surface of the cerebral hemisphere; to the anterior cingulate gyrus (area 24 of Brodmann) from the antero-medial nucleus; to the posterior cingulate gyrus (area 23 of Brodman) from the anteroventral nucleus and to the retrosplenial gyrus from the anterodorsal nucleus.

The dorsomedial nucleus of the thalamus

This nucleus consists of a parvicellular portion forming the greater part of the structure, and a magnicellular portion lying along the ventricular surface. Afferent fibres to the former are derived from other major thalamic nuclei and to the latter from the hypothalamus.

The efferent projection from the parvicellular portion of the nucleus passes to the granular cortex over the convexity of the frontal lobe (areas 8, 9 and possibly 10 of Brodmann), and from the magnicellular portion, fibres pass to the medial orbital cortex (Meyer and Beck, 1954).

The pulvinar of the thalamus

This structure forms the convex posterior portion of the thalamus. It receives afferent fibres from the pathways of visual and auditory sensation and its efferent fibres project to the posterior part of the convexity of the temporal lobe, the lower portion of the lateral aspect of the parietal lobe and the outer aspect of the occipital lobe anterior to the pole.

It must be stressed that, as far as the hippocampal formation and mammillary body are concerned, the information summarized in the above brief review is derived to a very large extent from studies in lower mammals. Powell (1959) has emphasized the dearth of information concerning the connections of the hippocampal formation, but the same is true of the distribution of the fibres of the fornix in Man. The only quantitative study of the fibres of the human fornix is that of Daitz (1953), who estimated that there were 2 000 000 fibres in the fornix just below the corpus callosum and 912 000 fibres just above the mammillary body. It was concluded that only one-third of the fibres of the human fornix reach the mammillary body, while this fraction is one-fourth in the macaca monkey.

Powell (1959) accepted that the septal region decreases in size with ascent of the phylogenetic scale but maintained that, in Man, this region receives the same proportion of fornix fibres as in lower forms. Adey (1964), in a discussion of the fornix fibres that terminate in regions other than the mammillary bodies stated that '. . . the proportion of them that terminate in this fashion increases the higher one goes in the phyletic scale'. In marked contrast to these views, Beck and Corsellis (1965) have failed to find evidence of degeneration in nerve fibres or in terminal synaptic boutons in the precommissural region of cases in which there had been a complete unilateral division of the posterior column of the fornix. These cases included two instances of temporal lobectomy and several of occlusion of the posterior cerebral artery.

As far as the body of the fornix is concerned, inspection of myelin-stained sections (in the coronal plane) of the cat, monkey and human brains reveals a consistent group of fibres that connect the dorsal aspect of each fornix to the under aspect of the corpus callosum. In Man, anterior to the interventricular foramen, these fibres lie within each lamina of the septum pellucidum. From the anterior limits of the latter back to the hippocampal commissure the total number of such fibres is unknown, but must be considerable, and may include:

(1) fibres of the 'fornix longus' from the cingulum; but according to Powell (1959), the existence of the former in Man is doubtful.

(2) fibres leaving the fornix to join or to perforate those of the corpus callosum, en route to the neocortex.

(3) Beck and Corsellis (1963) have tentatively suggested that the cortex of the frontal and parietal lobes may give rise to fibres which traverse the corpus callosum, enter the fornix and terminate in the hypothalamus, including the mammillary bodies.

Until neuroanatomical studies can provide a fuller understanding of the connections of the human hippocampal formation and of the fornix in particular, the assumption that the corresponding pattern of connections in lower mammals is applicable to Man has no justification.

DISCUSSION

The foregoing selective review of the neuropathological correlates of amnesia has indicated that the structures essential for the process of normal memorizing are the hippocampal formations within the temporal lobes, the mammillary bodies and, possibly, certain thalamic nuclei within the diencephalon. The anatomical connections of these two regions suggest that a continuous pathway might be traced along the afferent fibres from the hippocampal gyrus to the hippocampus and out, via its efferent pathway, the fornix, to the mammillary bodies. From these, the mammillothalamic tract leads to the anterior nuclear complex of the thalamus, which projects to the cingulate gyrus. The pathway is completed by the known connections between the cingulate and hippocampal gyri. This apparently continuous 'circuit' lies within the group of structures comprising the 'limbic lobe', to which Papez (1937) ascribed the elaboration of emotion and the control of visceral activity.

The most discrete anatomical link between the hippocampal and diencephalic regions is the fornix. It is surprising, therefore, that with the exception of the case reported by Sweet, Talland and Ervin (1959), bilateral division of the fornix (usually in the region of the interventricular foramen) has not resulted in a disorder of memorizing (Dott, 1938; Cairns and Mosberg, 1951; Garcia-Bengochea and his colleagues, 1954). This finding suggests that the two groups of structures linked by the fornix cannot be regarded as a unitary system subserving the process of memorizing, at least until major interconnections other than the fornix have been identified.

Evidence has now been presented to show that both a retrograde amnesia and a defect of memory for recent events can be symptoms of either bilateral hippocampal or bilateral diencephalic damage. The defect of recent memory implies that the establishment or consolidation of a recent sensory impression as a permanent memory trace or engram may be totally or partially deranged. While it is believed that the process of consolidation takes time, there is no general agreement as to the actual length of this period. It has been shown by Cronholm and Molander (1957) and Cronholm and Lagergren (1959) that recall of a sensory impression is severely impaired when an electrically induced seizure takes place a few minutes after the receipt of the impression, and that it is unaffected when this interval is one of a few hours. Whether a consolidation time of the same order is applicable to all new experiences seems improbable, and important and emotionally charged events may be established more rapidly than the less important and the emotionally neutral.

The view has been expressed by Milner (1962) and by Adams, Collins and Victor (1962) that the retrograde amnesia occurring in patients with hippocampal or diencephalic damage is evidence that the period of consolidation may be one of months rather than hours. According to Deutsch (1962), 'Compared with that from animals, the evidence from retrograde amnesia in Man suggests an entirely different time scale, that of years or a lifetime for the period of consolidation'. The shrinkage of a period of retrograde amnesia has been described only rarely in cases of proven brain damage (encephalitis: Adams, Collins and Victor, 1962), but was described in some detail in cases of head injury by Russell and Nathan (1946). Such shrinkage suggests that the memory trace had already been established but could not be revived. The fact that the presentation of appropriate associations may assist the recall of material that was apparently forgotten by patients with either hippocampal or diencephalic lesions, would also point to the participation of these structures in recall. On the other hand, the contrast between a severe defect of memory for recent events, and an apparently normal ability to recall those of the remote past, has often been invoked to justify the conclusion that the hippocampal-diencephalic structures play no part in recall. This conclusion could only be justified if an assessment of remote recall had been made before the onset of the amnesia, and could be shown to be unchanged after this event.

In the great majority of the cases that have been reviewed, the defect of memory for recent events has been so severe that retention was reduced to a few minutes. The importance of the report of Serafetinides and Falconer (1962) is that attention has been drawn to a qualitatively similar, but far less severe, impairment of memorizing. Further and more detailed study of similar cases may show that the retention span on the basis of bilateral temporal lobe lesions may range from a few minutes, as in Scoville's (1954) cases, through weeks and months, up to the proximal limit of the normal. Whether such a range exists in cases with diencephalic damage is not known, for reasons which have already been discussed. Further, in view of the fact that retention of progressively smaller fractions of the events of the present for progressively longer periods of time has already been noted as a feature of normal memorizing, there seems little reason to believe that the storage and recall of more recent memories is subserved by a neurophysiological process fundamentally different from that which subserves the storage and recall of memories that are more remote.

While all incoming general and specific sensory stimuli activate neurones within the corresponding areas of the cerebral cortex, there is no anatomical evidence to suggest that fibres from the sensory pathways pass directly to the hippocampal and diencephalic regions. Purely neurophysiological studies (reviewed by Green, 1964) have indicated that both regions can be influenced by the reticular formation of the brainstem. The sustained activity of these two regions that follows the receipt of a sensory impression and assures its consolidation as an engram, must imply the existence of reciprocal connections between them and many areas of the cerebral cortex. Knowledge of these connections is still meagre, and particularly so in respect of the hippocampal gyrus.

The role of the neuropathologist, up to the present time, has been to define with only limited precision those portions of the brain that appear to be essential to normal memorizing. It is the author's view that more precise 'localization' is an unrealistic goal, and one unlikely to be attained through further neuropathological studies, even of surgical material. Major contributions to the understanding of the mechanism of memorizing are more likely to be made by the neuropathologist, who studies selected cases of brain damage in order to increase neuro-anatomical knowledge of the connections of the hippocampal, hypo-thalamic and thalamic structures that have already been defined.

9 Psychogenic Loss of Memory

R.T.C. Pratt

It is natural but inaccurate to regard perfect reproduction of a perceived event as being the norm. Perception itself is highly individual and depends for example on interest and experience; the perception of a tracing of an EEG or of a seismograph is strikingly influenced by the training of the observer. Similarly remembering, as has been shown in particular by Bartlett (1932), is profoundly influenced and shaped by individual factors. It is likely that every memory is in some way a progressive distortion of the original event, and that many of the examples of the psychopathology of memory discussed in this chapter are exaggerations in one way or another of tendencies detectable in the errors of normal memory. Contrariwise, slips of the tongue and similar errors occurring in normal people may throw light on the mechanisms involved in more severe impairments of memory.

The title of this chapter requires that a brief consideration be given to the relationship between organic and functional disorders. It is not necessary to embark on the problem of the relationship between the brain and the mind: by the writer they are regarded as a single entity seen from different aspects (*see* Pratt, 1939), and their relationships have been illuminated particularly in Craik's (1943) monograph *The Nature of Explanation*. It follows that any organic disease of the brain is likely to impair cognitive functions, including memory. Furthermore, in instances of organic impairment there is no protection from the play of individual factors such as interest, experience and affect. In fact the reverse is the case; both Slater and Glithero (1965) and Merskey and Trimble (1977) have indicated that hysterical symptoms are facilitated and may be provoked by organic disease of the brain. Psychogenic influences therefore play a part in determining the nature of the memory impairment seen in patients with organic brain disease.

There is however a real distinction between organic and psychogenic memory loss; confusion has arisen because the relation between the two is not reciprocal: organic brain disease of necessity reflects psychogenic factors, whereas psychogenic amnesia may appear without any organic disease being present.

The motivation for psychogenic loss of memory is usually obvious when all the circumstances are known, and may plausibly be regarded as 'forgetting of the disagreeable'. Some authors have linked this with Freudian repression. However, in a critical review of the contributions of psychoanalysis Rapaport (1942) concludes: 'The survey of the pertinent psychoanalytic literature has shown us the fallacy of the widespread notion that Freud taught the forgetting of the disagreeable. What Freud discovered was the function preventing the emergence into consciousness of an unconscious idea which, if it became conscious, would give rise to conflict. This function, called repression, proved to be a specific and variable one, hardly amenable to the statistical treatment adopted by experimentalists'. One might add that the fact that the effects of repression in a particular individual are unpredictable means that the hypothesis is unscientific in the Popperian sense, namely incapable of refutation.

The connection between the superficial concept of forgetting of the disagreeable and the mechanism of repression has not been explored in respect of psychogenic loss of memory, nor have authors holding psychoanalytic views, such as Abeles and Schilder (1935), who claim deeper motives to be operative, shown that Oedipal conflicts are responsible. Neither is there a rival theory to explain the specificity of the symptom 'chosen' as a result of conflict, nor why amnesia rather than, for example, hysterical paralysis should appear.

The above considerations suffice to show that the clinical features displayed by patients with organic neurological disease may be expected to show little difference from those shown by patients with purely psychogenic amnesia; series of patients selected according to varying criteria usually contain a substantial proportion with organic cerebral disease. The time, place and circumstances of the selection of cases for publication will be seen to influence the composition of the series and the proportion with organic disease.

FUGUES AND LOSS OF MEMORY

A fugue is a state of clouding of consciousness in which the person wanders away from his normal surroundings. There are few reports of the mental state during a fugue; this suggests that the person is in good contact with his surroundings, and is able to act appropriately without drawing much attention to himself by any grossly abnormal behaviour. Evidence is conflicting over whether disinhibited behaviour is a feature of this period. During the fugue there is loss of personal identity, but no awareness of it, and usually a false identity is given. Patients often 'come to' long distances from their starting point and many days later, but they may be clean, tidy and well-fed; the inference is that clouding of consciousness is not severe, in contrast, as Rapaport (1942) points out, to somnambulism, where a lay observer promptly detects that the subject is behaving in an abnormal way.

Patients tend to emerge from the fugue in two ways — the first with a resumption of their identity and an amnesic gap covering the fugue, the second with an awareness of loss of personal identity, and an amnesia for their whole life.

Case History No. 1 A man of 45 was admitted to hospital for investigation of 'fits'. He said that 15 years previously he had been brought to a hospital unaware of his personal identity and of any event in his previous life. His amnesia persisted, and since he did not correspond to any notified missing person he had to select a name, which he did from a name above a shop opposite the hospital, James Williamson. He was able to relearn general information rapidly, and after two years was holding a responsible and well-paid foreman's post in engineering. His efforts to trace his relatives had been unsuccessful, but he was then found by his brother and learned that he had a wife and three young children, and, more remarkably, that his real name was William Jameson. He did not rejoin his family, nor resume his original name. By the age of 45 he was living with a partner who had adopted his surname by deed poll, but she reported that their relationship was a stormy one. His 'fits' were observed and considered to be non-organic. An explanation that they were due to tension, combined with superficial psychotherapy, resulted in their disappearance, even though his early amnesic gap persisted. Three years later he met, on the occasion of his mother's illness, his wife and children. At her deathbed the memory of his former life returned in full. He remained with his new partner, but his unkindness to her, together with his resumption of his original name in spite of her having taken his fictitious surname, induced her to leave him.

The striking features of this man's history are his choice of name, and the rapidity of his learning about the world about him. The learning of previously experienced information in such patients is now routinely tested quantitatively at the National Hospital. One test devised is a series of photographs of well-known personalities; information about the name and occupation of those not identified is given, and recall is then required. Usually recall is far more efficient than would be the case if the personalities had been encountered for the very first time.

Criteria for diagnosis of a fugue are somewhat variable between authors; Berrington, Liddell and Foulds (1956) required 'sudden onset of wandering with clouding of consciousness and a more or less complete amnesia for the event'. These authors compared 31 men and 6 women with controls. As with other series the average age was in the fourth decade, and males predominated. A definite association was found between fugues and, first, a reputation for lying, and, secondly, a mood of depression: further findings were a history of severe head injury in nearly one-half and significant precipitating factors in nearly all, the fugue usually leading to an escape from an intolerable situation. No fewer than two-thirds had experienced a prior fugue. The main diagnostic category was of psychopathy, in contrast to the predominance of depression in Stengel's series (*see below*). Berrington, Liddell and Foulds considered that head injury, with the associated concussion and subsequent amnesia, formed the basis for the suggestion of a psychogenic amnesia at a later date. Epilepsy would be a similar antecedent factor. The precipitating situation was essentially a state of depression in circumstances from which no rational escape was possible.

Abeles and Schilder (1935) described 63 patients (31 male, 32 female) seen at the Bellevue Hospital, New York, over 4 years, including 22 seen in a six-month period. The ages ranged from the second to the sixth decade, with a peak in the third. Several patients had had a preceding fugue and had 'come to' with the awareness of loss of personal identity; in others no account of a fugue state could be obtained. Previous episodes had occurred in nearly one-quarter. Most recovered spontaneously; the duration of the episode was less than a day in 27 patients, and less than a week in a further 30. Occasionally hypnosis was used to aid recovery, but often an amnesic gap remained covering the period from onset until declaration of loss of identity. A clear and obvious precipitating cause, often regarding family or finance, was usually present and organic disease occasionally present.

Stengel (1941) in his study of fugues restricted this term to patients who displayed compulsive wandering. In his 25 patients (full case histories are given) most had a history of recurrent depression, and in 12 there had been a suicidal attempt, although never in the fugue state. A tendency to compulsive lying was noted in 8 patients and a disturbed parent−child relationship was present in all save one. Five of his patients were epileptic. He suggested that 'going away' was a replacement for suicide, and depression in a predisposed personality was the most frequent diagnosis in his series. The concept of the occurrence of a fugue as a substitute for suicide in an attack of endogenous depression is an important contribution.

In very different circumstances were the wartime patients observed by Sargant and Slater (1941). Their series comprised the first thousand military admissions, many of whom had been evacuated from Dunkirk, to the neuropsychiatric unit of an emergency hospital near London. Of those thousand no fewer than 144 had loss of memory as a prominent symptom — a remarkably high proportion, especially as amnesia secondary to disease of the brain was excluded. The clinical features fell into two overlapping groups: one with fugues (usually wandering, always some impairment of consciousness, often with paranoid or hallucinatory experiences); and one with a retrospective forgetting of distressing events of the past occurring when the period of stress was over. Some patients had experienced only trifling stress (call-up and separation from home) and in them there was evidence of stronger constitutional predisposition to neurotic illness, and occasionally a strong presumption of malingering. In the remainder the military stress varied from occasional bombs to prolonged marching and fighting under heavy enemy action. The precipitating event did not always immediately antedate the fugue, which might occur some time after return to safe surroundings. Important antecedents were exhaustion, head injury, terror and exposure to bomb blast, a contrast to the situations in civilian life where the precipitating factor is often 'a criminal act or a situation from which an immediate, even though illusory, escape is desired'. Occasionally in soldiers the obvious precipitating event proved not to be the only pathogenic one and recovery might not occur until a further suppressed incident was uncovered. Treatment was directed towards restoring the lost memories with the aid of hypnosis or intravenous barbiturate. The outlook was not good in the sense that only about one-half returned to duty, but as the authors point out 'we have not as yet been able to tackle the pathogenic situation, that of the war'.

Of Parfitt and Gall's (1944) 30 patients who had episodes of amnesia in service life unrelated to action, 20 had a preceding fugue. The amnesia was so readily resolved by persuasion and suggestion that they categorized it as 'a refusal to remember'. It is likely that the relative lack of stress of their military service was responsible for the great frequency of malingerers in this series: Sargant commented in the discussion of this paper that malingering was rare in acute battle casualties. The theoretical distinction between malingering and hysteria is clear; in practice the full truth is not known for certain and the differential diagnosis is often very difficult. A final decision if necessary, may even require the resources displayed in the Grünthal–Störring case, summarized in Zangwill's (1967) entertaining account.

The onset of an amnesic state without a preceding fugue is more common in circumstances where a single dramatic event, such as a head injury or terror from a bomb explosion, crystallizes anxiety.

Case History No. 2   A peace-time soldier aged 23 was involved in a car accident on the night before he was due to fly abroad to a colony where terrorist attacks on soldiers and civilians were frequent. He regained consciousness after two minutes and had no focal neurological abnormality on examination, but he had lost not only personal identity and memory for the events of his life, but simple motor skills such as dressing and also the ability to recognize objects on the first occasion he encountered them after the accident. Progress over the next six months was rapid and he had relearned his technical skills and had retained information that had been given to him about his previous life, which remained a blank to him with no recollection of having experienced any of it. Suggestion under amylobarbitone narcosis led promptly to the recall of the circumstances of the accident which were personally stressful (quite apart from his impending service abroad); recall of his earlier life experiences followed immediately.

In this patient the discrepancy between the mild head injury with brief P.T.A., and the massive R.A. together with the rapid relearning, suggests that the head injury did not lead to organic brain damage, but merely provided the occasion for a motivated functional amnesia. As always, it is difficult in such circumstances to exclude malingering.

Kennedy and Neville (1957) reported 74 patients with sudden loss of memory, often with loss of personal identity. In all patients they found it possible either to arrive at a firm diagnosis of organic neurological illness (present in 36 of the 74), or to come to a definite conclusion about the influence of immediate psychological precipitants (26 patients showed clear psychogenesis without any organic disease and 5 were self-confessed malingerers). Recovery might follow after history-taking, hypnosis, narcotic abreaction, suggestion, 'discussion' (especially in malingerers), and treatment of an organic condition. The differential diagnosis of the organic from the functional patients did not depend on the features of the amnesia, but solely on the presence or absence of organic neurological disorder. Their conclusion was that their patients fell into three main categories: serious organic neurological disease, malingering, or flight from a severe depressive or anxiety state usually with obvious precipitants.

DUAL AND MULTIPLE PERSONALITIES

The literature on this subject (and on many other aspects of the influence of psychogenic factors on memory) has been ably reviewed by Rapaport (1942) in *Emotions and Memory*. The turn of the last century was the heyday of dual and multiple personalities, who conformed to and gave support to the concept of dissociation in the genesis of hysterical disorders. They are less frequent nowadays and it is likely that they were a product of the enthusiasm and credulity of the physician. It is appropriate that one recent instance made a greater impact on the entertainment world as a novel and a cinematograph film than it did on psychiatric thought. Abeles and Schilder (1935) considered that the emergence of a dual or alternating personality required the active co-operation of the physician. Rapaport pointed out that in many instances hypnosis was the occasion for the appearance of another personality: the view taken by Merskey (1971) of the nature of hypnosis is very pertinent here: 'Hypnosis is a manoeuvre in which the subject and hypnotist have an implicit agreement that certain events (e.g. paralysis, hallucinations, amnesias) will occur, either during a special procedure or later, in accordance with the hypnotist's instructions. Both try hard to put this agreement into effect and adopt appropriate behavioural rules and the subject uses mechanisms of denial to report on the events in accordance with the implicit agreement. This situation is used to implement various motives, whether therapeutic or otherwise, on the part of both participants. There is no trance state, no detectable cerebral physiological change, and only such peripheral physiological responses as may be produced equally by non-hypnotic suggestion or other emotional changes.'

THE GANSER STATE

The Ganser state has been reviewed with illustrative examples by Enoch, Trethowan and Barker (1967). The onset is sudden and the precipitating circumstances stressful, classically in prison. The central picture is that silly answers are given, after careful consideration, to simple questions, e.g. that a dog has five legs. This has been named as 'vorbeigehen', to pass by (the correct answer), the term used by Ganser, and also as 'vorbeireden', to talk beside the point. The setting is of a confusional state with a variety of accessory features such as hallucinations and somatic conversion symptoms. Both the circumstances and the bizarre answers give rise to a diagnosis of hysteria and a suspicion of malingering. The usual outcome is recovery with amnesia for the episode. The category is not a homogeneous one and an organic basis may be responsible.

PROLONGED RETROGRADE AMNESIA AFTER INTENSIVE ECT

Stengel (1951) reported four patients with massive retrograde amnesia (in one patient involving all the events of her previous life) after intensive

ECT (up to four treatments daily for a fortnight). Because of the severity of the R.A., previous hysterical symptoms and unimpaired current learning, these instances were regarded by Stengel as being hysterical. The usual form of amnesia after conventional bilateral ECT consists of: (1) permanent gaps for some episodes during the course of treatment; (2) some degree of transient ongoing learning impairment following the treatment; and (3) occasional gaps long antedating the ECT.

Case History No. 3 A woman of 50 seen three months after 9 bilateral ECT's had watched the previous night a cinematograph film taken on her summer holiday nine months earlier; she had recognized the members of her family and herself, but had no memory at all of the holiday.

Case History No. 4 A psychiatrist aged 35, two months after six ECT's (Anon., 1965), was asked if he was going to a lecture by Professor X; he did not recognize the name although he had spent a fortnight in Professor X's unit abroad six months earlier.

Such gaps for events long preceding the course of treatment used to occur commonly, and even more common was a failure to name or even recognize old acquaintances on return to work. The deleterious effect on memory of increasing amounts of electricity (Ottosson, 1960a) and of bilateral as contrasted with unilateral non-dominant ECT (Halliday *et al.,* 1968) was not appreciated at the time that intensive ECT was being given; it is possible that Stengel's patients had a considerable organic underlay. Now that unilateral non-dominant ECT with small measured amounts of electricity is replacing bilateral ECT, the amount of post-ECT amnesia has diminished enormously. It can be expected that with the general adoption of non-dominant unilateral ECT, the commonest and most disabling side-effect of the classic technique will disappear (Halliday *et al.,* 1975).

SLIPS OF THE TONGUE AND AMNESIA FOR WORD-FINDING

The psychoanalytical concept of repression has been used to explain not only the dissociative phenomena of conversion hysteria, but also errors in speech and recall such as misnaming and momentary amnesia for word-finding. Such an explanation is plausible and certainly has gained enormous popularity in lay circles, with the 'analysis' of such errors at times attaining the status of a party game. The psychoanalytical explanation is however not capable of refutation, for the action of repression is individual and specific, and not open to statistical treatment. A more mundane explanation derives from a consideration of the type of error made in recalling a string of words (Baddeley and

Patterson, 1971). If recall is required after a lapse of time during which the words are being held in the short-term memory store, say up to 30 seconds, errors tend to be acoustic, e.g. cat, mat, but if after five minutes, or indeed one month, when the words have been in the long-term memory store, errors are semantic, e.g. cat, dog. The notion that errors of naming depend on faulty retrieval from short- and long-term memory-stores is open to test, and indeed a few days of observation will show that most of such errors may be readily categorized as acoustic or semantic, and not infrequently as of combined type (Shallice and McGill, 1977). A more accurate if far less attractive monograph would be 'The Neuropsychology of Everyday Life'.

CONCLUSION

A sharp distinction between the various categories of psychogenic loss of memory discussed above seems unwarranted. Their explanation must be sought in psychological terms: the organic element is limited to providing a fertile ground for their growth.

Acknowledgement

Thanks are due to the H. J. Shorvon Memorial Fund for financial assistance concerned with the work described in this chapter.

10 Amnesia : A Psychoanalytic Viewpoint

M. M. Feldman

INTRODUCTION

It seems very natural to desire a unified theory of forgetting, whether one chooses to frame it in physiological terms, in terms of concepts like 'retroactive inhibition', or 'unconscious wishes'. The question arises, however, whether any such unitary model can fruitfully be applied to all types of amnesic phenomena. Specifically, when one asks the question 'Why did he forget this?', or 'What led to this being forgotten?', might it sometimes be appropriate and useful to answer in terms of 'unconscious' wishes, fears or processes? If so, are there specific kinds of 'forgetting' or specific instances of forgetting to which such an explanation best applies, or could one invoke psychodynamic factors in *all* kinds of forgetting? Finally, what *sorts* of psychodynamic explanations have been adduced to account for amnesic phenomena, and do these form part of a general theory of memory?

Peters (1958), in his study of the concept of motivation, has argued that when we ask a question like 'Why did Jones forget X?', we are in fact asking one of a number of different *types* of question. 'The particular formula employed in asking the question usually dictates the sort of answer which is expected and which counts as explanation'. The differences between these types of question are such that an all-embracing theory is inappropriate. To illustrate, when one asks 'Why has he forgotten the mathematics he learnt 15 years ago?', 'Why has he forgotten 75 per cent of the nonsense syllables in yesterday's experiment?', 'Why has he forgotten what happened just before his head injury?', 'Why has he forgotten his friend's name?', or 'Why has he forgotten his own name, and where he lives?', one is asking different *kinds* of question, and a different *kind* of explanation may be appropriate in each case.

People are likely, of course, to differ in the type or content of the explanation they consider satisfactory, and one may vary the kind of explanation given in the light of other evidence (such as evidence of progressive memory loss, or evidence that the memory loss was brief, transient, and occurred in circumstances that had special meaning for the subject). In some cases of forgetting, it seems appropriate to give a kind of 'normative' explanation such as 'He forgot because it was a long time ago', or 'Because he found it boring', or 'Because there was too much going on at the time'. This kind of explanation makes implicit reference to a 'normal', or 'understandable' process of forgetting. It often seems to imply that anyone would probably have not recalled such and such, given these conditions. This is not to deny that the patterns of normal forgetting, and the factors influencing it are of interest to the psychologist and the physiologist, but our 'explanations' of these are usually framed in terms of 'processes' rather than 'causes'. There are other instances of forgetting, however, where this type of explanation seems unsatisfactory, or inadequate, and one turns instead to a *causal* explanation, which is of a very different kind. This explanation might be framed, for example, in terms of organic brain dysfunction, or, as Freud suggested in some cases, in terms of unconscious forces or 'causes'. The kind of explanation that is felt to be appropriate is often implicit in our language, or our response to a piece of behaviour. One may say, for example, 'What *possessed* him to forget that important lecture?', 'What *drove* that out of his mind?', or 'What *made* him leave that at home?'. One might say he keeps forgetting things — his wife is worried, and wants him to see a doctor.

Now, as mentioned above, one may be mistaken in one's implicit or explicit classification of a piece of amnesic behaviour, and how to assign such behaviour may tax one's understanding. This is not different in principle, however, from the problem of knowing whether it is appropriate (or right) to say someone failed to do something because they couldn't be bothered, because they were depressed, or because they suffer from myxoedema. One of Freud's main contributions in this area was to link together, and give psychological explanations for classes of events which had previously been left to physiology, superstition, or disregarded as being of no importance whatever. He firmly believed in the principle of psychic determinism (1901), rejecting the notion that anything is due to chance or is incidental in psychic life. The theory that certain kinds of forgetting were not due to chance but strictly determined by unconscious motivation linked it with other inadequacies and unintentional activities in our psychic functions. He did not claim that explanations in terms of unconscious mental causes necessarily applied to *all* forgetting, but that they were particularly appropriate in some situations.

FREUD ON MEMORY

Freud saw the central importance of memory in any systematic general psychology, pointing out (1895) that 'Any psychological theory deserving consideration must provide an explanation of memory'. He was, at this time, exploring the explanatory potential of the concept of the repressed unconscious in relation to a wide variety of normal and pathological behaviour. He distinguished quite clearly, however, between the kinds of amnesic phenomena to which the concept of repression might be applicable, and those, which he termed the 'normal processes of forgetting', about which he claimed to know very little. Freud believed, though, that nothing was ever really forgotten: 'Since we overcame the error of supposing that the forgetting we are familiar with signified a destruction of the memory trace – that is, its annihilation – we have been inclined to take the opposite view, that in mental life nothing which has once been formed can perish – that everything is somehow preserved and that in suitable circumstances . . . it can once more be brought to light'. (Freud, 1930, p. 69).

Despite the fact that he did not try to elaborate a general theory of memory, Freud made some suggestions regarding the mechanism of 'forgetting in its proper sense'. 'Mnemic material is subject in general to two influences, condensation and distortion'. Memory traces that have remained affectively operative are subjected mainly to distortion, while 'The traces that have grown indifferent succumb unresistingly to the process of condensation . . .'. (By condensation he means the process whereby a single composite idea or compromise may come to represent several other more complex ideas, or associative chains). 'As these processes of condensation and distortion continue for long periods during which every fresh experience acts in the direction of transforming the mnemic content, it is generally thought that it is time which makes memory uncertain and indistinct. It is highly probable that there is no question at all of there being any direct function of time in forgetting' (Freud, 1901). Elsewhere, he says 'Normal forgetting takes place by way of condensation. In this way it becomes the basis for the formation of concepts'. Further, '. . . all impressions are preserved, not only in the same form in which they were first received, but also in all the forms which they have adopted in their further developments . . .' (Freud, 1901).

Thus Freud seems to be saying that 'normal' forgetting involves the continuous reorganization of existing memory traces, and that new memory input has the potential to affect the existing organization. This process does not seem to imply an intrinsic defensive purpose, or depend on unconscious motives. This desciption of the fate of the forgotten bears a striking resemblance to the model Henry Head (1926) used to describe the way in which proprioceptive impulses were dealt with. He developed the notion of the 'body schema', a complex, integrated organization, capable of being constantly modified by further input, and which in turn was used for reference in placing new sensations and initiating new movements (while not itself accessible to consciousness).

Oldfield and Zangwill (1942) point out that the concept of the 'schema' is used both in a *functional* sense (as a mediating mechanism), and in a *material* sense (involving some form of 'record' of past events). '. . . the first function of the schemata is to provide permanent, yet continuously modified physiological dispositions which, acting in co-operation with the immediate clues, can endow perception with the determinativeness of which we are in fact aware. The second function is the active one of mediating particular perceptions so determined'. However, they go on: '. . . It is scarcely possible to avoid the assumption that in some sense or other a record of past events or of the environment to which the organism reacts, is involved'.

Head's concept of the schema was elaborated by Bartlett (1926, 1932) who suggested that while on the one hand the schema is to be regarded as an arrangement of responses, '. . . it is also, regarded from another point of view, an arrangement of material sensory at a lowly level, affective at a perhaps slightly higher level, imaginal at a higher yet, and eventually ideational and conceptual. But its functions as arrangements of responses are not to be confused with its character and functions as arrangement of material'. These important contributions have led to the development of the more general concept of 'cognitive structures', which have been defined by Rapaport (1957) as '. . . both those quasi-permanent means which cognitive processes use and do not have to create *de novo* each time, and those quasi-permanent organizations of such means that are the framework for the individual's cognitive processes'. He points out that memory organizations are perhaps the most common 'cognitive structures'.

Such concepts are highly relevant to a discussion of the kind of 'forgetting' referred to above. The 'forgotten' content can be regarded as having become integrated into one or a set of 'cognitive structures' or 'schemata', having important adaptive functions. While it may not be possible to achieve the conscious recall of such content, and while considerable reorganization may have occurred, the suggestion is that such 'forgotten' material, as part of the schemata, plays a vital part in the organization of our mental activity, and in the reception of new material.*

Freud's main interest in the problem of amnesia was directed, however, not to the kind of processes referred to above, but to a rather special kind of forgetting. As a clinician he was confronted with lapses of memory which, while possibly serving an immediate defensive purpose, could be thought of as maladaptive. He studied these phenomena, and what were termed 'parapraxes' (apparently unimportant slips of the tongue, forgetting of names, etc.) as a means of elucidating psychic mechanisms of much wider psychopathological significance.

Thus psychoanalytic attention focused less on how memory traces were established, organized and recalled, than on the possible dynamic significance of the amnesia, and on ways of eliciting forgotten or 'repressed' memories which were thought to be functionally active and giving rise to symptoms or other interference with normal functioning. The paradox is, that 'In the case of *repressed* memory traces it can be demonstrated that they undergo no alteration even in the course of the longest period of time. The unconscious is quite timeless' (Freud, 1901, p. 275). In other words, while on the one hand normal forgetting can be seen as a necessary result of the reorganization of the working memory, and has an adaptive value, repression can be seen as a special form of memory. Though unavailable for conscious recall, that which is repressed is somehow preserved as a vivid and timeless memory. It implies a form of memory storage that violates all the principles of ordinary memory organization. In the early years of psychoanalysis, there was a belief that if these repressed memories could be brought into consciousness, they would cease to be troublesome. In the particular case of the 'parapraxes', the apparently unimportant forgetting of a name might indicate the presence of some dynamically significant repressed content, to which the name had become linked. The task here would be to elicit the repressed memories, thoughts or wishes, rather than simply the name itself.

Freud saw clearly the necessity for distinguishing the *kinds* of forgetting for which reference to the dynamic unconscious, and the mechanism of repression was appropriate. Although he attempted, in

---

*" 'Schema' refers to an active organisation of past reactions, or of past experience, which must always be supposed to be operating in any well-adapted organic response. That is, whenever there is any order or regularity of behaviour, a particular response is possible only because it is related to other similar responses which have been serially organised, yet which operate, not simply as individual members coming one after another, but as a unitary mass. Determination by schemata is the most fundamental of all the ways in which we can be influenced by reactions and experiences which occurred some time in the past." (Bartlett, 1932)).

the case of the parapraxes, to outline some criteria (*see below*), there is no simple way in which one might unequivocally distinguish between 'normal' forgetting and repression. The relevance and significance of unconscious dynamic factors in a given piece of behaviour will always be a matter of judgement, and open to doubt. Freud was suggesting, though, that the concept of forgetting brought about by unconscious wishes, conflicts or needs was of particular relevance in certain classes of phenomena. These were, firstly, the 'parapraxes' referred to above; secondly, the puzzling paucity of memories which his patients claimed for the period of life between about two and five years of age; thirdly, the 'forgetting' of certain disturbing experiences or events, which it might later be possible to recall with particular vividness, clarity, and affect.

The parapraxes

In *The Psychopathology of Everyday Life* (1901), Freud speaks of 'Certain shortcomings in out psychical functioning . . . and certain seemingly unintentional performances (which) prove, if psycho-analytic methods of investigation are applied to them, to have valid motives and to be determined by motives unknown to consciousness.' He included in this group '. . . the cases of forgetting, the errors in spite of better knowledge, the slips of the tongue, misreadings, slips of the pen, bungled actions and the so-called 'chance actions'.' Not all such failures of memory, speech or action were included, but only those meeting certain criteria. There must be a momentary, temporary, and apparently quite ordinary disturbance of a function the subject can normally perform successfully. If the parapraxis is pointed out by someone else, the subject immediately recognizes the failure or omission. In any case he is unaware of any motive, but tends to attribute it to inattentiveness, or chance.

Freud saw these failures as resulting from a conflict between unacceptable impulses seeking expression, and forces opposing them. The parapraxis, like the neurotic symptom, represents a more-or-less *unsuccessful* attempt at forgetting. The prohibited impulse asserts itself indirectly by causing the forgetting or distortion of a word or idea which is associatively linked with it. Freud gives a wealth of examples, illustrating different aspects of the mechanisms involved. Perhaps it will suffice to quote briefly one such example.

> A young man wished to end a rather intense exposition with a quotation from Virgil, but could not recall a missing word ('aliquis'). Freud completed the quotation, and accepted the challenge to find the reason for the omission, by

following the young man's associations to 'aliquis'. First, his subject thought of dividing the word into 'a' and 'liquis', then reliquien (relics), liquefying, fluidity, fluid, came to his mind. His next association was to relics in a particular church, and the accusation of ritual blood sacrifice. His thoughts then moved to an article 'What St. Augustine says about women'. Next he referred to a fine old gentleman, a real 'original', whose name was Benedict. He mentioned some saints' names, then St. Januarius, and the miracle of his blood came to his mind. He explained that on a particular holy day a phial of St. Januarius' blood miraculously liquefies. The people attach great importance to this miracle, and get very excited if it is delayed, as happened once when the French were occupying the town. The general in command, with an unmistakable gesture towards the soldiers posted outside, said he *hoped* the miracle would take place very soon.

After some hesitation the young man said he had been thinking about a young lady from whom he might hear 'a piece of news' that would be 'very awkward'. Freud indicated how the young man's anxiety over the cessation of her periods had been clearly indicated in the earlier associations. There was reference to 'the calendar saints, the blood that starts to flow on a particular day, the disturbance when the event fails to take place, the open threats that the miracle must be vouchsafed, or else . . .'

There was some further elaboration, but this fragment may serve to illustrate the way in which an idea associated with anxiety and conflict (the quotation from Virgil reads 'let someone (aliquis) arise from my bones as an avenger!') becomes associatively linked with an apparently innocuous indefinite pronoun which cannot then be recalled. Presumably the forgotten word has now acquired some 'signal value', and has itself the capacity to arouse the unwanted feelings. In this example, the analysis stops at the uncovering of the young man's conscious anxiety, but Freud's theory requires the assumption that in fact the parapraxis came about by the intercurrent conflict being somehow linked with a much deeper, repressed problem (for example, anxieties about parental sexuality, Oedipal fears, fantasies about mother's pregnancies, etc.)

The mechanism postulated in the case of the parapraxes are very similar to those operating in the apparently quite unrelated phenomenon of 'infantile amnesia'.

Infantile amnesia

Freud commented on '. . . the peculiar amnesia which, in the case of most people, though by no means all, hides the earliest beginnings of their childhood up to their sixth or eighth year. Hitherto it has not occurred to us to feel any astonishment at the fact of this amnesia, though we might have good grounds for doing so.' He goes on to say 'We have, on the contrary, good reason to believe that there is no period at which the capacity for receiving and reproducing impressions is greater than precisely during the years of childhood. On the other hand, we must assume, or we can convince ourselves by a psychological examination of other people, that the very same impressions that we have forgotten have none the less left the deepest traces on our minds and have had a determining effect upon the whole of our later development. There can, therefore, be no question of any real abolition of the impressions of childhood, but rather of an amnesia similar to that which neurotics exhibit for later events, and of which the essence consists in a simple withholding of these impressions from consciousness, viz., in their repression.' (Freud, 1905). He relates this repression to 'impressions of a sexual and aggressive nature, and . . . to early injuries to the ego (narcissistic mortifications)' (Freud, 1939). In other words, the repression is associated with the arousal of anxiety mainly connected with intense sexual or aggressive feelings, fantasies, wishes or experiences which the immature psyche is unable to deal with, and thus much of the content of these years is 'forgotten'. This infantile amnesia '. . . turns everyone's childhood into something like a prehistoric epoch and conceals from him the beginnings of his own sexual life . . .' (Freud, 1905). However, as in the case of the parapraxes, the forgetting is not complete. Freud refers to 'screen-memories', the few memories from this amnesic period that often seem rather insignificant. They are commonly visual, with a brightness or intensity contrasting with their relatively indifferent, innocuous or patently distorted content. The rememberer often seems detached and watches himself as a child performer.

Freud showed that here too, by following the associative links one might reach vividly retained experiences which had been accompanied (and might still be accompanied) by considerable conflict and anxiety. Like the forgetting of a name, a screen-memory indicates the presence of dynamically active, repressed content.

The mechanism of repression has been referred to a number of times. It is not only of central importance in understanding the psychoanalytic view of forgetting, but is a crucial concept in psychoanalytic theory.

Repression

In his early work with hysterical patients, Freud became convinced that the neurotic symptoms were connected with some antecedent psychic trauma (often of a sexual nature). Because the patient was not able to react to or cope with the disturbing thoughts and feelings associated with the experience, the memory of the trauma (and hence its capacity directly to evoke pain or anxiety) was 'repressed', or rendered unavailable to conscious recollection. These memories are, however, now no longer subject to normal processes of forgetting whereby '... the affect which was originally strong in his memory eventually loses intensity and that finally the recollection, having lost its affect, falls a victim to forgetfulness and the process of wearing away' (Freud, 1893). On the contrary, the repressed contents have not lost their affect, and if they are eventually able to be recalled, have a particular vividness.*

The importance of these repressed contents, for Freud, lay in his belief that although inaccessible to consciousness, they continued to exert a pathogenic effect. It is, to some extent, by virtue of its location in the Unconscious that the particular content has such a capacity to produce neurotic symptoms. Freud believed that to divest it of its force, it was necessary to alter its status of 'forgotten'. The dammed-up feelings might then be released, and the memory trace subject to normal processes of forgetting.

THE CONCEPT OF REPRESSION

To summarize briefly the classic concept of repression (*see* Freud, 1905; Brenner, 1957, 1966); it is seen as one of the mechanisms by which the ego defends itself against an unacceptable instinctual drive, or derivative of such drive, which might, were it to obtain conscious expression, give rise to anxiety. The postulated mechanism of repression is an active, dynamic force or 'counter-cathexis' which keeps the content out of consciousness, striving to protect the ego. The effects of this repression are that the drive and its derivatives are excluded from the ego, and hence from conscious awareness, but continue, at an unconscious level, to exert some pressure in the direction of emergence into consciousness and gratification. There is a tendency, however, for derivatives of the repressed drive to 'escape', and intrude into the functions of the ego, reaching consciousness, or being apparent in dreams, fantasies, slips and forgetting. These are seen as 'compromise formations', allowing a little of the repressed content to obtain disguised

---

*It sometimes appears that the 'motive' for such forgetting is the avoidance of 'unpleasure', but, as Rapaport (1942) points out, this formulation is unsatisfactory for two reasons. Firstly, it might be taken to imply that what is forgotten is consciously disagreeable, or unpleasant. Secondly, it implies that what is forgotten is *itself* disagreeable. Freud makes it clear that it is the threat of pain or anxiety at an unconscious level, which might be aroused by an idea or something associatively linked with such an idea, that leads to this kind of forgetting. That which is forgotten need not be unpleasant, and may be quite innocuous, but has become linked with some unconscious (i.e. repressed) conflict. If *this* were to impinge upon the individual's consciousness, it might give rise to feelings of anxiety or pain.

expression, and the term 'the return of the repressed' was used, implying a partial failure of repression.

Thus the classical view was that in so far as repression was successful, whatever mental elements have been repressed (e.g. memories) were effectively barred from access to consciousness and conscious behaviour. It is only when there is a return of the repressed (i.e. a partial failure of repression) that disguised and distorted derivatives of what has been repressed appear in conscious mental life. As has been indicated above, Freud invoked the concept of repression to account for, and link together phenomena such as the neurotic symptoms in his patients (where he initially believed the memory of some traumatic experience had been repressed), infantile amnesia, and some of the apparently unimportant 'forgetting' of names, etc. which he termed parapraxes. He inferred either from the *absence* of certain mental content or from the *presence* of certain phenomena, the operation of the mechanism of repression as a defence against unacceptable thoughts or feelings. Confirmation of this was sought both in the unravelling, as in a detective story, of the thread leading from the noticeably present or absent event, to the repressed idea, or impulse; and also in the response of the patient. An appropriate interpretation, or piece of work seemed to have the power to evoke 'forgotten' memories and affects.

However, as Brenner (1966) points out, it is probably an oversimplification to suggest that repressed mental elements are simply barred from access to conscious mental life. On the contrary, he suggests that, even though some content may be repressed, it can continue to exert an influence on conscious mental life. 'It plays its part, whether that part be obvious or obscure, in the creation of those compromise formations which are the stuff of conscious mental life and actions.' (The parallel with Head's concept of the schema, or Rapaport's 'cognitive structures' is very striking).

In the classic view of repression, emphasis seems to be placed on the notion of certain elements being barred from conscious mental life and action, except where this process fails and there occurs what Freud termed 'the return of the repressed'. Such failures are generally classed as pathological in waking life (neurotic symptoms, everyday psychopathology), though they occur normally as part of dreaming. Brenner stresses, however, that repression should not be regarded as a static, or once-and-for-all process, but a dynamic and shifting equilibrium between those forces which strive towards the conscious expression of some mental content, and those seeking to bar it from consciousness. (During an analytic session a patient may recall a previously repressed childhood memory or wish, only to 'forget' it shortly afterwards). He is thus emphasizing the view '. . . that repression results from an interplay of forces within the mind in which the balance is predominantly in favour of those forces which seek to bar one or several mental representations from expression in conscious mental life, usually with limited success. In other words, repressed mental elements usually play a part, in accordance with the principle of multiple function, in the phenomena of conscious mental life' (Brenner, 1966).

George Klein (1966) has somewhat broadened this argument, attempting to relate the concept of repression to some aspects of the memory process, as we now understand them. 'If remembering is conceived in terms of classes of function (tracemaking or registration; storage or retention; and retrieval), it is clear that forgetting need not itself be regarded as a unitary process; its behavioural meaning will be different in relation to each phase of the remembering process. In regard to retrieval, forgetting may mean loss of the remembering experience of a retrieved event, without implying that the memory is eliminated from storage or that retrieval through other modalities of experience, e.g. imagery, gesture or somatic displacements, is impossible. By the same token, forgetting may occur in the sense of an erasure that prevents long-term storage without loss of short-term utility. However, forgetting in the sense of erasure is entirely different from forgetting in the sense of transformation within or assimilation to existing schemata.'

With this in mind, Klein suggests one could look on repression as operating in respect of specific aspects of memory functions. It is possible, for example, to conceive of repression at the perceptual level — that is, in relation to the very process of registration (say, by means of efferent inhibitory circuits to receptors). On the other hand, it may be that the consolidation of stimuli which have been registered is interfered with, or repression can apply to transformations within the consolidation process of long-term storage itself. Finally, repression may affect the process of retrieval in specific ways.

Klein's is an interesting view, which stresses the 'necessity of viewing clinical phenomena of memory loss, remembering experience, and modes of retrieval within a broad perspective to memory, conceived as comprising a variety of adaptive functions.' One must note, however, that in suggesting that 'repression' might affect the processes of registration or consolidation, he is using the term in a special way. Generally the concept of repression implies no failure of registration or consolidation. On the contrary, the repressed persists as an unusually well preserved memory, which happens, for various dynamic reasons, to be unavailable to consciousness.

SUMMARY AND CONCLUSIONS

It thus seems that two main types of forgetting have been identified from the psychodynamic point of view. The first, or 'normal' process of forgetting consists in the 'forgotten' not being lost but somehow incorporated into the cognitive structures, or schemata which form the substrate of conscious thought, and co-ordinated actions. Some of this content is inevitably 'worn away', but on the other hand, it may be invoked as a self-conscious memory or image.

The other type of forgetting, which has been associated with the concept of repression, represents a paradox. Although that which is forgotten, in this second sense, is not available to consciousness, it is by no means lost. Indeed, as has been pointed out, the repressed content resists the normal processes of 'wearing away', or integration into other schemata, and retains not only a vividness and freshness, but considerable power to produce symptoms or interfere with the individual's functioning in various ways. The classic view of the parapraxes, or symptoms that often accompanied such repression, was that these represented the escape, or 'return of the repressed' – evidence of a partial failure of repression, though the repressed content could still not be recalled to consciousness without assistance. The mechanism was in operation to protect the psychic organization from intense pain or anxiety. The paradigm of this kind of forgetting was the traumatic experience, or the forbidden impulses or wishes, often of a sexual (or aggressive) kind. If the repressed or forgotten content *could* be recalled, the pressure giving rise to the symptoms or parapraxes would go, and that which had been repressed might now be subject to normal processes of forgetting.

Although it seems useful to delineate these two kinds of forgetting, the distinction may be difficult to make in practice, and is perhaps theoretically of less importance than it once appeared to be. Psychoanalysts are probably less concerned with specific repressed memories or impulses, and more with complex interactions of memories, wishes, fantasies and impulses.

As Brenner points out, it is perhaps not particularly useful to think in terms of a kind of locked storehouse of forbidden texts, from which material may occasionally 'escape' to cause trouble, but to see 'the repressed' as an essential substrate for normal conscious mental activity. Thus both in the case of 'normal forgetting' and in the case of 'repression', the most useful conceptual model may be that of 'the forgotten' not being lost but incorporated in one way or another into complex mental structures or 'schemata', upon which our mental processes depend, and by means of which we use past experience to organize and integrate the present.

11 Medicolegal Aspects of Amnesia

T.C.N. Gibbens and J.E. Hall Williams

Amnesia, or the disturbances of consciousness which lead to it, or surround and accompany it, has long been of great potential importance from the medicolegal point of view, but only recently has the matter become one of practical significance in decided cases. It may arise wherever the loss of consciousness is the cause of involuntary acts which amount to crimes or civil wrongs. Such involuntary acts arising in this way are often referred to in legal discussions as 'automatism', though this word is not in any sense a technical term of law. In Hill v Baxter ([1958] 1 Q.B. 277; [1958] 2 W.L.R. 76; [1958] 1 All E.R. 193), Lord Goddard referred to 'a state of automatism, or whatever term may be applied to someone performing acts in a state of unconsciousness'. He went on to say that this was the first time that the court had considered the question of automatism, but, in fact, there was a previous appeal case which turned on the rules of evidence R. v Harrison-Owen ([1951] 2 All E.R. 726), and there were several unreported cases where this issue had arisen. The medicolegal problems surrounding automatism have been the subject of growing attention in the literature and in the courts during the last twenty years. The whole question must be regarded as one of the 'growing points' in the relation between medicine and the law.

AMNESIA AS A MEDICAL CONDITION

Amnesia may occur as a result of disturbance of any of the stages of remembering — registration, retention and recall. A *failure of registration* due to inattention may be caused by any condition which affects the level of consciousness. Organic states, such as epilepsy, head injury, hypoglycaemia and intoxication with alcohol or other drugs, may produce varying degrees of clouding of consciousness; psychoses are commonly associated with periods of inattention, and acute emotional stress may so concentrate attention on particular events that other stimuli may pass unnoticed.

A *failure to retain* material which has been registered is typical of organic brain damage, and is accompanied by other signs of deterioration, such as disorientation, and typical disturbances of mood and personality. It especially affects recent rather than remote events. Failure either to register or retain the memory for events is necessarily permanent.

A *failure to recall* memories which have been registered and retained may be psychogenic, due to hysteria (that is, involuntary repression of the material into the unconscious mind) or simply malingering. Nowadays, it is generally regarded as fruitless to try to make a sharp distinction between the two; the difference is perhaps one of degree rather than of kind (Gillespie, 1936; Wexberg, 1960; Kanzer, 1939; Parfitt and Gall, 1944; Leitch, 1948; Wilson, Rupp and Wilson, 1950).

O'Connell (1960) has recently reviewed the extent of amnesia in 50 murderers; the subject has also been discussed by Leitch (1948) and Hopwood and Snell (1933). O'Connell found that 40 per cent had either no memory, or, at best, only the haziest recollection of the actions which had led to their arrest. When the amnesia cases were compared with the remainder, in many respects (including electro-encephalograph data) three factors especially distinguished them – low intelligence, an hysterical personality (immature, shallow, egocentric and histrionic, with a capacity to gain advantage from symptoms), and precipitating factors in the crime which would cloud or restrict attention such as alcoholic intoxication, sexual excitement and extreme rage reactions. Organic factors such as epilepsy, head injury or hypoglycaemia, with two possible exceptions, did not seem to account for the amnesia in this group. Among eight schizophrenics, three had amnesia, and of five established epileptics, three claimed amnesia and two did not.

In the diagnosis of the organic causes of amnesia, the physical and psychiatric signs, the degree of purposiveness and neatness of the act, the behaviour immediately before and after the act are of chief interest, since the state of mind at the time of the crime is the main issue. Those with psychogenic amnesia often give a clear impression that recovering the memory would be upsetting. 'My head bursts as the picture is getting clear, and that is what stops me getting it clear.' There may be variations in the account of the beginning and end of the amnesic period, evidence of an hysterical personality, dramatic recovery of memory and sometimes amnesia for large periods of a person's life. But many of these features of the history may initially give a wrong impression. As Hopwood and Snell point out (1933), a full memory may be feigned as well as an amnesia; some patients may hear details of the offence repeated to them so often that they come to believe that they remember them. An amnesia due to head injury may be prolonged by psychogenic factors.

AMNESIA, AUTOMATISM AND INVOLUNTARY CONDUCT IN THE CRIMINAL LAW

It is a fundamental principle of the criminal law that to be convicted of a crime a person must commit a voluntary act, and he must also have the necessary *mens rea* or guilty mind. It is not easy to know whether a state of automatism and amnesia should properly be regarded as negating the element of voluntariness in the requirement of an act, or as negating the requirement of a guilty mind. This may be more a matter of form and legal analysis than a matter of substance, though there are cases which show that it could make all the difference which classification or analysis is adopted (R. v Harrison-Owen [1951] 2 All E.R. 726). It must be observed that the requirement of *mens rea* is itself not a straightforward one and it is not always easy to separate the elements of intention from the requirements for an 'act'. There are undoubtedly some criminal offences for which it can be said that only a very slight degree of intention is required; all that is needed is that the act must be voluntary on the part of the accused, which some scholars regard as going to the requirement of an act rather than concerning intention. Thus, a person may be guilty of a minor traffic offence or a licensing contravention, without it being proved that he intended it. This is commonly exemplified by the case of the man driving without lights, who may not be aware that his lights are extinguished, but is nonetheless guilty of the offence. Such offences are known as offences of strict liability. A sane person who, it is shown, did not act voluntarily, must be acquitted. In this connection a man's conduct will normally be deemed to be voluntary on his part. If, however, there is evidence that consciousness was lost or grossly disturbed at the time of the act, this cannot be assumed. Where there is evidence that the offender 'did not know what he was doing' by reason of mental disease or illness, if the defence of insanity is raised and in certain other circumstances (*see below*), he may be dealt with as 'not guilty on the ground of insanity', and committed to a special hospital such as Broadmoor.

The real difficulty in this matter lies with the line between the sane person who is to be excused repsonsibility on the ground that he acted involuntarily in a state of clouded consciousness, and the sane person who must be held responsible for his conduct if the ordinary principles of responsibility are to be maintained. Lord Goddard in Hill v Baxter (1958 — *see* page 245) was clearly conscious of the dangers of allowing too much room for this kind of defence, and a fairly rigorous requirement of proof has been laid down. Otherwise scores of offenders might claim that they 'did not remember doing it' or 'did not mean to do it'.

It seems that there are two types of involuntary action which are now recognized by the criminal law as absolving from responsibility. The first concerns conscious involuntary movements, such as are involved in reflex or instinctive actions, or where there is physical compulsion or duress. An example of the first would be a sudden coughing or sneezing, a defensive gesture which is instinctive, or where a motor-cyclist is stung by a swarm of bees or hit by a stone and drives erratically; he might be exonerated on a charge of dangerous driving. This type of behaviour is irrelevant for our purpose, as the conduct in question would not be accompanied by, or followed by, amnesia. A marginal case which might belong in this category is where a person commits a crime under the influence of post-hypnotic suggestion; it might be agreed that he 'willed' the act, but that his will was under the control of another, and there might be amnesia for the event. Such cases do not appear to have occurred in the English courts, though there is a celebrated case occurring in Denmark (the case of Nielson), which went on appeal to the European Court of Human Rights. Glanville Williams (1961) takes the view that such a person might be excused from responsibility, just like any other person who acts under duress.

The second type of involuntary conduct occurs when an individual is unconscious or when his actions were 'purely automatic', to use the words of Barry J. in R. v Charlson ([1955] 1 All E.R. 859; [1955] 1 W.L.R. 317). These are our main concern, since there will usually be amnesia for the event, and the question is whether the person should be held legally responsible.

This form of involuntary act has been accepted in legal cases concerned with post-epileptic states, sleep-walking and, more recently, in cases of head injury, organic brain disease, anoxia, hypoglycaemia and intoxication with drugs.

Epileptic automatism has long been accepted as exempting from criminal responsibility. Indeed, the long history of the acceptance of this condition is a source of embarrassment today, since such offenders are customarily regarded as legally insane, and dealt with on that basis. In the well-known case cited by Hill and Sargant (1943), a murder was committed in a state of partial starvation and after four pints of beer. Simulating these conditions, it was possible to show that the accused's previous mildly abnormal EEG was grossly abnormal, and that overbreathing, such as must have been induced by the quarrel preceding the murder, would have produced a slight but definite impairment of consciousness. He was found guilty but insane. Such offenders fall under the M'Naghten Rules since, clearly, they do not know the nature and quality of their acts. But there may be many offences of epileptics, for example driving offences, which do not justify detention in a special hospital such as Broadmoor. As Glanville Williams remarks, it may be sufficient that the epileptic who drives dangerously should have his licence taken away (Glanville Williams, 1961, p. 485).

There have been several cases where people have killed while sleep-walking or waking from sleep, or where they have inflicted a serious wounding on another. Sometimes these situations have led to acquittals. Thus, in H.M. Advocate v Fraser (1878) (4 Couper 70), the accused person killed a child during sleep, thinking that he was struggling with a wild tiger, and was acquitted on the ground of mistake. In a South African case R. v Dhlamini (1955 (1) S.A.L.R. 120), a man killed under the influence of nightmares. He was acquitted on the ground that 'he acted mechanically without intention, volition or motive'. In R. v Price (1958) (Glanville Williams, 1961, p. 483, note 1) a marine was acquitted after attacking a corporal with a bayonet while in a twilight state of consciousness, not having fully recovered from a dream. In R. v Boshears (1961) (*The Times*, February 18th, 1961; Morris and Blom-Cooper, 1964, p. 177) an American airman was acquitted of the murder of a girl with whom he slept, the killing having taken place by strangulation. Glanville Williams comments that if EEG studies suggested that any of these persons had had nocturnal epilepsy, they might have been found not guilty on the ground of insanity (Glanville Williams, 1961, p. 484).

Though the law appears to take a common-sense view and exonerates such offenders, many psychiatrists might disagree with this result. Some of these offenders are only different in degree from others who commit crimes in a state of hysterical dissociation and are held responsible. Many murderers with subsequent amnesia probably commit their crimes in such a dissociated state, and are still regarded as responsible. In a case known to one of the present authors (Gibbens), a wife charged her husband before the magistrates' court because she had on several occasions been woken up by his attempts to strangle her or beat her up.

She said he seemed dazed during the attacks. On one occasion he nearly succeeded in throwing her downstairs. He had a history of a head injury at a time when he had suspected her of infidelity some years previously, and a vague history of subsequent blackouts. It was suspected that a feeling of hostile jealousy might have been 'built in' to epileptic attacks, as sometimes occurs. Prolonged EEG investigation day and night revealed no abnormality, however, and enquiry showed that he was an irritable, chronic alcoholic with hysterical tendencies. The court dismissed the case, but when the wife learned that no one felt able to guarantee that there would be no recurrence, she left him. Had he killed her, a simple acquittal would hardly have been the correct course.

The recent series of decisions with regard to automatism in criminal cases was initiated by R. v. Charlson (1955 – *see* page 248). The accused made a sudden assault with a wooden mallet on his young son, to whom he was devoted, picked him up and threw him out of the window; he fell into a river and was seriously hurt. It is not clear how much amnesia was present, but there was some clouding of consciousness afterwards, and he said he did not know why he had done it. The prison doctor gave evidence that the examination and history pointed to the possibility of the accused suffering from a cerebral tumour, in which case he would be liable to motiveless outbursts of violence over which he had no control. He was charged with causing grievous bodily harm (G.B.H.) with intent to murder, or with intent to cause G.B.H., or simply malicious wounding. The judge (Barry J.) pointed out that in order to support the first two charges, there must be evidence of the specific intent required; the third charge needed no such proof but depended solely on whether Charlson knew what he was doing, and it was his conscious act. If his actions were purely automatic, and his mind had no control over the movements of his limbs, he was like a person in an epileptic fit and not responsible. The jury acquitted him. It is important to note that no question of insanity was raised by the defence or the trial judge, and the result of this case has been criticized by Glanville Williams and Lord Denning. It was not followed in R. v Kemp (1956) where Devlin J. took a new line with regard to the effect of automatism on the issue of responsibility.

In R. v Kemp ([1956] 3 W.L.R. 724; [1956] 3 All E.R. 249) an elderly man of excellent character suddenly made an entirely motiveless and irrational attack on his wife during the night, striking her with a hammer and inflicting serious injury. Medical witnesses agreed that he suffered from arteriosclerosis, and that he did not know what he was doing. Argument developed as to the meaning of 'disease of the mind' under the M'Naghten Rules, and whether the accused came within them. The defence said that disease was limited to functional conditions such as schizophrenia or melancholia, but the prosecution argued that diseases of organic origin or those traceable to physical derangement, such as arteriosclerosis, were included. Devlin J. ruled that whichever view of the matter the jury accepted, they must bring in a verdict of 'guilty but insane'. He observed that the law 'is not concerned with the origin of the disease or the cause of it, but simply with the mental condition which has brought about the act'. He ruled that the whole question of the accused's sanity was before the court, even though it had not been the intention of the defence to raise this issue. The view taken by Devlin J. in this case has since been approved in the House of Lords by Lord Denning, and a similar situation which developed concerning the relation between the defence of diminished responsibility and insanity in cases of homicide, now provided for by statute, was resolved in a similar fashion by case law in R. v Bastian ([1958] 1 W.L.R. 413) and R. v Nott (1959) (43 Cr. App. R. 8).*

The defence counsel who wishes to raise a plea of automatism is now faced with the danger that it will be treated as evidence of insanity, leading to a M'Naghten verdict if the judge thinks that is the right course, and the jury agree. This is likely to be the case where there is some medical history of mental disease or where the circumstances strongly suggest it. The question of the degree of proof required for the defence of automatism has now been resolved by the House of Lords in Bratty v Attorney-General for Northern Ireland (1961). This will be separately discussed below (*see* p. 254).

Automatism in minor offences

When a crime is committed in a state of unconsciousness or automatism, it is often a trivial offence. Cases of serious violence or murder in this condition are rare, if one excludes those who are insane within the M'Naghten Rules. No doubt this is the reason for the surprising lack of major difficulties until recent years. Minor crimes, especially minor assaults and occasional cases of shop-lifting, in which there is something present which suggests a defence of automatism, are not uncommon, but in the higher courts the nature of the crime and the risk which exists of raising an issue of insanity means that it is simpler in most cases to plead guilty or be so found, and to use the medical features of the case in mitigation. Magistrates frequently impose a fine or otherwise take note of the circumstances in passing sentence. Offences

* See now Criminal Procedure (Insanity) Act, 1964, Section 6. Note that this Act, by Section 1, altered the form of verdict in insanity cases to 'not guilty by reason of insanity'.

involving amnesia, including hysterical fugues, and some offenders who must be regarded as mentally ill, and where there is real doubt about their legal responsibility, are commonly dealt with on the basis that there is no legal defence available, but the matter is one for the sentencing stage.

The case of Hill v. Baxter (1958 – *see* p. 245) was one of the first cases where an appellate court had considered the implications of the defence of automatism. The driver of a van was accused of dangerous driving and failing to stop at a halt sign, with the result that he ran into another car. He said that he remembered nothing of the events leading up to the accident, and that he had used a route which he would not normally have used if he had been aware of what he was doing. He was found by the police in a dazed condition after the accident. The magistrates dismissed the case on the ground that the accused person was not conscious of what he was doing, 'with the implication that he was not capable of forming any intention as to his manner of driving'. On appeal by way of case stated, the prosecution challenged this decision. The Divisional Court, in a reserved judgment, found the magistrates had erred in law.

Lord Goddard, C.J., observed that the offence of dangerous driving was one of absolute prohibition, and likewise the offence of failing to observe the traffic sign. This meant that no question of *mens rea* enters into the case at all, so that the justices' finding that he was not capable of forming any intention as to the manner of driving was immaterial. He was driving, and apparently exercising some skill. The onus of proof was on the defendant to prove that he was in a state of automatism; he had not provided sufficient evidence of this. Although there may be cases where it can be said that the accused was not driving at all, this was not one of them. The accused's evidence was 'quite inconsistent with being overcome with sleep or at least drowsiness . . . and it would be impossible as well as disastrous, to hold that falling asleep at the wheel was any defence to a charge of dangerous driving. If a driver finds that he is getting sleepy he must stop.' There was previous authority to this effect. In Kay v Butterworth (1945) (110 J.P. 75) a man coming off night-shift fell asleep at the wheel of a van, and ran into some soldiers. He was acquitted, but on appeal, Humphreys J. remitted the case to the magistrates for conviction on the ground that the accused should not have driven when he was drowsy.

The two other judges in Hill v Baxter (1958 – *see* p. 245) agreed with Lord Goddard, but gave separate judgments. Pearson J. said that the only question was whether the accused 'was driving at all'. One might not be responsible if one was unconscious as a result of an epileptic fit, a stroke or a heart attack. But even there, lack of volition might not always excuse the accused; one might have to consider the state of mind before the offence. An epileptic fit might render a driver irresponsible, but if he knew that he was liable to have epileptic fits or hypoglycaemic attacks, then driving itself would be dangerous, and he might have no defence if while driving he suffered an attack. Quite obviously, issues of this kind are likely to become increasingly important in the contemporary situation.

Devlin J., in a detailed judgment, observed that the part which automatism plays in determining liability for crime was 'a novel point', the answer to which depended on whether or not the temporary loss of consciousness was attributable to a disease of the mind within the M'Naghten Rules, and on the nature of the liability which the prosecution had to establish. This latter point refers to the necessity or otherwise of proving full *mens rea*. He dealt with the problem of the difficult borderline between automatism and insanity by saying 'for the purposes of the criminal law, there are two categories of mental irresponsibility, one where the disorder is due to disease, and one where it is not . . . if there is some temporary loss of consciousness arising accidentally, it is reasonable to hope that it will not be repeated, and that it is safe to let an acquitted man go entirely free.'

This judgment went to the heart of the practical problem: the choice lies between two different sorts of acquittal, one involving complete release and the other involving a finding of insanity, leading to committal to Broadmoor on an indefinite basis. This choice should depend upon the likelihood of further crime being committed and the need for some form of social control. The same judge had shown himself to be very conscious of the latter consideration in R. v Kemp (1956 –*see* p. 250) and, as we shall see, in Bratty v Attorney-General for Northern Ireland (1961) –*see below*) Lord Denning went even further.

Glanville Williams has suggested that it would be logical to separate the trial of responsibility from the trial of insanity; or even that once irresponsibility has been decided, the question of insanity should be left to the civil processes of medical certification (Glanville Williams, 1961, p. 484). This is one of the many issues on the modern legal scene which seem to point to the need for some aspects of sentencing to be remitted to some new form of tribunal after the decision about guilt. It does seem, however, that to leave the disposal to be judged according to the civil criteria of medical certification would not be a satisfactory solution. Doctors cannot be expected to weigh up the risks which society should be prepared to take, in the same way as judges. As Prevezer observes, one can classify automatism for legal purposes into three types, when considering disposition: (1) With a likelihood of recurrence. (2) With no risk of recurrence. (3) With some risk of recurrence, but not perhaps a further crime (Prevezer, 1958). In cases of epilepsy or hypoglycaemia involved in motoring offences, it would often be enough to take away the driving licence. In the U.S.A. it has been suggested that epileptics may, with treatment, be made fit to drive, and insurance companies are willing to cover them with a 5 per cent increase in premium. In such cases, it would be sufficient if the court had means of assuring itself that appropriate action had been taken. Cross (1961) has suggested that in many serious cases the court should be able to detain the accused until suitable action had been taken.

The burden of proof of automatism

Because of the dangers inherent in any defence of this kind, it has been cautiously approached by the courts, and hedged around with various safeguards. The principal one has been the requirement of .proof, and resting the burden of establishing the condition on the accused. Until Bratty v Attorney-General for Northern Ireland ([1961] 3 W.L.R. 965; [1961] 3 All E.R. 523), this might have been thought to apply to all claims of automatism, following Hill v Baxter (1958 — *see* p. 245), but we now have to separate off sane and insane automatism, and different rules apply. Bratty killed a girl whom he had taken for a ride in his car. It was said that, at the time, a blackness came over him, so that he did not know what he was doing. There was evidence of previous episodes of 'blackness', of backwardness, headaches, religious inclinations and odd behaviour. The question of psychomotor epilepsy was raised, though without conclusive evidence. The jury was invited by the defence to consider a verdict of manslaughter, or automatism leading to an acquittal, or guilty but insane, but the judge withdrew the plea of automatism from the jury, and the accused was convicted of murder. On appeal to the House of Lords, it was held that in law there were two types of automatism, namely insane and non-insane automatism; that a judge was only under a duty to leave the issue of automatism of either type to the jury, where the defence had laid a proper foundation for so doing by adducing positive evidence in respect of it, which was a question of law for the judge to decide. In this way, the jury would no longer be exposed to frivolous or exaggerated claims of automatism as a legal defence to crime. Where the only evidence supporting the defence of automatism concerns the presence of M'Naghten insanity, that is, a defect of reason from disease of the mind, it must be considered on the basis of the insanity rules alone. 'A rejection by the jury of this defence of insanity necessarily implies that they reject this possibility (of automatism)', said Viscount

Kilmuir (Prevezer, 1958). But where there might be a divergence of view as to the cause of the involuntary conduct, so that sane automatism might be the explanation, the jury should be told that the defence do not have to prove this even on balance, because it is for the Crown to prove their case beyond reasonable doubt, and if the jury are left in doubt about the matter, they must be told to acquit. This alters substantially the position with regard to the defence of automatism. Where it rests on evidence of a disease of the mind, the defence must satisfy the jury on a balance of probabilities, as in the case of a defence of insanity. But where it rests on other evidence, it is sufficient if the defence raise a doubt in the minds of the jury, when they should acquit.

Lord Denning went further and remarked that 'any mental disorder which has manifested itself in violence and is prone to recur, is a disease of the mind' (Prevezer, 1958, p. 981), which means that the danger of recurrence may be taken as one of the criteria for dealing with the matter, as Devlin J. did in R. v Kemp (*see* p. 250), on the basis of the insanity rules rather than as leading to an acquittal.

Since Bratty v Attorney-General for Northern Ireland, 1961, (*see* p. 254) there have been several other cases which demonstrate the wisdom of the solution reached. In R. v Harvey (unreported case), for example, the accused awoke in the early hours of the morning to the sound of screaming. He found himself standing by his bed, his hands were sticky, and on turning on the light he found he had blood on them and a hammer in his hands. He had seriously injured his wife with blows about the face. His attitude of amazement never varied subsequently. He had been out of work for some time and on the previous day had been told that he was to be evicted. He had gone to bed in great conflict about how he was to tell his wife, with whom he had had no differences, but had no recollection after going to sleep at 2 a.m. The medical evidence was that there was no clinical or EEG evidence of epilepsy, that he was unlikely to be malingering, and that hysteria was the probable diagnosis. The judge ruled that there was sufficient evidence for the jury to consider, and the accused was acquitted (Russell v Barton, personal communication).

Since Bratty, although the law has been clearer, in practice there has been some difficulty in knowing when the defence of automatism is likely to be available as distinct from the defence of insanity. Such a situation arose in R. v Quick, R. v Paddison [1973] 3 W.L.R. 26, where one of the defendants, Quick, called medical evidence to show that at the material time when it was alleged that, while employed as a male nurse at a mental hospital, he assaulted a patient, he was suffering from hypoglycaemia. The trial judge ruled that the proper course would be to invite the jury to bring in a verdict of insanity, which is what the prosecution had suggested. The defence counsel contended that there should be a complete acquittal, but in the end, in the light of the judge's ruling, he pleaded guilty to one of the two counts. The other defendant Paddison was then tried and convicted for his part in aiding and abetting Quick. Both defendants appealed and their convictions were quashed, it being held that, in respect of Quick, the trial judge incorrectly applied the ruling in Bratty [1961], and that on these facts it was open to the defendant to raise a defence of automatism without being in peril of a finding of insanity.

In the course of his judgment, Lord Justice Lawton gave some very useful guidance about the correct approach in situations of this kind. He first reviewed the authorities, including some Commonwealth cases from Australia and New Zealand, culminating in Bratty's case [1961]. 'This quagmire of law', he said, is 'seldom entered nowadays save by those in desperate need of some kind of defence.' Bratty's case provided 'the only firm ground'. Looking at the question of what the law now means by the words 'disease of the mind' for the purpose of resolving these matters, Lord Justice Lawton came to the conclusion that 'the fundamental concept is of a malfunctioning of the mind caused by disease'*. Then comes the crux of his decision: 'A malfunctioning of the mind of transitory effect caused by the application to the body of some external factor such as violence, drugs (including anaesthetics), alcohol and hypnotic influences cannot fairly be said to be due to disease.' He went on to explain that such malfunctioning will not always relieve a person from criminal responsibility. Difficult border-line cases are to be resolved by asking whether the mental condition can fairly be regarded as amounting to or producing a defect of reason from disease of the mind. In this particular case, Quick's condition was caused by his own behaviour as a diabetic in using the insulin prescribed by his doctor; 'such malfunctioning of the mind as there was, was caused by an external factor and not by a bodily disorder in the nature of a disease which disturbed the working of his mind'. It followed that he was entitled to have his defence of automatism left to the jury. If that had been done, a number of other questions would have had to be taken into account, such as Quick's consumption of alcohol and his neglect of his doctor's instructions about taking regular meals, and whether he had any advance warning of getting into a hypoglycaemic

* This distinction was recognized by the Butler Committee on Mentally Abnormal Offenders, and they recommended the express exclusion of transient states of mind not related to other forms of disorder from the legal provisions governing the defence of mental disorder (*see* discussion on pp. 224, 225 of the Report, 1975, Cmnd. 6244).

state. Commenting on this case, Jennifer Temkin has remarked that insofar as the judgment may be said to have put a stop to any further attempts to expand the M'Naghten Rules, it is a truly welcome one. So far as the automatism defence is concerned, however, the judgment 'exhibits the traditional judicial reserve'. This is the first occasion on which it has been suggested that fault might preclude the defence of automatism, apart from the case of Kay v Butterworth in 1945. There is however some authority for the fault proposition, as Temkin observes, in the Canadian case of Hartridge [1967] 57 D.L.R. (2d.) 332, in which it was stated that the automatism defence would apply where there was an unconscious act ensuing 'from the taking or administration of a drug when the effect thereof was unknown to the recipient or of the effects of which he had not been advised.' Temkin argues that this new restriction places an unwarranted limitation upon the ambit of the defence which runs counter to its whole rationale; for there is no justification for denying the defence of automatism on the ground of the accused's negligence.

Two Canadian cases show how far the courts might be tempted to stray in expanding the notion of automatism, though in the event it appears that a more restricted interpretation was adopted. In R. v K. (1970) a devoted father and husband, suffering from a mild neurotic depression, was informed by a family friend by telephone that his wife intended to leave him. A few moments later Mrs K entered the room, and K in a dazed condition embraced his wife and implored her not to leave him. Some fifteen minutes later K emerged from a blackout to find his wife asphyxiated by his forceful and extended embrace. The judge, after hearing the evidence of a distinguished psychiatrist to the effect that K has suffered 'a tremendous emotional blow, as forceful as any external blow to the head', left it for the jury to decide whether there was a state of automatism produced by a severe psychological blow, so that the accused had a diminished awareness of what was going on because of his unconscious and involuntary state. The jury acquitted K. In R. v Parnerkar [1972] 1 W.W.R. 161 a Hindu who killed a woman he was hoping to marry, put up the defence that he had suffered a psychological blow when she told him she could not marry him and tore up his letters in his presence, which was sufficient to bring about a period of dissociation or automatism or to produce hysterical amnesia after the event. The trial judge instructed the jury with regard to the defence of automatism and the defence of provocation. The jury convicted of manslaughter. On appeal it was held that there must be a new trial, for the judge had erred in putting to the jury the defence of automatism. The only possible defence was that of insanity in accordance with the ruling in Hartridge (*see above*).

Other cases of automatism

The question of automatism has arisen in several other cases, both in the United Kingdom and in the Commonwealth. This study is mainly confined to a selection of the former, and for details of the latter, reference should be made to Morris and Howard (1964). A list of such cases is contained in an Appendix.

The case of Watmore v Jenkins ([1962] 3 W.L.R. 463; [1962] 2 All E.R. 868; [1962] 2 Q.B. 572) showed the courts getting into further difficulties in reconciling the medical evidence with the tests of legal responsibility. It showed also the problem of communicating medical opinion satisfactorily to the courts. The defendant was a diabetic recovering from an attack of infective hepatitis. He had been obliged to give himself higher doses of insulin than usual to counteract the effect of raised blood cortisone content caused by the infection. He drove for some miles in an erratic manner and collided with a stationary car. He was found in a dazed condition, and claimed that he had no memory for the last five miles of his drive. The justices acquitted him of the charge of dangerous driving and driving under the influence of drugs, but on appeal the plea of automatism was accepted only as a defence to the charge of driving under the influence of drugs, and not as a defence to the charges of driving dangerously and driving without due care and attention.

The Divisional Court was of the opinion that the evidence that the accused had driven some miles and shown some degree of control, was incompatible with automatism, and 'there was no complete destruction of voluntary control such as could constitute automatism in law' (at p. 474). The evidence here showed that the accused did not experience the normal sweating reaction which would have warned him that his blood sugar was low, probably because the liver glycogen was depleted by his illness.

This case demonstrates the difficulty of convincing courts that a fairly orderly sequence of behaviour, especially when habitual, does not necessarily indicate that an individual is fully conscious. This has always been recognized in relation to sleepwalking, but has not been accepted in relation to other circumstances. One of the difficulties of motoring offences is that driving is precisely the sort of semi-automatic act which can be carried out with little conscious awareness. How far this may apply to other acts which have been carried out on numerous previous occasions is a difficult question. For example, a man of 30 with 13 previous convictions for house-breaking had a head injury at nine years of age and developed jerkings and cramp of the right leg at 15 years, leading occasionally to fits. He claimed to be so embarrassed that he took to going out only at night, and lived by burglary. On the last offence he was 'awakened' by a policeman on the steps of a house he had burgled. He knew he had not been in his right mind because he had burgled the house previously (he never revisited a house), had been wearing his best clothes and had no instruments or gloves. He pleaded guilty 'to save time' and received a four-year sentence but was referred by the medical officer. He had wasting of the right leg and arm. On operation a scar was excised from the superior margin of the left hemisphere. Five years later he had a subsequent fit associated with drinking excessively. Follow-up ten years after the operation showed that he had not been reconvicted.

The influence of alcohol and other drugs upon consciousness and in the production of amnesia is an important matter affecting responsibility. If alcoholic intoxication causes a psychosis, such as delirium tremens, there is no difficulty in including such a condition within the framework of the M'Naghten Rules. Alcoholic intoxication in other respects is only a defence to a criminal charge, if of such degree as to render the accused incapable of forming the intent required by the law. The ordinary person is assumed to know what effect alcohol is likely to have, and to be able to act according to this knowledge. Similarly, with regard to other drugs such as insulin, the individual should know and guard against the possible consequences of intoxication. The case of Lipman [1969] 3 W.L.R. 819 raised in an acute form the relationship between the legal rules governing the defence of drunkenness and the factual state of being under the influence of drugs. An American killed a girl while suffering from the effect of drugs. He imagined he was struggling with snakes and struck her several blows on the head, then asphyxiated her by stuffing a sheet down her throat. He was charged with murder, but was convicted of manslaughter (by a majority verdict) and sentenced to six years' imprisonment and recommended for deportation. The appeal was based on the contention that the trial judge misdirected the jury about the relevant law. It was held that the appellant's arguments (which we need not go into) were unacceptable. It was also pointed out (and here is the relevancy of the case) that there is no reason in law to distinguish between the effect of drugs voluntarily taken and drunkenness voluntarily induced. For the purpose of criminal responsibility, they are to be treated alike. This means that only when drink or drugs render a person incapable of forming the required intention to commit a crime will they act as a legal defence. In this case, the crime of manslaughter did not require the formation of an intention to kill or to do grievous bodily harm (unlike murder). A person could be guilty for grossly negligent behaviour involving the risk of death, or unlawful behaviour which a sober and responsible person would recognize involved that risk. It was on the latter basis that Lipman was convicted, and the conviction was upheld on appeal.*

So far as motoring offences are concerned, the intoxicated person should stop driving if he is feeling in any way affected by a drug; it would seem that no defence is available unless consciousness is sufficiently affected that one can say he had no volition and is 'not driving', and this occurs without any premonition. In cases where a driver has been affected by drugs whose effects he could not anticipate, and prescribed by a doctor, the justices have dismissed charges on the basis that the accused was 'not driving'. Unconsciousness coming on insidiously as a result of carbon monoxide poisoning has been accepted as a defence. In the case of Padgett (*The Times*, May 18th, 1962; Whitlock, 1963, pp. 120 and 123), the defence claimed that the accused killed in a condition of partial anoxia due to chronic lung disease — pneumoconiosis; but the judge withdrew the plea of automatism from the jury (*compare* Bratty, 1961, p. 254) and the accused was found guilty but insane.

AMNESIA AND FITNESS TO PLEAD

There is one other way in which amnesia may affect the proceedings in a criminal trial, and that is on the preliminary issue of fitness to plead. Until the case of Podola ([1959] 3 W.L.R. 718; [1959] 3 All E.R. 418), there was hardly any authority on the question of how far amnesia, if established as genuine, might afford a basis for a finding of unfitness to plead. In that case, it was contended that as a result of a head injury, the accused had a total amnesia for the circumstances of his offence, and was, therefore, unable to instruct counsel or in other ways prepare his own defence. After much medical argument as to whether the amnesia was organic, hysterical or feigned, the jury found that it was not genuine, and the trial proceeded to conviction. On appeal, the question of the relevance of amnesia, assuming it had been genuine, was considered, and the appeal court held that this was no bar to the accused person being tried. Many trials proceed in the absence of a witness whom the accused considers essential for his defence, or without the assistance of the evidence of the accused himself. Amnesia would therefore not appear to be relevant on this preliminary issue, except insofar as it might point to some other underlying condition affecting fitness to plead.

* See also R. v Majewski [1976] 2 W.L.R. 263 for the effect of drink on responsibility in common law.

AMNESIA IN CIVIL ACTIONS

If it is true to say that the criminal courts have been slow to recognize the relevance of amnesia and involuntary conduct in relation to criminal charges, the civil courts have as yet scarcely begun to grapple with the problem as affecting civil liability, and much of what we shall say must necessarily be speculative. There have been few discussions of this aspect of the matter in legal journals. One particularly helpful paper by Fitzgerald (1961), entitled 'Voluntary and Involuntary Acts', has been of great assistance.

Divorce law

Since 1969, all the old grounds for divorce have been abolished and replaced by one ground, that the marriage has irretrievably broken down. This however may be established only by proof of one or more of five facts set out in the Divorce Reform Act 1969. As Bromley points out, 'the old bars to divorce, both absolute (like condonation) and discretionary (like the petitioner's own adultery), are abolished, but various safeguards are to be found to protect the spouse whose conduct has not, on the face of it, brought about the breakdown'.

Of these five statutory facts, the first, adultery, is governed by the same rules which applied before the reform was introduced. But adultery, if proved, is treated rather as a symptom of the breakdown of the marriage than as a cause of breakdown, and an isolated act of adultery may not be sufficient. This is because the proof of one of the five facts raises no more than a presumption of breakdown of the marriage, and it is open to the respondent in a defended suit to show that the marriage has not broken down irretrievably. The statutory requirement is not just that the respondent has committed adultery but also that the petitioner finds it intolerable to live with the respondent.

A second statutory fact which may be proved relates to the respondent's behaviour. If it is such that the petitioner cannot reasonably be expected to live with the respondent, then it raises a presumption of breakdown of the marriage. This is primarily designed to cover cruelty as defined in Gollins v Gollins [1964] A.C. 644 and Williams v Williams [1964] A.C. 698. These cases established that, where the respondent was mentally ill, the presence of an intention to injure the other spouse was not essential in order to establish cruelty, nor was there any requirement of proof that the conduct of the respondent was aimed at the other spouse. The test of cruelty was wholly objective so that proof that the respondent was insane was not necessarily an answer to the charge of cruelty, as had been previously thought. Under the new law, this test is adopted, in that the court must be satisfied that the petitioner cannot *reasonably* be expected to live with the respondent.

The other three facts relate to desertion and separation, and are unlikely to involve questions of amnesia or automatism, since the conduct must last for years.

A person suffering from amnesia or in a state of automatism might conceivably commit adultery, or commit acts of cruelty on the other spouse. In this event, the courts might be persuaded to grant a divorce on the ground that the marriage had broken down irretrievably. In doing so, the court will have regard to the state of the respondent's mind, and, to quote Bromley, 'his knowledge, belief, motive and intention all become relevant'.

Taking the first situation, adultery, since this requires a voluntary act of sexual intercouse, someone who is insane within the M'Naghten Rules (not knowing what he was doing) could not commit adultery. It is difficult to imagine automatism in this connection. Amnesia may occur of course without the conduct itself being involuntary, in which case it is of little or no avail. With regard to the second situation, objectionable behaviour, we have the precedents from the old law relating to cruelty as reinterpreted in Gollins and Williams, and as has been said, because the test is wholly objective, the mere fact that the respondent did not intend to be objectionable is no bar to relief. It follows that a person in an amnesic state or in a state of automatism whose conduct might amount to cruelty is not necessarily excused by reason of his mental condition.

The law of tort

Most of the civil wrongs for which actions for damages or other remedies lie in the civil courts, require either intentional or negligent conduct on the part of the wrongdoer before there is any liability. It would seem to follow that proof that the acts were done under conditions of loss of consciousness (whether or not accompanied by amnesia) would excuse from liability. This might apply to the torts of trespass and negligence, and it has been suggested that a man would not be held liable for slander by defamatory words spoken in his sleep. Generally, there would be no civil liability for an act or omission which a person could not help. Even the so-called torts of strict liability (rule in Rylands v Fletcher [1868] L.R. 3 H.L. 330) seem to require, at the very least, some power of control excercisable at some stage by the defendant before liability will be held to exist, though this cannot be said to be clearly established (Fitzgerald, 1961).

Testamentary law and management of affairs

Defective memory for recent events, such as may occur in old age or in a number of diseases or injury of the brain, may make or appear to make an individual incompetent to manage his own affairs. Defect of memory alone need not necessarily produce this result, provided there is no loss of general intelligence, reasoning and judgment. Thus, the medicolegal decision in this setting has to depend on a wider assessment of mental competence, of which defective recent memory is only one aspect.

A sound disposing mind is a necessary prerequisite for making a will. A testator whose mind was affected by physical or mental illness or senility, to the point where he could no longer think rationally about his affairs, might be held to have been incapable of will-making. But the test is a severe one for anyone seeking to upset the will on the ground of incapacity to satisfy. Chief Justice Cockburn in Banks v Goodfellow (1870, L.R. 5 Q.B. 549, at p. 565)* thought that a testator should 'understand the extent of the property of which he is disposing ... be able to comprehend and appreciate the claims to which he ought to give effect'. Presumably, the presence of amnesia would be a factor to consider in this connection.

Contracts

In order to enter a contract there must be a meeting of the minds of the parties in an agreement. This does not mean, however, that an insane person can avoid his contracts. He can only do so if he can show that the other party was aware of his insanity at the time of the contract. Again, the presence of amnesia or clouded consciousness might be a factor. There is one contract which is rather special, the contract of marriage. Here it might be that a person who married without being conscious of a prior subsisting marriage (because he had forgotten about it and was in a genuine state of amnesia), might have a good defence to bigamy. But the second marriage contracted in these circumstances would not be valid if there was a prior subsisting marriage.

Damages

One further connection which amnesia might have with the civil law is in connection with the law of damages. Liability to blackouts or fits or bouts of amnesia, resulting from some injuries received, would undoubtedly be a factor to be considered in the assessment of damages.

---

* See also Swinfen v Swinfen (1858) 1 F. and F. 584. Bellis, Polson v Parrott (1929) 141 L.T. 245.

Summary of the civil law position

Broadly speaking, one might enunciate the following principle as a guide to the position concerning amnesia and involuntary conduct in the civil law. 'Insofar as liability depends on fault, clearly involuntary acts or omissions on the part of the defendant should not render him liable, for a person is not at fault for doing what he cannot help doing' (Fitzgerald, 1961). It may well be that with the advance of medical and psychiatric knowledge we shall have to modify the rather primitive notions of legal liability which stem from analytical philosophy but which may no longer fit the facts of common and scientific experience.

APPENDIX

Further English cases not discussed in this chapter:

R. v Sell [1962] Crim L.R. 463; Whitlock, 1963, p. 123.
R. v Sibbles [1959] Crim L.R. 660; Whitlock, 1963, p. 125.
R. v Bentley [1960] Crim L.R. 777; Glanville Williams, 1961, pp. 485 and 887.
R. v Martin (*The Times,* October 25, 1957); Glanville Williams, 1961, p. 488.
R. v Paltridge (*Daily Telegraph,* February 20, 1952); Glanville Williams, 1961, p. 483.
Police v Beaumont [1958] Crim L.R. 620.
R. v Coster (*The Times,* December 4, 1959).

Further Commonwealth cases not discussed in this chapter:

R. v Cottle (1958) N.Z.L.R. 999
R. v Carter (1959) V.R. 105
Queen v Meddings (1966) V.R. 306
Cooper v McKenna (1960) Qd.R. 406
R. v Foy (1960) Qd.R. 225
R. v Tsigos (1964–65) N.S.W.R. 1607
R. v Minor 112, C.C.C. 29 (1955)
R. v King 38 C.R. 52
Bleta v Queen (1965) 1 C.C.C. 1
R. v O'Brien (1966) 3 C.C.C. 284
R. v Szimszak (1972) 19 C.R.N.S. 373
R. v Sproule (1972) 19 C.R.N.S. 384
R. v Kasparek (1951) O.R. 776
R. v Baker (1969) 7 C.R.N.S. 298

References

Abeles, M., and Schilder, P. (1935). Psychogenic loss of personal identity. *Archs Neurol. Psychiat. Chicago*, **34**, 587

Abrams, R. (1974). Multiple ECT: What have we learned? In *The Psychobiology of Convulsive Therapy*. Ed. M. Fink. New York: John Wiley

− and Taylor, M. A. (1973). Anterior Bifrontal ECT: a clinical trial. *Br. J. Psychiat.* **122**, 587

Adams, J. A. (1967). *Human Memory*. New York: McGraw-Hill

Adams, J. H., Brierley, J. B., Connor, R. C. R. and Treip, C. (1966). The effects of systemic hypotension upon the human brain. Clinical and neuropathological observations in 11 cases. *Brain*, **89**, 235

Adams, R. D. (1969). The anatomy of memory mechanisms in the human brain. In: *The Pathology of Memory*. Edited by G. A. Talland and N. C. Waugh, pp. 91−106, New York and London: Academic Press

− Collins, G. H. and Victor, M. (1962). Troubles de la mémoire et de l'apprentissage chez l'homme; leurs relations avec dés lesions des lobes temporaux et du diencéphale. In *Physiologie de l'Hippocampe*, pp. 273−296. Paris: Centre National de la Récherche Scientifique

Adey, W. R. (1964). Hippocampal mechanisms in processes of memory; thoughts on a model of cerebral organization in learning. In *Brain Function*, Vol. II: *RNA and Brain Function, Memory and Learning*. Ed. by M. A. B. Brazier, Berkeley: University of California Press

− and Meyer, M. (1952). Hippocampal and hypothalamic connections of the temporal lobe of the monkey. *Brain*, **75**, 358

Ajuriaguerra, J. de and Hécaen, H. (1960). *Le Cortex Cerebral*. Paris: Masson

− and Rouault de la Vigne, A. (1946). Troubles mentaux de l'intoxication oxycarbonée. *Sem. Hôp. Paris,* **22**, 1950

− Hécaen, H. and Sadoun, R. (1954). Les troubles mentaux au cours des tumeurs de la region meso-diencephalique. *Encéphale*, **43**, 406

Alexander, L. (1939). Topographic and histologic identity of the experimental (avitaminotic) lesions of Wernicke with lesions of hemorrhagic polioencephalitis occurring in chronic alcoholism in Man. *Archs Neurol. Psychiat., Chicago*, **42**, 1172

− (1940). Identity of lesions produced experimentally by B_1 avitaminosis in pigeons with haemorrhagic polioencephalitis in chronic alcoholism in Man. *Am. J. Path.*, **16**, 61

− (1953). *Treatment of Mental Disorders*. Philadelphia: W. B. Saunders

- Pijoan, M. and Meyerson, A. (1938). Beri-beri and scurvy. *Trans. Am. Neurol. Ass.* **64**, 135
Allen, I. M. (1930). Tumours involving occipital lobe. *Brain,* **53**, 194
Allison, R. S. (1961). Chronic amnesic syndromes in the elderly. *Proc. R. Soc. Med.,* **54**, 961
Aminoff, M. J., Marshall, J., Smith, E. M. and Wyke, M. A. (1975). Pattern of intellectual impairment in Huntington's chorea. *Psychol. Med.* **5**, 169
Angelergues, R. (1958). *Le Syndrome Mental de Korsakow.* Paris: Masson
Annett, M., Hudson, P. and Turner, A. (1973). Effects of right and left unilateral ECT on naming and visual discrimination analysed in relation to handedness. *Br. J. Psychiat.* **123**, 73
Anon. (1965). The experience of electro-convulsive therapy. *Br. J. Psychiat.* **111**, 365
Aszkanazy, C. L., Tom, M. I. and Zeldowicz, L. R. (1958). Encephalitis presumably of viral origin, associated with massive necrosis of the temporal lobe. *J. Neuropath. exp. Neurol.,* **17**, 565
Atkinson, R. C. and Shiffrin, R. M. (1968). Human memory. A proposed system and its control process. In *The Psychology of Learning and Motivation.* K. W. Spence and J. T. Spence (Eds.) pp. 89–195. New York: Academic Press
Baddeley, A. D. (1973). Theories of amnesia. Paper presented at the Dundee Conference on *Current Research in Aspects of Long-term Memory.*
- (1975). Theories of amnesia. In *Studies in Long-Term Memory.* Ch. 17. Ed. A. Kennedy and A. Wilkes. New York: John Wiley
- and Patterson, K. (1971). The relationship between long-term and short-term memory. *Br. med. Bull.* **27**, 237
- and Scott, D. (1971). Short-term forgetting in the absence of pro-active interference. *Q. Jl exp. Psychol.* **23**, 275
- - Drynan, R., and Smith, J. C. (1969). Short-term memory and the limited capacity hypothesis. *Br. J. Psychol.* **60**, 51
- and Warrington, E. K. (1970). Amnesia and the distinction between long-and short-term memory. *J. Verb. Learn. Verb. Behav.* **9**, 176
- - (1973). *Neuropsychologia,* **11**, 159
Bailey, F. W. (1946). Histopathology of Polioencephalitis Hemorrhagica Superior (Wernicke's Disease). *Archs Neurol. Psychiat., Chicago,* **56**, 609
Barbizet, J. (1964). *Etudes sur la Mémoire.* Paris: L'Expansion Scientifiques Francaise
- (1970). *Human Memory and its Pathology.* Transl. D. K. Jardine. San Francisco: W. H. Freeman
- and Cary, E. (1970). A psychometric study of various memory defects associated with cerebral lesions. In *The Pathology of Memory.* G. A. Talland and N. C. Waugh, (Eds). New York: Academic Press
Bartlett, F. C. (1926). Review of Henry Head's 'Aphasia and kindred disorders of speech.' *Brain,* **49**, 581
- (1932). *Remembering.* Cambridge University Press
Bechterew, W. V. Von. (1900a). Demonstration eines Gehirns mit Zerstörung der vorderen und inneren Theile der Hirnrinde beider Schläfenlappen. *Neurol. Zentbl.,* **19**, 990
- (1900b). Uber periodische Anfälle retroactiver Amnesie. *Mschr. Psychiat. Neurol.* **8**, 353
Beck, E. and Corsellis, J. A. N. (1960). Pathological and anatomical aspects of orbital undercutting *Proc. R. Soc. Med.* **53**, 737
- - (1963). Das Fornixsystem des Menschen im Lichte anatomischer und pathologischer Untersuchungen. *Zbl. ges. Neurol. Psychiat.* **173**, 220

– – (1965). Personal communication

Bedford, P. D. (1955). Adverse cerebral effects of anaesthesia on old people. *Lancet*, 2, 259

Bender, M. B. (1956). Syndrome of isolated episode of confusion with amnesia *J. Hillside Hosp*, 5, 212

– (1960). Single episode of confusion with amnesia. *Bull. N. Y. Acad. Med.* 36, 197

Benedek, L. and Juba, A. (1944). Beiträge zur Pathologie des Diencephalon. III. Histologische Befunde beim chronischalkoholischen Korsakoff-Syndrom. *Z. ges. Neurol. Psychiat.*, 177, 282

Bennett, R., Hughes, G. R. V., Bywaters, E. G. and Holt, P. J. L. (1972). Neuropsychiatric problems in systemic lupus erythematosus. *Br. med. J.*, 4, 342

Benson, D. F. and Geschwind, N. (1967). Shrinking retrograde amnesia. *J. Neurol. Neurosurg. Psychiat.*, 30, 539

Benton, A. L. and Van Allen, M. W. (1968). Impairment in facial recognition in patients with cerebral disease. *Trans. Am. neurol. Ass.*, 93, 38

Berent, S., Cohen, B. D. and Silverman, A. J. (1975). Changes in verbal and non-verbal learning following a single left or right unilateral electroconvulsive treatment. *Biol. Psychiat.* 10, 95

Berger, H. (1936). Uber des Elektrenkephalogram des Menschens. XI. *Arch. Psychiat. NervKrankh.*, 104, 678

Berlyne, N. and Strachan, M. (1968). Neuropsychiatric sequelae of attempted hanging. *Br. J. Psychiat.*, 114, 411

Berrington, W. P., Liddell D. W., and Foulds, G. A. (1956). A re-evaluation of the fugue. *J. ment. Sci.* 102, 280

Bickford, R. G., Mulder, D. W., Dodge, H. W., Svien, H. J. and Rome, P. R. (1958). Changes in memory function produced by electrical stimulation of the temporal lobe in Man. *Res. Publs Ass. Res. nerv. ment. Dis.*, 36, 227

Blakemore, C. and Falconer, M. A. (1966). Personal communication

– Ettlinger, G. and Falconer, M. A. (1966). Cognitive abilities in relation to frequency of seizures and neuropathology in the temporal lobe. *J. Neurol. Neurosurg. Psychiat.*, 29, 268

Bleuler, M. (1951). Psychiatry of cerebral diseases. *Br. med. J.*, 2, 1233

Bloomfield, S. and Marr, D. (1970). How the cerebellum may be used. *Nature, Lond.* 227, 1244

Bolwig, T. G. (1968). Transient global amnesia. *Acta neurol. scand.* 44, 101

Bonhoeffer, K. (1899). Pathologisch-anatomische Untersuchungen an Alkohol-deliranten *Mschr. Psychiat. Neurol.*, 5, 265

– (1901). *Die akuten Geisteskrankheiten der Gewohnheitstrinker.* Jena: Fisher

– (1904) Die Korsakowsche Symptomenkomplex in seinen Beziehungen zu den verschiedenen Krankheitsformen. *Allg. Z. Psychiat.*, 61, 744

Bousfield, W. A. (1953). The occurrence of clustering in the recall of randomly arranged associates. *J. gen. Psychol.* 9, 229

Bowman, K. M., Goodhart, R. and Jolliffe, N. (1939). Observations on the role of Vitamin B₁ in the etiology and treatment of Korsakoff's psychosis. *J. nerv. ment. Dis.* 90, 569

Braceland, F. J. (1942). Mental symptoms following carbon disulphide intoxication. *Ann. intern. Med.*, 16, 246

Brengelman, J. C. (1959). *The Effect of Repeated Electrical Shocks on Learning.* Berlin: Springer

Brenner, C. (1957). The nature and development of the concept of repression in Freud's writings. *Psychoanal. Study Child.* XII

- (1966). The mechanism of repression. In: *Psychoanalysis – a general psychology*. Ed. R. M. Loewenstein, *et al*. New York: International University Press
Brett, E. M. (1966). Minor epileptic status. *J. neurol. Sci.*, 3, 52
Brierley, J. B. (1961). Clinico-pathological correlations in amnesia. *Geront. clin.*, 3, 97
- (1965). The influence of brain swelling, age and hypotension upon the pattern of cerebral damage in hypoxia. *Proc. Fifth Int. Congr. Neuropathol.*, Zürich.
- Corsellis, J. A. N., Hierons, R. and Nevin, S. (1960). Subacute encephalitis of later adult life mainly affecting the limbic areas. *Brain*, 83, 357
Brindley, G. S. and Janota, I. (1975). Observations on cortical blindness and on vascular lesions that cause loss of recent memory. *J. neurol. neurosurg. Psychiat.* 38, 459
Brion, S. (1969) Korsakoff's syndrome: clinico-anatomical and physiological considerations. In: *The Pathology of Memory*. Edited by G. A. Talland and N. C. Waugh, pp. 29–40, New York and London: Academic Press
Brody, H. (1955). Organization of the cerebral cortex. III. A study of ageing in the human cerebral cortex. *J. comp. Neurol.*, 102, 511
Brody, M. B. (1944). Prolonged memory defect following ECT. *J. ment. Sci.*, 90, 51
Bromley, P. M. (1971). *Family Law* 4th ed.
Brook, C. G. D. (1969). Psychosis in systemic lupus erythematosus (SLE) and the response to cyclophosphamide. *Proc. R. Soc. Med.*, 62, 912
Brooks, D. N. (1976). Wechsler memory scale performance and its relation to brain damage after severe closed head injury. *J. Neurol. Neurosurg. Psychiat.* 39, 593
- and Baddeley, A. D. (1976). What can amnesic patients learn? *Neuropsychologia*, 14, 111
Brown, J. (1958). Some tests of the decay theory of immediate memory. *Q. Jl exp. Psychol.* 10, 12
- (1964). Short-term memory. *Br. med. Bull.*, 20, 8
Brunschwig, L., Strain, J. J., and Bidder, T. G. (1971). Issues in the assessment of post ECT memory changes. *Br. J. Psychiat.* 119, 73
Bumke, O. (1931). Proceedings of the Association of Bavarian Psychiatrists. *Allg. Z. Psychiat.*, 94, 217
- (1947). Quoted by Lotmar (1958)
Bürger, H. (1927). Zur Psychologie des amnestischen Symptomenkomplex. *Arch. Psychiat. NervKrankh.*, 81, 348
Bürger-Prinz, H. and Kaila, M. (1930). Uber die Struktur des amnestischen Symptomenkomplex. *Z. ges. Neurol. Psychiat.*, 124, 553
Busch, E. (1940). Psychical symptoms in neurosurgical disease. *Acta psychiat. neurol. scand.*, 15, 257
Busse, E. W. (1962). *Medical and Clinical Aspects of Ageing*. p. 115. Ed. H. T. Blumenthal. New York' Columbia University Press
Butters, N., and Cermak, L. S. (1974). The role of cognitive factors in the memory disorders of alcoholic patients with the Korsakoff syndrome. *Ann. N. Y. Acad. Sci.* 233, 61
- - (1975). Some analyses of amnesic syndromes in brain-damaged patients. In *The Hippocampus*. Eds. K. Pribram, and R. L. Isaacson
- - Jones, B. and Glosser, G. (1975). Some analyses of the information processing and sensory capabilities of alcoholic Korsakoff patients. In *Experimental Studies of Alcohol Intoxication and Withdrawal*. M. G. Gross (Ed.) New York: Plenum Press

- Lewis, R., Cermak, L. S. and Goodglass, H. (1973). Material-specific memory deficits in alcoholic Korsakoff patients. *Neuropsychologia* 11, 291
Cairns, H. (1950). Personal communication
- and Mosberg. W. H. (1951). Colloid cysts of the third ventricle *Surgery Gynec. Obstet.*, 92, 545
Cajal, S. R. (1909). *Histologie du Système Nerveux de l'Homme et des Vertébrés.* Paris: Maloine.
Campbell, A. C. P. and Biggart, J. H. (1939). Wernicke's encephalopathy (Polioencephalitis Haemorrhagica Superior); its alcoholic and non-alcoholic incidence *J. Path. Bact.*, 48, 245
- and Russell, W. R. (1941). Wernicke's encephalopathy. *Q. Jl. med.* 10, 41
Cannicott, S. M. (1962). Unilateral ECT. *Post-grad. med. J.* 38, 451
Carmichael, E. A. and Stern, R. D. (1931). Korsakoff's syndrome; its histopathology. *Brain*, 54, 189
Carney, M. W. P. (1971). 'Five Cases of Bromism.' *Lancet*, 2, 523
Cermak, L. S. (1972). *Human Memory:Research and Theory.* New York: Ronald
- (1975). Imagery as an aid to retrieval for Korsakoff patients. *Cortex* 11, 163
- (1976). The encoding capacity of a patient with amnesia due to encephalitis. *Neuropsychologia.* 14, 311
- and Butters, N. (1972). The role of interference and encoding in the short term memory deficits of Korsakoff patients. *Neuropsychologia* 10, 89
- Butters, N. and Gerrein, J. (1973). The extent of the verbal encoding ability of Korsakoff patients. *Neuropsychologia* 11, 85
- - and Goodglass, H. (1971). The extent of memory loss in Korsakoff patients. *Neuropsychologia* 9, 307
- - and Moreines, J. (1974). Some analyses of the verbal encoding deficit of alcoholic patients. *Brain Lang.* 1, 141
Chaslin, P. (1895). *La Confusion Mentale Primitive.* Paris; Asselin a Houzean.
- and Portocalis (1908). Un cas de Syphilis Cérébrale avec Syndrome de Korsakoff à Forme Amnesique Pure. *J. Psychol. norm. path.*, 5, 303
Claparède, E. (1911). Recognition et moiité. *Archs Psychol., Genève,* 11, 79
Clark, W. E. le Gros., Beattie, J., Riddoch, G. and Dott, N. M. (1938). *The Hypothalamus.* Edinburgh: Oliver and Boyd.
Clarke, A. D. B. (1969). *Recent Advances in the Study of Subnormality.* Revised edition. London: National Association for Mental Health
Clarke, P. R. F., Wyke, M. and Zangwill, O. L. (1958). Language disorders in a case of Korsakoff's syndrome. *J. Neurol. Neurosurg. Psychiat.*, 21, 190
Cloake, P. C. P. (1951). In *Modern Trends in Neurology*, p. 468. Ed. A. Feiling. London: Butterworths
Clunie, G. J. A., Gunn, A. and Robson, J. B. (1967). Hyperparathyroid crises. *Br. J. Surg.*, 54, 538
Clyma, E. A. (1975). Unilateral electroconvulsive therapy. *Br. J. Psychiat.* 126, 372
Cohen, B. D., Noblin, C. D., Silverman, A. J. and Penick, S. B. (1968). Functional asymmetry of the human brain. *Science, N. Y.* 162, 475
Conrad, K. (1953a). Zur Psychopathologie des amnestischen Symptomenkomplex. Gestaltanalyse einer Korsakowschen Psychose. *Deutsche Z. NervHeilk.*, 190, 471
- (1953b) Uber einen Fall von "Minuten Gedächtnis". *Arch. Psychiat. u. Z. Neurol.*, 190, 471
Corkin, S. (1965a). Tactually-guided maze learning in man: effects of unilateral cortical excisions and bilateral hippocampal lesions. *Neuropsychologia* 3, 339

– (1965b). Acquisition of Motor Skill after Bilateral Medial Temporal-lobe Excision *Neuropsychologia*, **6**, 255
– (1968). Acquisition of motor skill after bilateral medial temporal lobe excision *Neuropsychologia* **6**, 255
Correll, R. E. and Scoville, W. B. (1970). Relationship of ITI to acquisition of serial visual discrimination following temporal rhinencephalic resection in monkeys. *J. comp. physiol. Psychol.*, **70**, 464
Corsellis, J. N. A. (1970). The limbic areas in Alzheimer's disease and in other conditions associated with dementia. In *Alzheimer's Disease and Related Conditions*, Ciba Foundation Symposium. (Eds: G. O. W. Wolstenholme, and M .O'Connor), London: Churchill.
– Goldberg, G. J. and Norton, A. R. (1968). Limbic encephalitis and its association with carcinoma. *Brain*, **91**, 481
Corsi, P. M. (1972). Human memory and the medial temporal region of the brain. Unpublished Ph.D. thesis for McGill University
Costello, C., Belton, G., Abra, J. and Dunn, B. (1970). The amnesic and therapeutic effects of bilateral and unilateral ECT. *Br. J. Psychiat.* **116**, 69
Cotman, C. W., Banker, G., Zornetzer, S. F. and McGaugh, J. L. (1971). Electroshock effects on brain protein synthesis: relation to seizures and retrograde amnesia. *Science,* **173**, 454
Cragg, B. G. (1961). Olfactory and other afferent connections of hippocampus in the rabbit, rat and the cat. *Expl. Neurol.,* **3**, 588
Craik, F. I. M., and Lockhart, R. S. (1972). Levels of processing: a framework for memory research. *J. Verb. Learn Verb. Behav.* **11**, 671
Craik, K. J. W. (1943). *The Nature of Explanation.* Cambridge: University Press
Crewel, H. van (1969). Transient global amnesia. *Psychiat. Neurol. Neurochir,* **72**, 319
Cronholm, B., and Blomquist, C. (1959). Memory disturbances after ECT. *Acta psychiat. neurol. scand.,* **34**, 18
– and Lagergren. Å. (1959). Memory disturbances after ECT. *Acta psychiat. neurol. scand.* **34**, 283
– and Molander, L. (1957). Memory disturbances after ECT. *Acta psychiat. neurol. scand.,* **32**, 280
– – (1960). Memory disturbances after ECT. *Acta. psychiat. neurol. scand.* **36**, 83
– – (1964). Memory disturbances affter ECT. *Acta psychiat. neurol. scand.,* **40**, 211
– and Ottosson, J–0. (1961). "Countershock" in ECT. *Archs gen. Psychiat.* **4**, 254
– – (1963a). The experience of memory functions after ECT. *Br. J. Psychiat.* **109**, 251
– – (1963b). Ultrabrief stimulus technique in ECT. *J. nerv. ment. Dis.* **137**, 117, 268
– and Schalling, D. (1963). Intellectual deterioration after focal brain injury. *Archs Surg., Chicago,* **86**, 670
– Eriksson, I., and Lindgren, A. (1961). Memory and concentration after exposure to carbon monoxide. *Acta psychiat. neurol. scand.* **37**, 127
Cross. R. (1961). The Defence of Automatism. *The Listener,* December 7th, p. 967
Cruickshank, E. K. (1961). *Psychiatrie der Gegenwart.* Vol. 3, p. 807. Berlin, Göttingen, Heidelberg: Springer.
Curran, F. J. (1944). Neuropsychiatric effects of barbiturates and bromides. *J. nerv. ment. Dis.,* **100**, 142
Daily Telegraph, February 20th, 1952
Daitz, H. (1953). Note on the fibre content of the fornix system in Man. *Brain,* **76**, 509

Davison, C. and Demuth, E. L. (1946). Disturbances in sleep mechanism: a clinicopathological study. *Archs Neurol. Psychiat., Chicago,* 55, 111

Dee, H. L. and Fotenot, D. J. (1973). Cerebral dominance and lateral differences in perception and memory. *Neuropsychiatry.* 11, 167

De Jong, R. N., Tabashi, H. H. and Olson, J. P. (1969). Memory loss due to hippocampal lesions. *Archs. Neurol.* 20, 339

Delay, J. (1942). *Les Dissolutions de la Memoire.* Paris: P.U.F.

  – and Brion, S. (1954). Syndrome de Korsakoff et corps mamillaires. *L'Encéphale,* 43, 193

  – – (1969). *Le Syndrome de Korsakoff.* Paris: Masson et Cie

  – – and Elissalde, B. (1958). Corps mamillaires et syndrome Korsakoff. Étude anatomique de huit cas de syndrome de Korsakoff d'origine alcoolique sans altérations significative du cortex cérébral. I. Etude anatomo-clinique. *Presse méd.,* 66, 1849–1852 (a). II. Tubercules mamillaires et mécanisme de la memoire. *Presse méd.,* 66, 1965–1968 (b)

  – Boudin, G., Brion, S. and Barbizet, J. (1956). Etude anatomoclinique de huit encèphalopathies alcooliques; encéphalopathie de Gayet-Wernicke et syndromes voisins. *Rèvue Neurol.,* 94, 596

d'Elia, G. (1970). Unilateral electro-culvulsive therapy. *Acta psychiat. scand.* 46, (suppl. 215). 1

  – (1974). Unilateral ECT. In *The Psychobiology of ECT.* (Ed.) M. Fink. New York: Wiley

  – Lorentzson, S., Raotma, H. and Widepalm, K. (1976). Comparison of unilateral dominant and non-dominant ECT on verbal and non-verbal memory. *Acta psychiat. scand.* 53, 85

De Nosaquo, N. (1969). The hallucinatory effect of Pentazocine (Talwin). *J. Amer. med. Ass.,* 210, 502

De Renzi, E. (1968). Non verbal memory and hemispheric side of lesion. *Neuropsychologia,* 6, 181

  – and Spinnler, H. (1966). Facial recognition in brain-damaged patients. *Neurology,* 16, 144

  – Faglioni, P. and Scotti, G. (1970). Hemispheric contribution to exploration of space through the visual and tactile modalities. *Cortex,* 6, 191

  – – – (1971). Judgement of spatial orientation in patients with focal brain lesions. *J. Neurol. Neurosurg. Psychiat.* 34, 489

  – – and Spinnler, H. (1968). The performances of patients with unilateral brain damage on face recognition tasks. *Cortex,* 4, 17

Deutsch, J. A. (1962). Higher nervous function; the physiological basis of memory. *A. Rev. Physiol.,* 24, 259

Dimsdale, H. B. (1971). Transient global amnesia. *Ann. R. Coll. Phys. Surg. Can.* 3, 41

  – Logue, V. and Piercy, M. (1964). A case of persisting impairment of recent memory following right temporal lobectomy. *Neuropsychologia,* 1, 287

Dorff, J. F., Mirsky, A. F. and Mishkin, M. (1965). Effects of unilateral temporal lobe lesions. *Neuropsychologia,* 3, 39

Dornbush, R. L., Abrams, E., and Fink, M. (1971). Memory changes after unilateral and bilateral ECT. *Br. J. Psychiat.* 119, 75

  – and Williams, M. (1974). Memory after ECT. In *The Psychobiology of ECT.* Ed. M. Fink. N.Y.: J. Wiley & Sons

Dott, N. M. (1938). Surgical aspects of the hypothalamus. In *The Hypothalamus,* p. 131. Ed. by W. E. Le Gros Clark. London: Oliver and Boyd

Drachman, D. A. and Adams, R. D. (1962). Acute herpes simplex and inclusion body encephalitis. *Archs. Neurol., Chicago,* 7, 45

– and Arbit, J. (1966). Memory and hippocampal complex, II. *Archs Neurol. Chicago,* **15,** 52

Ebtinger, R. (1958). *Aspects Psychopathologiques du Post-électrochoc.* Colmar. Imprimerie Asatie

Edwards, J. L. J. (1958). Automatism and criminal responsibility. *Modern Law Review,* **21,** 375

Elsom, K. O., Lewy, F. H. and Heublein, G. W. (1940). Clinical studies of experimental human vitamin B complex deficiency. *Amer. J. med. Sci.,* **200,** 757

Ely, F. A. (1922). Memory defect of Korsakoff type observed in multiple neuritis following toxaemia of pregnancy. *J. nerv. ment. Dis.,* **56,** 115

Enoch, M. D., Trethowan W. H., and Barker J. C. (1967). *Some Uncommon Psychiatric Syndromes.* Bristol: John Wright

Ettlinger, G. (1962). Relationship between test difficulty and the visual impairment in monkeys with ablations of temporal cortex. *Nature Lond.* **196,** 911

Evans, J. H. (1966). Transient loss of memory: an organic mental syndrome. *Brain,* **89,** 539

Ewald, G. (1930). Review of Grünthal and Störring's Report. *Zentbl. ges. Neurol. Psychiat.,* **57,** 473

– (1940). Zur Frage der Lokalisation des amnestischen Symptomenkomplexes. *Allg. Z. Psychiat.,* **155,** 220

Falconer, M. A. (1965). Personal communication

Feindel, W. and Penfield, W. (1954). Localization of discharge in temporal lobe automatism. *A. M. A. Archs neurol. psychiat.,* **72,** 605

Fenton, G. W. (1972). Epilepsy and automatism *Brit. J. Hosp. Med.* **7,** 57

Ferraro, A. and Roizin, L. (1941). Neuropathological findings in experimental starvation. Preliminary report. *Trans. Am. neurol. Ass.,* **67,** 177

Fields, W. S. and Blattner, R. J. (1958). *Viral Encephalitis.* Springfield, Illinois: Thomas

Fink, M. (1974). Clinical progress in convulsive therapy. In *The Psychobiology of ECT.* Ed. M. Fink. New York: J. Wiley & Sons

Fisher, C. M. (1966). Concussion amnesia. *Neurology (Minneap.)* **16,** 826

– and Adams, R. D. (1958). Transient global amnesia. *Trans. Am. neurol. Ass.,* **83,** 143

– – (1964). Transient global amnesia. *Acta neurol. scand.* **40,** Suppl. 9

Fitzgerald, P. J. (1961). Voluntary and involuntary acts. In *Oxford Essays in Jurisprudence,* p. 1. Ed. by A. G. Guest. London: Oxford University Press

Flatau, E. (1921). Sur le Haemorrhagies Meningées Idiopathiques. *Gaz. Hôp. civ. milit. Paris,* **94,** 1077

Fleminger, J., Thorpe, D. and Nott, P. (1970). Unilateral ECT and cerebral dominance: effect of right and left sided electrodes placement on verbal memory. *J. Neurol. Neurosurg. Psychiat.* **33,** 408

Fletcher, R. F., Henly, A. A., Sammons, H. G. and Squire, J. R. (1960). A case of magnesium deficiency following massive intestinal resection. *Lancet,* **1,** 522

Fodor, I. E. (1972). Impairment of memory functions after acute head injury. *J. Neurol. Neurosurg. Psychiat.* **35,** 818

– and Bever, T. G. (1965). The psychological reality of linguistic segments. *J. Verb. Learn. Verb. Behav.* **4,** 414

Frazier, C. H. (1936). A review, clinical and pathological, of parahypophyseal lesions. *Surgery Gynec. Obstet.,* **62,** 158

– and Waggoner, R. W. (1929). Tumours of the occipital lobe: a review of forty cases. *Archs Neurol. Psychiat., Chicago,* **22,** 1096

Freud, S. (1893). *The Mechanism of Hysterical Phenomena*. Standard Edition III. London: The Hogarth Press, (1962)
– (1895). *Project for a Scientific Psychology*. Standard Edition I. London: The Hogarth Press, (1966)
– (1901). *The Psychopathology of Everyday Life*. Standard Edition VI. London: The Hogarth Press, (1960)
– (1905). *Repression*. Standard Edition XIV. London: The Hogarth Press (1957)
– (1930). *Civilisation and its Discontents*. Standard Edition XXI. London: The Hogarth Press (1961)
– (1939). *Moses and Monotheism*. Standard Edition XXIII. London: The Hogarth Press (1964)
Gaffan, D. (1972). Loss of recognition memory in rats with lesions of the fornix. *Neuropsychologia* 10, 327
Gamper, E. (1928). Zur Frage der Polioencephalitis haemorrhagica der chronischen Alkoholiker. Anatomische Befunde beim alkoholischen Korsakow und ihre Beziehungen zum klinischen Bild. *Dt. Z. NervHeilk.*, 102, 122
Garcia-Bengochea, F., de la Torre, E., Esquival, O., Vieta, R. and Fernandez, C. (1954). The section of the fornix in the surgical treatment of certain epilepsies. *Trans. Am. neurol. Ass.*, 79, 176
Gascon, G. G. and Gilles, F. (1973). Limbic dementia. *J. neurol. neurosurg. psychiat.* 36, 421
Gellerstedt, N. (1933). Zur Kenntnis der Hirnveränderungen bei der normaler Altersinvolution. *Uppsala LäkFör. Förh.*, 38, 193
Geschwind, N. & Fusillo, M. (1966). Color-naming defects in association with dexion. *Archs. Neurol.* 15, 137
Gilbert, J.J. (1972). Transient global amnesia: 2 cases with definite aetiology. *J. nerv. ment. Dis.* 154, 461
Gilbert, P. (1975). How the cerebellum could memorise movements. *Nature Lond.* 254, 688
Gillespie, R. D. (1936). Amnesia: component functions in remembering. *Br. med. J.*, 2, 1179
Glanzer, M. and Cunitz, A. R. (1966). Two storage mechanisms in free recall. *J. Verb. Learn. Verb. Behav.* 5, 351
Glaser, G. H. and Pincus, J. H. (1969). Limbic encephalitis. *J. nerv. ment. Dis.*, 149, 59
Glees, P. and Griffith, H. B. (1952). Bilateral destruction of hippocampus (cornu Ammonis) in case of dementia. *Mschr. Psychiat. Neurol.*, 123, 193
Glowinski, H. (1973). Cognitive deficits in temporal lobe epilepsy. An investigation of memory functioning. *J. nerv. ment. Dis.*, 157, 129
Goddard, G. V. and Douglas, R. M. (1975). Does the engram of kindling model the engram of normal long term memory? *Canad. J. neurol. Sci.* 2, 385
– McIntyre, D. and Leech, C. (1969). A permanent change in brain function resulting from daily electrical stimulation. *Expl. Neurol.* 25, 295
Godlewski, S. (1968). Les episodes amnestique (transient global amnesia). *Sem. Hôp, Paris.* 44, 553
Gollin, E. S. (1960). Developmental studies of visual recognition of incomplete objects. *Percept. Mot. Skills* 11, 289
Goodhart, A. L. (1963). Cruelty, Desertion and Insanity in Matrimonial Law. *Law Quarterly Review,* 79, 98
Goodwin, D. W., Crane, J. B. and Guze, S. B. (1969a) Alcoholic blackouts: a review and clinical study of 100 alcoholics. *Amer. J. psychiat.,* 126, 191
– – – (1969b). Phenomenological aspects of the alcoholic 'blackout'. *Br. J. psychiat.,* 115, 1033

Gottlieb, B. (1944). Acute nicotine acid deficiency (amiacinosis). *Br. med. J.* **1**, 392

Granville-Grossman, K. (1971). Symptomatic mental disorders. In *Recent Advances in Clinical Psychiatry*. London: Butterworths

Green, J. D. (1964). The hippocampus. *Physiol. Rev.* **44**, 561

Gregor, A. and Römer, H. (1907). Beiträge zur Psychopathologie des Gedächtnisses. *Mschr. Psychiat. Neurol.,* **25**, 218, 330

Gruner, J. E. (1956). Sur la pathologie des encéphalopathies alcooliques. *Révue Neurol.,* **94**, 682

Grünthal, E. (1930). Die pathologische Anatomie der senilen Demenz und der Alzerheimerschen Krankeit (mit besonderer Berücksichtigung der Beziehungen zur Klinik). In *Handbuch der Geisteskrankheiten XI. Spezieller Teil VII,* p. 638. Berlin: Springer

— (1947). Über das klinische Bild nach umschriebenem beiderseitigem Ausfall der Ammonshornrinde; ein Beitrag zur Kenntnis der Funktion des Ammonshorns. *Mschr. Psychiat. Neurol.,* **113**, 1

— and Störring, G. E. (1930a). Uber das Verhalten bei umschriebener, völliger Merkunfähigkeit. *Mschr. Psychiat. Neurol.,* **74**, 354

— — (1930b). Ergänzende Beobachtungen zu den beschreiben Fall mit reiner Merkunfähigkeit. *Mschr. Psychiat. Neurol.,* **77**, 374

— — (1950). Völliger isolierter Verlust der Merkfähigkeit: Organische Schädigung oder hysterische Verdrängung? *Nervenarzt,* **21**, 522

— — (1956). Abschliessende Stellungnahme zu den vorstehenden Arbeit von H. Vökel und R. Stolze über den Fall *B. Mschr. Psychiat. Neurol.* **132**, 309

Gudden, H. (1896). Klinische und anatomische Beitrage zur Kenntnis der multiplen Alkoholneuritis nebst Bemarkungen über die Regenerationsvorgänge im peripheren Nervensystem. *Arch. Psychiat. NervKrankh.* **28**, 643

Guyotat, J. and Courjon, J. (1956). Les Ictus Amnesiques. *J. Med. Lyon.* **37**, 697

Halliday, A. M., Davison, K., Browne, M. N., and Kreeger, L. C. (1968). A comparison of the effects on depression and memory of bilateral ECT and unilateral ECT to the dominant and non-dominant hemispheres. *Br. J. Psychiat.* **114**, 997

— Merskey, H., Pratt, R. T. C., and Warrington, E. K. (1975). (Letter) Unilateral ECT. *Br. J. Psychiat.,* **127**, 416

Hassler, F. (1962). In *Frontiers in Brain Research,* p. 242. Ed. J. D. French. New York: Columbia University Press

Head, H. (1926) *Studies in Neurology,* Vol. I. Cambridge University Press

Heathfield, K. W. G., Croft, P. B., and Swash, M. (1973). The syndrome of transient global amnesia. *Brain* **96**, 729

Hebb, D. D. (1961). Distinctive features of learning in the higher animals. In *Brain Mechanisms and Learning.* J. F. Delafresnaye (Ed.) pp. 37–46. London and New York: Oxford University Press

Hécaen, H. and Ajuriaguerra, J. de (1956). *Troubles Mentaux au Cours de Tumeurs Intracraniennes.* Paris: Masson

Helweg-Larsen, P., Hoffmeyer, H., Kieler, J., Thayson, E. H., Thygesen, P. and Wulff, M. H. (1952). Famine disease in German concentration camps. *Acta psychiat. scand.,* Suppl. 83

Hetherington, R. (1956). The effects of ECT on efficiency and retentivity. *Br. J. Med. Psychol.* **29**, 258

Hill, D. and Sargant, W. (1943). A case of matricide. *Lancet,* **1**, 526

Himmelhoch, J., Pincus, J. H., Tucker, G. and Detre, T. (1970). Subacute encephalitis: behavioural and neurological aspects. *Brit. J. psychiat.,* **116**, 531

Hines, D., Satz, P. and Clementino, T. (1973). Perceptual and memory components of the superior recall of letters from the right visual half-fields. *Neuropsychologia,* **11**, 175

Holmberg, G. (1955). The effect of certain factors on the convulsions in ECT. *Acta psychiat. neurol. scand.* **30**, 98

Hooper, R., McGregor, J. M. and Nathan, P. W. (1945). Explosive rage reactions following head injury. *J. ment. Sci.,* **91**, 458

Hopwood, J. S. and Snell, H. K. (1933). Amnesia in relation to crime. *J. ment. Sci.,* **79**, 27

Hossain, M. (1970). Neurological and psychiatric manifestations in idiopathic hypoparathyroidism: response to treatment. *J. Neurol. neurosurg. psychiat.,* **33**, 153

Hosslin, R. von. (1905). Die peripheren Schwangerschaftlähmungen der Mutter. *Archs Psychiat. NervKrankh.,* **40**, 445

Huppert, F. A. and Deutsch, J. A. (1969). Improvement in memory with time. *Q. Jl. exp. Psychol.,* **21**, 267

— and Piercy, M. (1976). Recognition memory in amnesic patients: effect of temporal context and familiarity of material. *Cortex* **12**, 8

Hutt, S. J. (1967). Epilepsy and education. In *Proceedings of the First International Conference of the Association for Special Education.* Stanmore: Association for Special Education

Inglis, J. A. (1962). Effects of age on responses to dichotic stimulation. *Nature, Lond.* **194**, 1101

— (1969). Electrode placement in ECT and its effect. *Can. Psychiat. Ass. J.* **14**, 463

— (1970). Shock, surgery and cerebral asymmetry. *Br. J. Psychiat.* **117**, 143

Iversen, S. D. (1976). Do hippocampal lesions produce amnesia in animals? *Int. Rev. Neurobiology*

Jackson, J. Hughlings (1932). *Selected Writings,* Vol. 1, p. 399. Ed. Taylor. London: Hodder and Stoughton

Jaffe, R. and Bender, M. B. (1966). E.E.G. studies in the syndrome of isolated episodes of confusion with amnesia, 'transient global amnesia'. *J. Neurol. Neurosurg. Psychiat.* **29**, 472

James, W. (1890). *The Principles of Psychology,* Vol. 1. Ch. 16. Holt

Janis, I. L. (1950). Psychological effects of ECT. *J. nerv. ment. Dis.* **111**, 359, 383

Jarho, L. (1973). Korsakoff-like amnesic syndrome in penetrating brain injury. *Acta Neurol. Scand. Suppl. 54,* Vol. 49, pp. 156

Jellinek, E. M. (1952). Phases of alcohol addition. *Q. J. Stud. Alcohol.* **13**, 673

Jolliffe, N., Wortis, H. and Fein, H. D. (1941). The Wernicke Syndrome. *Archs Neurol. Psychiat., Chicago,* **46**, 569

Jolly, F. (1897). Quoted by Talland (1965)

Jones, M. K. (1974). Imagery as a mnemonic aid after left temporal lobectomy: contrast between material-specific and generalized memory disorders. *Neuropsychologia* **12**, 21

Jus, A. and Jus, K. (1962). Retrograde amnesia in petit mal. *Archs gen. Psychiat.,* **6**, 163

Kalinowsky, L. B., and Hoch, P. H. (1961). *Somatic Treatments in Psychiatry.* (Revised ed.). New York: Grune and Stratton

Kant, F. (1932). Die pseudoencephalitis Wernicke der Alkoholiker (Polioencephalitis haemorrhagica superior acuta). Ein Beitrag zur Klinik der Alkoholpsychosen. *Arch. Psychiat. NervKrankh.,* **98**, 702

Kanzer, M. (1939). Amnesia: a statistical study. *Am. J. Psychiat.* **96**, 711

Kehlet, H., and Lunn, V. (1951). Retrograd amnesi ved electrochockbehandlung. *Nord. psykiat. Medlemsbl.* **5**, 51

Kelly, D., Richardson, A., Mitchell-Heggs, N., Greenup, J., Chen, C. and Hafner, R. J. (1973). Stereotactic limbic leucotomy: a preliminary report on forty patients. *Brit. J. psychiat.* **13**, 141

Kennedy, A., and Neville, J. (1957). Sudden loss of memory. *Br. med. J.* **ii**, 428

Keppel, G. and Underwood, B. J. (1962). Proactive inhibition in short-term retention of single items. *J. Verb. Learn. Verb. Behav.*, **1**, 153

Kesner, R. P., Dixon, D. A., Pickett, D. and Berman, R. F. (1975). Experimental animal model of transient global amnesia: the role of the hippocampus. *Neuropsychologia* **13**, 465

Kimura, D. (1963). Right temporal lobe damage. *Archs Neurol.* **8**, 264

– (1966). Dual functional asymmetry of the brain in visual perception. *Neuropsychologia* **4**, 275

Kintsch, W. (1970). *Learning, Memory and Conceptual Processes* New York: Wiley

Kirby, G. H. and Davis, T. K. (1921). Psychiatric aspects of epidemic encephalitis. *Archs Neurol. Psychiat., Chicago,* **5**, 491

Klein, G. S. (1966). The several grades of memory. In *Psychoanalysis – a general psychology.* Ed. R. M. Loewenstein, *et al.* New York: Int. Univ. Press

Klein, R. (1952). Immediate effects of leucotomy on cerebral functions and their significance. A preliminary report. *J. ment. Sci.,* **98**, 60

Kleist, K. (1934). Joint Proceedings of the South-West German and Bavarian Psychiatric Associations. *Allg. Z. Psychiat.,* **102**, 127

Knowles, F. W. (1973). Anterior bifrontal ECT. *Br. J. Psychiat.* **123**, 376

Kohn, E. and Crosby, E. C. (1972). Korsakoff's syndrome associated with surgical lesions involving the mamillary bodies. *Neurology, (Minneap.),* **22**, 117

Kolodny, A. (1928). The symptomatology of tumours of the temporal lobe. *Brain,* **51**, 385

Konorski, J. (1959). A new method of physiological investigation of recent memory in animals. *Bull. Acad. Pol. Sci.* **7**, 115

Körner, G. (1935). Zur Psychopathologie des amnestischen Syndroms. *Mschr. Psychiat. Neurol.,* **90**, 177

Környey, K. (1938). Wernicke-Korsakoff prozess als Komplikation Bösartiger extraneuraler Geschwülste. *Dt. Z. NervHeilk.,* **144**, 241

Korsakoff, S. S. (1887). Troubles de l'activité psychique dans la paralysie alcoolique et leurs rapports avec les troubles de la sphère psychique dans la névrite multiple d'origine non alcoolique. *Vest. Psichiatrii,* **4**, Fasc. 2

– (1889a). *See under* Victor and Yakovlev (1955)

– (1889b). Etude Médico-psychologique sur une forme des maladies de la mémoire. *Revue Philosophique,* **28**, 501

– (1889c). Psychic disorders in conjunction with multiple neuritis (Psychosis Polyneuritica Cerebropathia Psychica Toxaemia). *Medizinskioje Obozrenije,* **31**, No. 13

– (1889d). A few cases of peculiar cerebropathy in the course of multiple neuritis. *Yejenedelnaja Klinicheskaja Gazeta,* No. **5**, 5, 7

Kossman, C. E. (1947). Severe anoxia follow-up report of case with recovery. *J. aviat. Med.,* **18**, 465

Kral, V. A. (1958). Neuropsychiatric observations in an Old Peoples Home. *J. Gerontol.,* **13**, 169

– and Durost, H. B. (1953). A comparative study of the amnesic syndrome in various organic conditions. *Am. J. Psychiat.*, **110**, 41

Krauss, S. (1930). Untersuchungen über Aufbau and Störung der menschlichen Handlung. I. Die Korsakowsche Störung. *Arch. ges. Psychol.*, **77**, 649

Lackner, J. R. (1974). Observations on the speech processing capabilities of an amnesic patient: several aspects of H. M.'s language function. *Neuropsych.* **12**, 199

Lancaster, D. P., Steinart, R. R., and Frost, I. (1958). Unilateral ECT. *J. ment. Sci.*, **104**, 221

Laurell, B. (1970). Flurothyl convulsive therapy. *Acta psychiat. scand.* Suppl. 213

Leitch, A. (1948). Notes on amnesia in crime for the general practitioner. *Med. Press*, **219**, 459

Levin, J. (1970). The Divorce Reform Act, 1969. *Modern Law Review*, **33**, 632

Lewis, A. (1953). Hysterical dissociation in dementia paralytica. *Mschr. Psychiat. Neurol.*, **125**, 589

– (1954). In *Ciba Foundation Colloquia on Ageing.* Vol. 1, p. 32. London: Churchill

– (1961). Discussion on amnesic syndromes: the psychopathological aspect. *Proc. R. Soc. Med.*, **54**, 955

Lhermitte, F. and Signoret, J. L. (1972). Analyse neuropsychologique et differenciation des syndromes amnésiques. *Revue neurol.* **126**, 161

Lidz, T. (1942). The amnesic syndrome. *Archs Neurol. Psychiat.*, *Chicago*, **47**, 586

Liebaldt, G. P. and Scheller, M. (1971). Amnestisches Syndrom und Korsakoff Syndrom – Zwei auch anatomisch-lokalisatorisch unterscheidbare Syndrome? *Nervenarzt.* **42**, 402

Loess, H. and Waugh, N. C. (1967). Short-term memory and inter-trial interval. *J. Verb. Learn. Verb. Behav.* **6**, 455

Logue, V., Durward, M., Pratt, R. T. C., Piercy, M. and Nixon, W. C. B. (1968). The quality of survival after rupture of an anterior cerebral aneurysm. *Br. J. psychiat.*, **114**, 137

Lopez, R. I. and Collins, G. M. (1968). Wernicke's encephalopathy; a complication of chronic haemodialysis. *Archs Neurol. Chicago*, **18**, 248

Lorente de No, R. (1934). Studies on the structure of the cerebral cortex. II. Continuation of the study of the ammonic system. *J. Psychol. Neurol.*, **46**, 113

Lotmar, F. (1954). Zur psycho-physiologischen Deuten "isolierten" dauernden Markfähigkeitsverlustes von extremer Grade nach initialer Kohlenoxydschädigung eines Unfallversicherten. *Schweizer Arch. Neurol. Psychiat.*, **73**, 147

– (1958). Uber die abschliessende Stellungsnahme Grünthals und Störrings zu der auf den Fall B. Sekundengedächtnis bezüglichen Arbeit von Völkel und Stolze (1956). *Schweizer Arch. Neurol. Psychiat.*, **81**, 203

Lou, H. O. C. (1968). Repeated episodes of transient global amnesia. *Acta neurol. scand.*, **44**, 612

Love, J. G. and Marshall, T. M. (1950). Cranio-pharyngiomas (Pituitary Adamantinomas). *Surgery Gynec. Obstet.* **90**, 591

Luria, A. R. (1971). Memory disturbances in local brain lesions. *Neuropsychologia*, **9**, 367

– and Karraseva, T. A. (1968). Disturbances of auditory speech memory in focal lesions of the deep regions of the temporal lobe. *Neuropsychologia*, **6**, 97

Lynch, S. and Yarnell, P. R. (1973). Retrograde amnesia: delayed forgetting after concussion. *Am. J. Psychol.* **86**, 643

Mabille, H. and Pitres, A. (1913). Sur un cas d'amnesie de fixation post-apoplectique ayant persisté pendant 23 ans. Mort-Autopsie-Reflexions. *Revue Med.,* **33,** 257

MacCurdy, J. T. (1928). *Common Principles in Psychology and Physiology.* (Cambridge University Press)

McEntee, W. J., Biber, M. P., Perl, D. F. and Benson, D. F. (1976). Diencephalic amnesia: a reappraisal. *J. Neurol. Neurosurg. Psychiat.,* **39,** 436

McFie, J. and Piercy, M. F. (1952). The relation of laterality of lesion to performance on Weigl's Sorting Test. *J. ment. Sci.,* **98,** 299

McGaugh, J. L. (1966). Time dependent processes in memory storage. *Science, N.Y.* **153,** 1351

— (1974). ECS: effects on learning and memory in animals. In *The Psychobiology of ECT.* Ed. M. Fink. N.Y. J. Wiley & Sons

Mackay, H. A. and Inglis, J. A. (1963). The effect of age on a short-term auditory storage process; *Gerontologia,* **8,** 193

McMenemy, W. H. (1963). The dementias and progressive diseases of the basal ganglia. In *Greenfield's Neuropathology,* pp. 520–580. Ed. R. M. Norman. London: Edward Arnold.

McNeill, D. L., Tidmarsh, D. and Rastall, M. L. (1965). A case of dysmnesic syndrome following cardiac arrest. *Br. J. Psychiat.* **111,** 697

Malamud, N. and Skillicorn, S. A. (1956). Relationship between the Wernicke and the Korsakoff syndrome. *Archs. Neurol. Psychiat., Chicago,* **76,** 585

Mandleberg, I. A. and Brooks, D. N. (1975). Cognitive recovery after severe head injury. *J. Neurol. Neurosurg. Psychiat.* **38,** 1127

Marr, D. (1969). A theory of cerebellar cortex. *J. Physiol.* **202,** 437

Marslen-Wilson, W. D. (1974). The implications of anterograde amnesia for the structure of human memory. Paper read at the Eastern Psychological Association Symposium on *Brain Mechanisms and Memory Processes*

— and Teuber, H. L. (1975). Memory for remote events in anterograde amnesia: recognition of public figures from news photographs *Neuropsychologica* **13,** 353

Martin, E. A. (1971). Transient global amnesia. *Irish J. med. Sci.,* **3,** 331

Mason, S. T. and Iversen, S. D. (1976). An investigation of the role of cortical and cerebellar noradrenaline in associative motor learning in the rat. *Brain Res.* In Press

Mayer-Gross, W. (1944). Retrograde amnesia. Some experiments. *Lancet,* **2,** 603

— Slater, E., and Roth, M. (1960). *Clinical Psychiatry.* London: Cassell

Meggendorfer, E. G. (1928). Intoxikationspsychosen. Die exogen Reaktionsformen und die organische Psychosen. In *Handbuch der Geisteskrankheiten.* Spezieller Teil 3. Ed. by O. Bumke. Berlin: Springer

Melton, A. W. (1963). Implications of short-term memory for a general theory of memory. *J. Verb. Learn. Verb. Behav.* **2,** 1

Merskey, H. (1971). An appraisal of hypnosis. *Postgrad. Med. J.* **47,** 572

— and Trimble, M. (1977). In preparation

Meyer, V. (1956). Cognitive changes following temporal lobectomy for relief of Ed. by R. M. Norman. London: Edward Arnold

— and Beck, E. (1954). Prefrontal leucotomy and related operations: anatomical aspects of success and failure. *The Henderson Trust Lectures,* No. XVII. London: Oliver and Boyd

Meyer, V. (1956). Cognitive changes following temporal lobectomy for relief of temporal lobe epilepsy. *Archs. Neurol. Psychiat. Chicago,* **81,** 299

— and Yates, A. J. (1955). Intellectual changes following temporal lobectomy for psychomotor epilepsy; preliminary communication. *J. Neurol. Neurosurg. Psychiat.,* **18,** 44

Miller, E. (1970). The effect of ECT on memory and learning. *Br. J. med. Psychol.* **43**, 57
– (1973). Short and long-term memory in patients with presenile dementia. (Alzheimer's Disease). *Psychol. Med.* **3**, 221
– (1975). Impaired recall and the memory disturbance in presenile dementia. *Br. J. soc. clin. psychol.*, **14**, 73
Milligan, W. L. (1946). Psychoneuroses treated with ECT. *Lancet*, **2**, 516
Milner, B. (1958). Psychological defects produced by temporal lobe excision. *Res. Publ. Ass. Res. nerv. ment. Dis.* **36**, 244
– (1962). Les troubles de la memoire accompagnant des lesions hippocampiques bilaterales. In *Physiologie de L'hippocampe (Colloques Internationaux du C.N.R.S. No. 107)*. p. 257
– (1963). Effects of different brain lesions on card sorting. *Archs, Neurol.* **9**, 90
– (1965). Visually-guided maze learning in man: effects of bilateral frontal and unilateral cerebral lesions. *Neuropsychologia* **3**, 317
– (1966). Amnesia following operation on the temporal lobes. In: *Amnesia.* Ed. C. W. M. Whitty and O. L. Zangwill. London: Butterworths, pp. 109–133
– (1968a). Disorders of memory after brain lesions in Man. *Neuropsychologia*, **6**, 175
– (1968b). Visual recognition and recall after right temporal-lobe excision in man. *Neuropsychologia*, **6**, 191
– (1969). Residual intellectual and memory deficits after head injury. In: *The Late Effects of Head Injury*. Eds. A. Earl Walker, W. F. Caveness and MacDonald Critchley. Springfield, Illinois: Charles C. Thomas. pp. 84–97
– (1970). Memory and the medial temporal regions of the brain. In *Biology of Memory*, Eds. K. H. Pribram and D. E. Broadbent. New York: Academic Press, p. 29
– (1971). Interhemispheric differences and psychological processes. *Br. Med. Bull.* **27**, 272
– (1973). Hemispheric specialisation: scope and limits. In: *The Neurosciences: Third Study. Program.* Eds P. O. Schmitt and F. G. Worden. pp. 75–89. Boston: M.I.T.
– (1975). Psychological aspects of focal epilepsy and its neurosurgical management. *Adv. Neurol.* **8**, 299
– and Penfield, W. (1955). The effect of hippocampal lesions on recent memory. *Trans. Am. Neurol. Ass.*, **80**, 42
– and Taylor, L. (1972). Right-hemisphere superiority in tactile pattern-recognition after cerebral commissurotomy: excellence for non-verbal memory. *Neuropsychologia*, **10**, 1
– and Teuber, A-L. (1968). Alteration of perception and memory in man: reflections on methods. In: *Analysis of Behavioural Change*. Ed: L. Weiskrantz. pp. 268–375. New York: Harper and Row
– Branch, C. and Rasmussen, T. (1962). Study of short-term memory and intracarotid injection of Sodium Amytal. *Trans. Am. Neurol. Assoc.* **87**, 224
– Corkin, S. and Teuber, H-L. (1968). Further analysis of the hippocampal amnesic syndrome: 14-year follow-up study of H.M. *Neuropsychologia* **6**, 215
Mirsky, A. and Van Buren, J. (1965). On the nature of the absence in centrencephalic epilepsy: a study of some behavioural, electroencephalographic and autonomic factors. *Electroenceph. clin. Neurophysiol.*, **18**, 334
Moersch, F. P. (1924). Psychic manifestations in migraine. *Am. J. Psychiat.*, **3**, 697
Morris, N. and Howard, C. (1964). *Studies in Criminal Law*. London: Oxford University Press

Morris, T. P. and Blom-Cooper, L. (1964). *A Calendar of Murder.* London: Michael Joseph

Mumenthaler, M. and von Roll, L. (1969). Amnestische Episoden. *Schweiz. med. Wschr.* 99, 133

Nadel, L. and O'Keefe, J. (1974). The hippocampus in pieces and patches: an essay on modes of explanation in physiological psychology. In *Essays on the Nervous System.* Eds. R. Bellairs and E. G. Gray, Clarendon Press: Oxford, p. 367

Narabayashi, H., Nagao, T., Saito, Y, Yoshida, M. and Nagahata, M. (1963). Stereotaxic amygdalectomy for behaviour disorders. *Archs Neurol.* 9, 1

Nelson, N.C. and Becker, W. F. (1969). Thyroid crisis: diagnosis and treatment. *Ann. Surg.,* 170, 263

Neubürger, K. (1931). Uber Hirnveränderungen nach Alkoholmissbrauch (unter Berüchsichtigung einiger Fälle von Wernickescher Krankheit mit anderer Atiologie). *Z. ges. Neurol. Psychiat.,* 135, 159

— (1936). Uber die nichtalkoholische Wernickesche Krankheit, insbesondere über ihr Vorkommon beim Krebsleiden. *Virchows Arch. path. Anat.,* 298, 68

— (1937). Wernickesche Krankheit bei chronischer gastritis. *Z. ges. Neurol. Psychiat.,* 160, 208

Newcombe, F. and Russell, J. C. (1969). Immediate recall of 'sentences' by subjects with unilateral cerebral lesions. *Neuropsychiatry,* 5, 329

Nielsen, J. M. (1958). *Memory and Amnesia.* Los Angeles: San Lucas Press

Norman, D. A. and Rumelhart, D. E. (1970). A system for perception and memory. In *Models of Human Memory.* Ed. D. A. Norman. New York: Academic Press

O'Connell, B. A. (1960). Amnesia and homicide. *Br. J. Crim.* 10, 262

O'Connor, N. and Hermelin, B. (1971). Cognitive deficits in children. *Br. med. Bull.* 27, 227

Oldfield, R. C. and Zangwill, O. L. (1942). I. Head's concept of the schema and its application in contemporary British psychology. II. Critical analysis of Head's concept of the schema. III. Bartlett's theory of memory. *Br. J. Psychol.* 33, 58–64, 113–129

Olsen, P. Z. and Torning, K. (1968). Isoniazid and loss of memory. *Scand. J. resp. Dis.,* 49, 1

Orbach, J., Milner, B. and Rasmussen, T. (1960). Disturbances in learning and retention following bilateral resection of the amygdala-hippocampus complex in monkeys. (Institute for Psychomatic and Psychiatric Research and Training, Chicago, and Montreal Neurological Institute, Montreal). *Archs Neurol.* 3, 230

Örthner, von H. (1957). Pathologische Anatomie der vom Hypothalamus ausgelösten Bewusstseinsstörungen. *P.C.I. Int. Congr. neurol. Sci. II,* pp.77–96

Oscar-Berman, M. (1972). Hypothesis testing and focusing behaviour during concept formation by amnesic Korsakoff patients. *Neuropsychologia* 11, 191

— Goodglass, H. and Cherlow, D. G. (1973). Perceptual laterality and iconic recognition of visual materials by Korsakoff patients and normal adults. *J. comp. physiol. Psychol.* 82, 316

Ottosson J. O. (1960a). Experimental studies of the mode of action of electroconvulsive therapy. *Acta psychiat. scand.* Suppl. 145

— (1960b). Effect of intensity of stimulus on memory. *Acta Psychiat. Neurol. Scand.* 145, 103

— (1970). Age and memory impairment after ECT. *Acta psychiat. scand.* Suppl. 219

Owen, G., and Williams, M. (1977). The effect of verbal cues on the recall of pictures. (In press)

Paivio, A. (1969). Mental imagery in associative learning and memory. *Psychol. Rev.* 76, 241

Papez, J. W. (1937). A proposed mechanism of emotion. *A.M.A. Archs Neurol. Psychiat.*, 38, 725

Parfitt, D. N., and Gall, C. M. C. (1944). Psychogenic amnesia: the refusal to remember. *J. Ment. Sci.*, 90, 511

Paterson, A. and Zangwill, O. L. (1944). Recovery of spatial orientation in the post-traumatic confusional state, *Brain*, 67, 54

Patrick, J. and Whitty, C. W. M. (1965). Recurrent cerebral emboli and the diagnosis of focal epilepsy. *Lancet*, 1, 1291

Penfield, W. (1958). Functional localization in temporal lobe and deep sylvian areas. *Proc. Ass. Res. nerv. ment. Dis.* 36, 210

– and Mathieson, G. (1974). Memory: autopsy findings and comments on the role of hippocampus in experiential recall. *Archs Neurol.* 31, 145

– and Milner, B. (1958). Memory deficit produced by bilateral lesions in the hippocampal zone. *A.M.A. Arch Neurol. Psychiat.* 79, 475

– and Perot, P. (1963). The brain's record of auditory and visual experience. *Brain*, 86, 595

Penry, J. K. (1973). Behavioural correlates of generalised spike-wave discharge in the electroencephalogram. In: *Epilepsy, its Phenomena in Man*, Ed. Brazier, M. New York: Academic Press

Perlson, J. (1945). Studies of a patient who received 248 shock treatments. *Archs Neurol. Psychiat. Chicago*, 54, 409

Peters, R. S. (1958). *The Concept of Motivation.* London: Routledge and Kegan Paul

Petersen, P. (1968). Psychiatric disorder in primary hyperparathyroidism. *J. Clin. Endocr.*, 28, 1491

Peterson, L. R. (1966). Short-term verbal memory and learning. *Psychol. Rev.* 73, 193

– and Peterson, M. J. (1959). Short-term retention of individual verbal items. *J. exp. Psychol.* 58, 193

Petit-Dutaillis, D., Christophe, J., Pertuiset, B., Dreyfus-Brisac, C. and Blanc, C. (1954). Lobectomie temporale bilaterale pour epilepsie; évolution des perturbations fonctionneles post-operatoires. *Révue Neurol.*, 91, 129

Pick, A. (1903). Clinical studies: III. On reduplicative paramnesia. *Brain*, 26, 260

– (1915). Beitrag zur Pathologie des Denkverlaufes beim Korsakow. *Z. ges. Neurol. Psychiat.*, 28, 344

Piercy, M. (1964). The effect of cerebral lesions on intellectual functions: a review of current research trends. *Br. J. Psychiat.*, 110, 310

Poser, C. M. and Ziegler, D. K. (1960). Temporary amnesia as a manifestation of cerebrovascular insufficiency. *Trans. Am. Neurol. Ass.* 85, 221

Posner, M. I. (1966). Components of skilled performance. *Science N.Y.* 152, 1712

Postman, L. (1969). Mechanisms of interference in forgetting. In *The Pathology of Memory*. Eds G. A. Talland and N. C. Waugh. New York: Academic Press p. 195

Powell, T. P. S. (1959). The organization and connexions of the hippocampal and intralaminar systems. In *Recent Progress in Psychiatry*, Vol. 3, p. 54. Ed. by C. W. T. H. Fleming and A. Walk. London: Churchill

Pratt, C. C. (1939). *The Logic of Modern Psychology.* New York: Macmillan

– and Warrington, E. K. (1972). The assessment of cerebral dominance with unilateral ECT. *Br. J. Psychiat.* 121, 327

Pratt, R. T. C., Warrington, E. K., and Halliday, A. M. (1971). Unilateral ECT as a test for cerebral dominance. *Br. J. Psychiat.* **119,** 79

Prescott, L. F. (1972). In *Side Effects of Drugs,* Vol. 7. Eds. L. Mayler, and A. Herxheimer. *Excerpta. med.(Amst.)* 1972, p. 158

Prickett, C. O. (1934). The effect of a deficiency of vitamin B₁ upon the central and peripheral nervous systems of the rat. *Am. J. Physiol.,* **107,** 459

Prevezer, S. (1958). Automatism and involuntary conduct. *Criminal Law Review,* pp. 261 and 440

Prisko, L. (1963). Short term memory in cerebral damage. Unpublished Ph.D. thesis for McGill University.

Pugh, L. G. C. and Ward, M. P. (1956). Some effects of high altitude on Man. *Lancet,* **2,** 1115

Quillian, M. R. (1968). In *Semantic Information Processing* Ed. M. Minsky. Boston, Mass: M.I.T. Press

Rapaport, D. (1942). *Emotions and Memory.* The Menninger Clinic Monograph Series No. 2. 5th Ed. 1971. New York: International Universities Press

— (1957). Cognitive structures. In: *The Collected Papers of David Rapaport.* Ed. M. M. Gill. New York: Basic Books

Rémy, M. (1942). Contribution a l'étude de la maladie de Korsakow. Étude anatomo-clinique. *Mschr. Psychiat. Neurol.,* **106,** 128

Rennick, P. M., Nolan, D. C., Baner, R. B. and Lerner, A. M. (1973). Neuropsychologic and neurologic follow-up after herpes virus hominis encephalitis. *Neurology,* **23,** 42

Reynolds, E. H. (1971). Anticonvulsant drugs, folic acid metabolism, fit frequency and psychiatric illness. *Psychiat. Neurol. Neurochir.,* **74,** 167

— (1975). Chronic anti-epileptic toxicity: a review. *Epilepsia,* **16,** 319

Ribot, T. (1882). *Diseases of Memory.* London: Kegan Paul, Trench & Co.

Riggs, H. E. and Boles, H. S. (1944). Wernicke's disease; a clinical and pathological study of 42 cases. *Q. Jl Stud. Alcohol,* **5,** 361

Rochford, G., and Williams, M. (1962). Development and breakdown of the use of names. *J. Neurol. Neurosurg. Psychiat.* **25,** 222

Rodnick, E. H. (1942). Effect of metrazol on habits. *J. abnorm. soc. Psychol.* **37,** 560

Romano, J. and Coon, G. P. (1942). Physiologic and psychologic studies in spontaneous hypoglycaemia. *Psychosom. Med.,* **4,** 283

Rose, F. C. and Symonds, C. P. (1960). Persistent memory defect following encephalitis. *Brain,* **83,** 195

Ross, E. J., Marshall-Jones, P. and Friedman, M. (1966). Cushing's syndrome: diagnostic criteria. *Q. Jl. Med.,* **35,** 149

Ross, R. R. (1958). Use of pyridoxine hydrochloride to prevent isoniazid toxicity. *J. Am. med. Ass.,* **168,** 273

Russell, J. R., and Jillett, R. L. (1953). Intensified ECT. Review of five years' experience. *Lancet,* **2,** 1177

Russell, W. R. (1935). Amnesia following head injuries. *Lancet,* **2,** 762

— (1948). Studies in amnesia. *Edin. med. J.* **55,** 92

— (1971). *The Traumatic Amnesias.* London: Oxford University Press

— and Espir, M. L. E. (1961). *Traumatic Aphasia: A Study of War Wounds of the Brain.* Oxford University Press

— and Nathan, P. W. (1946). Traumatic amnesia. *Brain,* **69,** 280

Rylander, G. (1939). Personality changes after operations on the frontal lobes. *Acta psychiat. scand.,* Suppl., **20**

Sachs, E. (1927). Symptomatology of a group of frontal lobe lesions. *Brain,* **50,** 474

Sanders, H. I. and Warrington, E. K. (1971). Memory for remote events in amnesic patients. *Brain,* **94,** 661

– – (1975). Retrograde amnesia in organic amnesic patients. *Cortex,* **11,** 397

Sano, K. and Malamud, N. (1953). Clinical significance of sclerosis of the cornu ammonis. *Archs Neurol. Psychiatry.* **70,** 40

Sargant, W. and Slater, E. (1941). Amnesic syndromes in war. *Proc. R. Soc. Med.* **34,** 757

– – (1963). *Physical Methods of Treatment in Psychiatry.* London: Livingstone

Scheller, H. (1950). Völliger isolierter Verlust der Merkfähigkeit-Organische CO-Schädigung oder hysterische Verdrängung. Nachuntersuchung des Falles Br. von Grünthal and Störring. *Nervenarzt,* **21,** 49

– (1956). Ein Sekunden Gedächtnis? Kritische Beobachtungen and neue Ermittlung zum Fall. Br. von Grünthal und Störring. *Nervenarzt,* **27,** 216

– (1957). Personal communication

Schenk, V. W. D. (1955). Syndrome d'Alzheimer. Étude anatomoclinique de 35 cas. *Folia psychiat. neurol. neurochir. neerl.,* No. 5/6, 422

Schlesinger, B. (1950). Mental changes in intracranial tumours, and related problems. *Confinia neurol.,* **10,** 225, 322

Schulman, H. G. (1971). Similarity effects in short-term memory. *Psychol. Bull.* **75,** 399

Schwartz, M. S. and Scott, D. F. (1971). Isolated petit mal status presenting de novo in middle age. *Lancet,* **2,** 1399

Scoville, W. B. (1954). The limbic lobe in Man. *J. Neurosurg.,* **11,** 64

– and Milner, B. (1957). Loss of recent memory after bilateral hippocampal lesions. *J. Neurol. Neurosurg. Psychiat.,* **20,** 11

Seltzer, B. and Benson, D. F. (1974). The temporal pattern of retrograde amnesia in Korsakoff's disease. *Neurology, Minneap.* **24,** 527

Serafetinides, E. A. and Falconer, M. A. (1962). Some observations of memory impairment after temporal lobectomy for epilepsy. *J. Neurol. Neurosurg. Psychiat.,* **25,** 251

Shallice, T. and McGill, J. (1977). In *The Origins of Mixed Errors. Attention and Purpose,* 7. Ed. Requin, J. and Bertelson, P. Academic Press (In press)

Shallice, T. and Warrington, E. K. (1970). Independent functioning of verbal memory stores: a neuropsychological study. *Q. Jl. exp. Psychol.,* **22,** 261

– – (1974). Further tests of STM in left preoccipital lesions. *Neuropsychologia.* **12,** 553

– and McGill, J. (1977). *The Origins of Mixed Errors. Attention and Purpose,* 7. Ed. Requin, J. and Bertelson, P. Academic Press (In press)

Shankweiler, D. (1966). Defects in recognition and reproduction of familiar tunes after unilateral temporal lobectomy. Paper read at 37th Ann. Meeting East. Psychological Ass. New York

Shapiro, M. B., Pote, F., Lofving, B. and Inglis, J. (1956). Memory function in psychiatric patients over sixty. *J. ment. Sci.,* **102,** 233

Sherman, I. and Mergener, J. (1942). The effect of convulsive treatment on memory. *Am. J. Psychiat.* **98,** 401

Shillito, F. H., Drinker, C. K. and Shaughnessy, T. J. (1936). Problem of nervous and mental sequelae in carbon monoxide poisoning. *J. Am. med. Ass.,* **106,** 669

Shuttleworth, E. C. and Morris, C. E. (1966). The transient global amnesia syndrome: a defect in the second stage of memory in man. *Archs Neurol. (Chicago)* **15,** 515

Sidman, M., Stoddard, L.T. and Mohr, J. P. (1968). Some additional quantitative observations of immediate memory in a patient with bilateral hippocampal lesions. *Neuropsychologia* **6,** 245

Slater, E. and Glithero, E. (1965). A follow-up of patients diagnosed as suffering from 'hysteria'. *J. Psychosom. Res.* **9, 9**

Small, I. F. (1974). Inhalant convulsive therapy. In *Psychobiology of ECT.* Ed. M. Fink. (New York: J. Wiley & Sons)

Small, J. G. and Small, I. F. (1972). Indoklon versus ECT. *Seminars in Psychiatry.* **4, 13**

Smith, J. S. and Brandon, S. (1973). Morbidity from acute carbon monoxide poisoning at three year follow-up. *Br. med. J.,* **1, 318**

Smythies, J. R. (1970). *Brain Mechanisms and Behaviour.* Oxford: Blackwell

Spiegel, E. A., Wycis, H. T. Orchinik, C. W. and Freed, H. (1955). The thalamus and temporal orientation. *Science, N.Y.* **121, 771**

– – – – (1956). Thalamic chronotaraxis. *Am. J. Psychiat.,* **113, 97**

Spielmeyer, W. (1930). The anatomic substration of the convulsive state. *Archs Neurol. Psychiatry.* **23, 869**

Spillane, J. D. (1947). *Nutritional Disorders of the Nervous System.* Edinburgh: Livingstone

Spratling, W. P. (1902). Epilepsy in relation to crime. *J. nerv. ment. Dis.,* **29, 481**

Sprofkin, B. E. and Sciarra, D. (1952). Korsakoff psychosis associated with cerebral tumours. *Neurology,* **2, 427**

Squire, L. (1974). Remote memory as affected by ageing. *Neuropsychologia,* **12, 429**

Starr, A. and Phillips, L. (1970). Verbal and motor memory in the amnesic syndrome. *Neuropsychologia* **8, 75**

Stein, J. A. and Tschudy, D. P. (1970). Acute intermittent porphyria: a clinical and biochemical study of 46 patients. *Medicine (Baltimore),* **49, 1**

Stengel, E., (1941). The aetiology of fugue states. *J. ment. Sci.,* **87, 572**

– (1951). Intensive electro-convulsant therapy. *J. ment. Sci.* **97, 139**

Stones, M. J. (1970). The effect of attention on memory following ECT. Dissertation for BA at Brunel University, London

– (1973). ECT and short-term memory. *Br. J. Psychiat.* **122, 591**

Stores, G. (1975). Behavioural effects of anti-epileptic drugs. *Devl. Med., child neurol.* **17, 647**

– and Hart, J. A. (1976). Reading skills in children with generalised or focal epilepsy attending ordinary school. *Devl. Med. Child Neurol.* **18, 705**

Storey, P. B. (1967). Psychiatric sequelae of sub-arachnoid haemorrhage. *Br. med. J.,* **3, 261**

Störring, G. E. (1931). Uber den ersten reinen Fall eines Menschen mit völligen, isolierten Verlust der Merkfähigkeit. *Arch. ges. Psychol.,* **81, 257**

– (1936). *Gedächtnisverlust durch Gasvergiftung. Ein Mensch ohne Zeitgedächtnis.* Leipzig: Akademie Verlag

Strachan, R. and Henderson, J. (1965). Psychiatric syndromes due to avitaminosis B12 with normal blood marrow. *Q. Jl. Med.,* **34, 303**

– – (1967). Dementia and folate deficiency. *Q. Jl. Med.,* **36, 189**

Strich, S. J. (1956). Diffuse degeneration of the cerebral white matter in severe dementia following head injury. *J. Neurol. Neurosurg. Psychiat.,* **19, 163**

Strickland, N. J., Bold, A. M. and Medd, W. E. (1967). Bronchial carcinoma with hypercalcaemia simulating cerebral metastases. *Br. med. J.,* **3, 590**

Summerskill, W. H. J., Davidson, E. A., Sherlock, S. and Steiner, R. E. (1956). Neuropsychiatric syndrome associated with hepatic cirrhosis. *Q. Jl. Med.,* **25, 245**

Sutherland, E., Oliver, J. and Knight, D. (1969). EEG, memory and confusion in dominant, non-dominant and bitemporal ECT. *Br. J. Psychiat.* **115, 1059**

Sweet, W. H., Talland, G. A. and Ervin, F. R. (1959). Loss of recent memory following section of the fornix. *Trans. Am. neurol. Ass.*, **84**, 76

Sydenstricker, V. P. (1943). Neurological complications of malnutrition. *Proc. R. Soc. Med.*, **36**, 169

Symonds, C. P. (1940). In *Injuries of the Skull, Brain and Spinal Cord*. Ed. by S. Brock. Baltimore: William Wood
– (1960). Concussion and contusion of the brain and their sequelae. In: *Injuries of the Brain and Spinal Cord*. Edited by S. Brock. 4th Ed. London: Cassell
– (1962). Concussion and its sequelae. *Lancet*, **1**, 1
– (1966). Disorders of memory. *Brain*, **89**, 625

Symposium on Brain Research in Neurosciences: Kindling, (1975). *Can. J. neurol. Sci.* **2**, 385

Syz, H. (1937). Recovery of loss of mnemic retention after head trauma. *J. gen. Psychol.*, **17**, 355

Talland, G. A. (1959). Psychological studies of Korsakoff's psychosis. III. Concept formation. *J. nerv. ment. Dis.*, **128**, 214
– (1961). Confabulation in the Wernicke-Korsakoff Syndrome. *J. nerv. ment. Dis.*, **132**, 361
– (1965). *Deranged Memory: A Psychonomic Study of the Amnesic Syndrome.* New York and London; Academic Press
– and Ekdall, M. (1959). Psychological studies of Korsakoff's psychosis. IV. The rate and mode of forgetting narrative material. *J. nerv. ment. Dis.*, **129**, 391

Tarachow, S. (1939). The Korsakoff Psychosis in spontaneous subarachnoid haemorrhage. Report of three cases. *Am. J. Psychiat.*, **95**, 887

Temkin, Jennifer. (1974). Automatism and proper precautions. *Mod. Law Rev.* **37**, 199

Terzian, H. and Ore, G. D. (1955). Syndrome of Klüver and Bucy reproduced in Man by bilateral removal of the temporal lobes. *Neurology*, **5**, 373

Teuber, M. L., Milner, B. and Vaughan, H. G. Jr. (1968). Persistent anterograge amnesia after stab wound of the basal brain. *Neuropsychologia*, **6**, 267

Tharp, B. R. (1969). EEG in transient global amnesia. *Electroenceph. clin. Neurophysiol.* **26**, 96

The Times, October 25th, 1957
– December 4th, 1959
– February 18th, 1961
– May 18th, 1962

Thorpe, J. G. (1959). Learning ability during a course of 20 ECT's. *J. ment. Sci.* **105**, 1017

Tiling, T. (1890). Über die bei alkoholischen Neuritis multiplex beobachtete Geistesstörung. *Allg. Z. Psychiat.*, **46**, 233
– (1892). Über die amnestische Geistesstörung. *Allg. Z. Psychiat.*, **48**, 549

Tolstoy, D. (1963). *The Law and Practice of Divorce and Matrimonial Causes,* 5th ed. London: Sweet and Maxwell

Tonks, C. M. (1964). Mental illness in hypothyroid patients. *Br. J. Psychiat.*, **110**, 706

Tulving, E. (1973). Episodic and semantic memory. In *Organisation of Memory.* Academic Press: New York

Underwood, B. J. (1957). Interference and forgetting. *Psychol. Rev.* **64**, 49
– (1965). False recognition by implicit verbal responses. *J. exp. Psychol.* **70**, 122

Van Buren, J. M. and Borke, R. C. (1972). The mesial temporal substratum of memory. *Brain* **95**, 599

Victor, M. (1964). In *Brain Function,* Vol. II: *RNA and Brain Function, Memory and Learning.* Ed. M. A. B. Brazier. Berkeley: University of California Press
– and Adams, R. D. (1953). Effect of alcohol on the nervous system. *Res. Publs. Ass. Res. nerv. ment. Dis.,* **32**, 526
– and Yakovlev, P. I. (1955). S. S. Korsakoff's psychic disorder in conjunction with peripheral neuritis. A. translation of Korsakoff's original article with brief comments on the author and his contribution to clinical medicine. *Neurology,* **5,** 394
– Adams, R. D. and Collins, G. H. (1971). *The Wernicke-Korsakoff Syndrome. A Clinical and Pathological Study of 245 Patients, 82 with Post-mortem Examinations.* Oxford: Blackwell
– Talland, G. A. and Adams, R. D. (1959). Psychological studies of Korsakoff's psychosis. I. General intellectual functions. *J. nerv. ment. Dis.* **128,** 528
– Angevine, J. B., Mancall, E. L. and Fisher, C. M. (1961). Memory loss with lesions of hippocampal formation. *Archs. Neurol. Psychiat., Chicago,* **5,** 244
Völkel, M. and Stolze, R. (1956). Nachuntersuchung und Versuch einer epikritischen Deutung des Falles B. von E. Grünthal und G. E. Störring. *Mschr. Psychiat. Neurol.,* **132,** 291
Walker, A. E. (1957). Recent memory impairment in unilateral temporal lesions. *Archs, Neurol. Psychiat., Chicago,* **78,** 543
– (1958). *Discussion on Temporal Lobe Epilepsy.* Eds. Baldwin, M. and Bailey, P. Springfield, Illinois: C. C. Thomas
de Wardener, H. E. and Lennox, B. (1947). Cerebral beri-beri. *Lancet,* **1,** 11
Warrington, E. K. (1971). Neurological disorders of memory. *Brit. Med. Bull.,* **27,** 243
– and Baddeley, A. D. (1974). Amnesia and memory for visual location. *Neuropsychologia* **12,** 257
– and James, M. (1967a). An experimental investigation of facial recognition in patients with unilateral cerebral lesions. *Cortex* **3,** 317
– – (1967b). Disorders of visual perception in patients with localized cerebral lesions. *Neuropsychologia* **5,** 253
– and Rabin, P. (1970a). Perceptual matching in patients with cerebral lesions. *Neuropsychologia* **8,** 475
– – (1970b). A preliminary investigation of the relation between visual perception and visual memory. *Cortex* **6,** 87
– and Shallice, T. (1969). The selective impairment of auditory verbal short term memory. *Brain,* **92,** 885
– and Silberstein, M. (1970). A questionnaire technique for investigating very long term memory. *Q. Jl. Exp. Psychol.* **22,** 508
– and Taylor, A. M. (1973). Immediate memory for faces: long or short-term memory? *Q. Jl. Exp. Psychol.* **25,** 316
– and Weiskrantz, L. (1968a). A study of learning and retention in amnesic patients. *Neuropsychologia* **6,** 283
– –(1968 b). A new method of testing long-term retention with special reference to amnesic patients. *Nature, Lond.* **217,** 972
– – (1970). Amnesic syndrome: consolidation or retrieval? *Nature, Lond.* **228,** 628
– – (1971). Organisational aspects of memory in amnesic patients. *Neuropsychologia* **9,** 67
– – (1973). An analysis of short-term and long-term memory defects in man. In: *The Physiological Basis of Memory.* J. A. Deutch (Ed.) New York: Academic Press

– – (1974). The effect of prior learning on subsequent retention in amnesic patients. *Neuropsychologia* 12, 419
– Logue, V. and Pratt, R. T. C. (1971). The anatomical localisation of selective impairment of auditory verbal short-term memory. *Neuropsychologia*, 9, 377
Wasterlain, C. G. (1971). Are there two types of post-traumatic retrograde amnesia? *Europ. Neurol.* 5, 225
Watkins, E. S. and Oppenheimer, D. R. (1962). Mental changes after thalamolysis. *J. Neurol. Neurosurg. Psychiat.*, 25, 243
Waugh, N. C. and Norman, D. A. (1965). Primary memory. *Psychol. Rev.*, 72, 89
Weingartner, H. (1968). Verbal learning in patients with temporal lobe lesions. *J. verb. learn. verb. Behav.* 7, 520
Weinstein, E. A. and Kahn, R. L. (1950). Syndrome of anosognosia. *Archs Neurol. Psychiat.*, Chicago, 64, 772
– – (1951). Patterns of disorientation in organic brain disease. *J. Neuropathol. clin. Neurol.*, 1, 214
– – (1952). Nonaphasic misnaming (paraphasia) in organic brain disease. *A.M.A. Archs. Neurol. Psychiat.*, 67, 72
– – (1953). Personality factors in denial of illness. *A.M.A. Archs Neurol. Psychiat.*, 69, 355
– – (1955). *Denial of Illness.* Springfield, Ill.: Thomas
– and Sugarman, L. A. (1952). Phenomena of reduplication. *A.M.A. Archs Neurol. Psychiat.*, 67, 808
Weisenburg, T. H. (1911). Tumours of the third ventricle with the establishment of a symptom-complex. *Brain*, 33, 236
Weiskrantz, L. (1966). Experimental studies of amnesia. In *Amnesia*. Ed. C. W. M. Whitty and O. L. Zangwill. pp. 1–35. London: Butterworth
– (1968). Memory. Chap. 8 in *Analysis of Behavioural Change*. Ed. L. Weiskrantz. New York: Harper and Row
– (1971). Comparison of amnesic states in monkey and man. In *Cognitive Processes of Non-human Primates*. Ed. L. E. Jarrard. New York: Academic Press
– and Warrington, E. K. (1970a). A study of forgetting in amnesic patients. *Neuropsychologia*, 8, 281
– – (1970b). Verbal learning and retention by amnesic patients using partial information. *Psychonom. Sci.* 20, 210
Welford, A. T. (1958). *Ageing and Human Skill*. Oxford: Nuffield Foundation
Wernicke, C. (1881). *Lehrbuch der Gehirnkrankheiten*, Vol. II, p. 229. Berlin
Wexberg, L. E. (1960). *Individual Psychology Publications* (Pamphlet). London: Medical Society for Individual Psychology
White, J. C. and Cobb, S. (1955). Psychological changes associated with giant pituitary neoplasms. *Archs Neurol. Psychiat.* Chicago, 74, 383
Whitehead, A. (1973). Verbal learning and memory in elderly depressives. *Br. J. Psychiat.*, 123, 203
Whitlock, F. A. (1963). *Criminal Responsibility and Mental Illness*. London: Butterworths
Whitty, C. W. M. (1962). The neurological basis of memory. In *Modern Trends in Neurology*. p. 314. Ed. D. Williams. London: Butterworths
– and Lewin, W. (1960). A Korsakoff syndrome in the post-cingulectomy confusional state. *Brain*, 83, 648
– and Zangwill, O. L. (1966). (Editors) *Amnesia*. London: Butterworths
Whybrow, P. C., Prange, A. J. and Treadway, C. R. (1969). Mental changes accompanying thyroid gland dysfunction. *Archs gen. Psychiat.*, 20, 48

Wickelgren, W. A. (1968). Sparing of short-term memory in an amnesic patient: Implications for strength theory of memory. *Neuropsychologia.* **6**, 235
– (1970). Multitrace strength theory. In *Models of Human Memory.* Ed. D. A. Norman. New York: Academic Press
– (1973). The long and the short of memory. *Psychol. Bull.,* **80,** 425
– and Norman, D. A. (1966). Strength models and serial position in short-term recognition memory. *J. Ment. Psychol.* **3,** 316
Wickens, D. D. (1970). Encoding categories of words: an empirical approach to meaning. *Psychol. Rev.* **77,** 1
– and Clark, S. E. (1968). Osgood dimensions as an encoding class in short-term memory. *J. exp. Psychol.* **78,** 580
– Born, D. G. and Allen, C. K. (1963). Proactive inhibition and item similarity in short-term memory. *J. Verb. Learn. Verb. Behav.,* **2,** 440
Williams, D. (1953). Study of thalamic and cortical rhythms in petit mal. *Brain,* **76,** 50
Williams, Glanville, L. (1961). *Criminal Law – the General Part.* 2nd ed. London: Stevens
Williams, M. (1950). Memory studies in ECT. *J. Neurol. Neurosurg. Psychiat.* **13,** 30, 314
– (1952). A case of displaced affect following ECT. *Br. J. med. Psychol.* **25,** 156
– (1953). Investigations of amnesic defects by progressive prompting. *J. Neurol. Neurosurg. Psychiat.,* **16,** 14
– (1973). Errors in picture recognition after ECT. *Neuropsychologia.* **11,** 429
– (1975). Retrograde amnesia. Ch. 16. in *Studies in Long-term Memory* Eds Kennedy and Wilkes. New York: Wiley
– (1977). Word vs picture recognition in amnesic and aphasic patients. *Neuropsychologia* **15,** 357
– and Pennybacker, J. (1954). Memory disturbances in third ventricle tumours. *J. Neurol. Neurosurg. Psychiat.,* 17, 115
– and Smith, H. V. (1954). Mental disturbances in tuberculous meningitis. *J. Neurol. Neurosurg. Psychiat.,* **17,** 173
– and Zangwill, O. L. (1950). Disorders of temporal judgement in amnesic states. *J. ment. Sci.* **94,** 484
– – (1952). Retrograde amnesia following head injury. *J. Neurol. Neurosurg. Psychiat.,* **15,** 54
Williams, M. W. and Rupp, C. (1938). Observations on confabulation. *Am. J. Psychiat.,* **95,** 395
Williams, R. D., Mason, H. L., Power, M. H. and Wilder, R. M. (1943). Induced thiamine deficiency in Man. *Archs intern. Med.,* **71,** 38
Wilson, G., Rupp, C. and Wilson, W. (1950). Amnesia. *Am. J. Psychiat.,* **106,** 481
Winocur, G. and Weiskrantz, L. (1976). An investigation of paired-associate learning in amnesic patients. *Neuropsychologia,* **14,** 97
Woods, R. T. and Piercy, M. (1974). A similarity between amnesic memory and normal forgetting. *Neuropsychologia* **12,** 437
World Health Organisation (1955). Alcohol and alcoholism. *Tech. Rep. Ser. Wld. Hlth. Org.* No. 94
Wyke, M. and Warrington, E. (1960). An experimental analysis of confabulation in a case of Korsakoff's syndrome using a tachistoscopic method. *J. Neurol. Neurosurg. Psychiat.,* **23,** 327
Zangwill, O. L. (1941). On a peculiarity of recognition in three cases of Korsakoff's psychosis. *Br. J. Psychol.,* **31,** 230

– (1943). Clinical tests on memory impairment. *Proc. R. Soc. Med.,* 36, 576
– (1946a). Some qualitative observations on verbal memory in cases of cerebral lesion. *Br. J. Psychol.,* 37, 8
– (1946b). Some clinical applications of the Rey–Davis Performance Test. *J. ment. Sci.,* 92, 19
– (1953). Disorientation for Age. *J. ment. Sci.,* 99, 698
– (1961). Psychological studies of amnesic states. *Proc. III Wld. Congr. Psychiatry,* 3, 219
– (1964). Psychological studies in amnesic states. *Proc. Third Wld. Congr. Psychiat.* 3, 219
– (1967). The Grünthall-Störring case of amnesic syndrome. *Br. J. Psychiat.,* 113, 113
Zinkin, S., and Birchnell, J. (1968). Unilateral ECT – its effect on memory. *Brit. J. Psychiat.* 114, 973
Zubin, J., and Barrera, S. E. (1941). Effects of ECT on memory. *Proc. Soc. exp. Biol. & Med.* 48, 596

Index

SUBJECT/AUTHOR

Brown, J., 199, 268
Browne, M. N., 180, 188, 191, 231, 274
Brown–Peterson procedure, 12, 14,
15, 17, 20
Brunschwig, L., 187, 268
Bumke, O., 111, 268
Bürger, H., 105, 268
Bürger-Prinz, H., 105, 268
Busch, E., 81, 268
Busse, E. W., 88, 268
Butters, N., 4, 9, 10, 11–24, 28, 31,
32, 43, 50, 145, 147, 157, 167,
268, 269
Bywaters, E. G., 69, 267

Cairns, H., 88, 222, 269
Cajal, S. R., 218, 269
Campbell, A. C. P., 61, 203, 269
Cannicott, S. M., 190, 269
Capacity of short-term memory, 8, 9
Carbon monoxide poisoning, 215
amnesia following, 111, 112, 196
transient amnesic states caused by,
57–59
Cardiac arrest, 215
Cardiazol, 196
Carmichael, E. A., 202, 269
Cary, E., 83, 266
Cerebellum noradrenergic innervation
of, 161
Cerebral (*see also* headings beginning
Brain)
Cerebral aneurysms, 79
Cerebral anoxia, transient amnesic
states caused by, 57–61
Cerebral arteriosclerosis, 88
Cerebral artery aneurysms, 80
Cerebral beriberi, 61
Cerebral commissure section, 141
Cerebral cortex, 202
ageing effects, 216, 217
damage to, 138, 202
Cerebral disease,
amnesia in, 52–92
toxic and metabolic factors, 54–57
transient states, 54–75
persistent amnesia in, 75–92
site of lesion, amnesia and, 81
Cerebral thrombo-angiitis obliterans, 69
Cerebropathia toxaemia psychica, 104

Cermak, L. S., 4, 9, 10, 11, 15–24,
26, 28, 31, 32, 43, 47, 50, 98,
146, 147, 148, 150, 157, 164,
167, 168, 269
Chaslin, P., 104n, 106, 269
Chen, C., 86, 276
Cherlow, D. G., 145, 280
Christophe, J., 210, 281
Cingulate gyrus, lesions of, 215
Claparède, E., 115, 185, 269
Clark, S. E., 21, 288
Clark, W. E. le Gros, 88, 269
Clarke, A. D. B., 91, 269
Clarke, P. R. F., 113, 269
Clementino, T., 175, 275
Click distraction, test, 150
Clunie, G. T. A., 55, 269
Clyma, E. A., 191, 269
Cobb, S., 208, 287
Cognitive defects in Korsakoff syn-
drome, 105
Cognitive structures, 236, 242
Cohen, B. D., 180, 267, 269
Collins, G. H., 77, 106, 205, 206, 208,
216, 222, 265, 286
Collins, G. M., 61, 277
Coma, 122
Concentration, impairment of, 57
Concept formation, 161–164
Conceptual weakness, 105
Confabulation, 57
content of, 125
Korsakoff syndrome, in, 105, 108,
112, 113, 203
meningitis, in, 67
post-traumatic amnesia, in, 124
Confusional states,
causes of, 55
toxic, 56
Connor, R. C. R., 215, 265
Conrad, K., 65, 106, 269
Consolidation hypothesis, 8, 47, 49,
170, 222, 223
Continuous amnesia, 106
Continuous memory following post-
traumatic amnesia, 123
Coon, G. P., 55, 282
Corkin, S., 6, 31, 33, 34, 114, 115,
137, 138, 139, 141, 144, 145,
146, 159, 160, 161, 174, 269,
270, 279
Corpus callosum tumours, 83

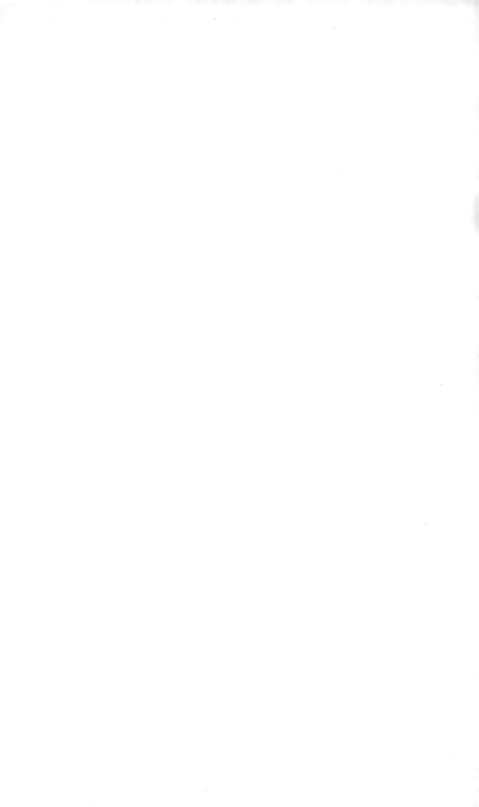